Achieving
Service
Excellence
Strategies for Healthcare

SECOND EDITION

Myron D. Fottler

Robert C. Ford

Cherrill P. Heaton

Achieving Service Excellence

Strategies for Healthcare

SECOND EDITION

ACHE Management Series

Your board, staff, or clients may also benefit from this book's insight. For more information on quantity discounts, contact the Health Administration Press Marketing Manager at (312) 424–9470.

14   13   12   11   10   5   4   3   2   1

Library of Congress Cataloging-in-Publication Data

Fottler, Myron D.
  Achieving service excellence : strategies for healthcare / Myron D.
Fottler, Robert C. Ford, and Cherrill P. Heaton. -- 2nd ed.
    p. cm.
  Includes index.
  ISBN 978-1-56793-327-7 (alk. paper)
  1. Medical care--Customer services. 2. Patient satisfaction. 3.
Customer relations. I. Ford, Robert C. (Robert Clayton), 1945- II.
Heaton, Cherrill P. III. Title.
  R727.F684 2010
  362.1068--dc22

                    2009037788

The paper used in this publication meets the minimum requirements of American National Standard for Information Sciences—Permanence of Paper for Printed Library Materials, ANSI Z39.48-1984. ♾ ™

Acquisitions editor: Eileen Lynch; Project manager: Jane Calayag; Cover designer: Gloria Chantell; Layout: BookComp

Found an error or a typo? We want to know! Please e-mail it to hap1@ache.org, and put "Book Error" in the subject line.

For photocopying and copyright information, please contact Copyright Clearance Center at www.copyright.com or at (978) 750–8400.

Health Administration Press
A division of the Foundation of the American
      College of Healthcare Executives
One North Franklin Street, Suite 1700
Chicago, IL 60606–3529
(312) 424–2800

Contents

Foreword

Quint Studer, Founder, The Studer Group

WHEN MYRON FOTTLER and Bob Ford asked me to write the Foreword for this book, just as I had for the first edition seven years ago, I agreed. This second edition of *Achieving Service Excellence* has been substantially updated to reflect the new realities in the healthcare industry. While healthcare workers still need to feel a sense of purpose, still seek opportunities to do worthwhile work, and still desire to make a difference, the environment in which they deliver the healthcare experience has changed.

Direct caregivers and support staff share a great feeling of accomplishment in seeing a patient get better, in being recognized by family members for preserving the dignity of their ill or dying loved one, and in hearing positive comments in the community about their work particularly and their organization generally. Conversely, each healthcare worker feels great sadness in knowing that a patient, a family member, or another customer is not satisfied with the service provided. Although patients today may find it difficult, if not impossible, to measure the effectiveness of clinical interventions, they know what to expect from all other aspects of the care experience. Patients and families scrutinize the courteous manner of the staff, the length of wait times, the speed of admission or discharge, the responsiveness to questions and complaints, the quality of the food, the cleanliness of the facility, and the instructions and information given for self-care.

In the last 20 years or so, something happened to the essence of healthcare. Formerly focused on caregiving, healthcare is now caving to the pressures of the bottom line. On a daily basis, healthcare leaders are bombarded with reimbursement cuts, labor shortages, revenue losses, complicated regulations, and medical staff challenges, among a multitude of crises. Boards of directors can go for months without discussing patient issues at their meetings.

At the beginning of the movie "It's a Wonderful Life," two characters in heaven are talking. One says to the other, "You have to go down to earth and help George Bailey." The other replies, "Why, is he in trouble?" The first responds, "Even worse. He is discouraged." In my travels around the country to help healthcare organizations improve their delivery of the patient experience, the word *discouraged* seems an appropriate description for how patients, families, physicians, leaders, and staffs feel about the state of healthcare service today. We all wonder, "What happened to healthcare's core function?" What role did cuts in Medicare reimbursement, the introduction of HIPAA, increases in pharmaceutical costs, and other issues play in this imbalance?

All of these factors have had an impact, but the number one culprit, in my opinion, has been the failure of healthcare's leaders to make patient, employee, and physician satisfaction a priority. Maybe many executives did not adopt this focus because it seemed to be common sense for a hospital or clinic to pay attention to these three groups. But common sense is often very uncommon. I know it was for me.

As a healthcare leader, I was guilty of moving away from patient and staff interaction. Managed care negotiations, program development, mergers, consolidations, cash collection, and debt financing all crowded out my time, providing me with rationalizations. In 1993, as the senior vice president and chief operating officer of an inner-city hospital in Chicago called Holy Cross Hospital, I was put in charge of patient satisfaction. After some false starts, I surrendered, not knowing what to do, so I sought help. I visited nonhealthcare companies with great service reputations, but most important of all, I asked the staff what to do and listened. Those steps kick-started my journey back to why I entered healthcare.

At first I was worried that our satisfaction efforts would take away from our bottom line. But soon, I realized that our new focus led us to a better understanding of employees and physicians and that in order to achieve great patient satisfaction, we first had to address employee and physician issues. As each month went by, I learned more. As employee satisfaction increased, employee turnover decreased. A stable workforce reduced the length of stay and improved both patient and physician satisfaction. These outcomes boosted our patient volume and gave us better leverage with managed care companies. Most surprising of all my discoveries was that not focusing on the bottom line increased the bottom line, and did so dramatically. The results our team at Holy Cross achieved garnered the hospital numerous awards, including the American Hospital Association's Great Comeback Award in 1994.

In June 1996, I took the lessons learned at Holy Cross and other hospitals to Baptist Hospital, Inc. (now Baptist Health Care) in Pensacola, Florida. At Baptist, the approach of focusing on satisfaction rather than on the bottom line also worked. As more hospitals benchmarked our practices at Baptist and as I spoke about our achievements throughout the country, I began to put together the "must haves" for patient satisfaction. These pillars or principles produced tremendous results for Baptist: It ranked in the top 1 percent of organizations for patient satisfaction, and it placed first in employee satisfaction and quality. In 2000, Baptist received *USA Today's* Quality Cup. In 2002, Baptist was named by *Fortune* as one of the "Top 10 Places to Work," showing that service principles stick if hardwired into the culture. While at Baptist, I developed a seminar to give myself an opportunity to share my ideas with other leaders. This seminar led me to establish a coaching business, which allows me to make an even greater difference in the field of patient satisfaction.

What I have learned and continue to learn is this: Leadership matters a lot, a truth detailed in my recent book *Results That Last*. Every healthcare organization must identify and then study the causes of its success. Its leaders must realize that to improve patient, staff, and physician satisfaction, the organization must return to its core values of serving a purpose, doing worthwhile work, and making a difference. This book, as was the last edition, is deceptive because although it is easy and fun to read, it is filled with customer satisfaction theories and applications. It presents current examples and trends and offers the latest research. I especially appreciate the Service Strategies sections, which enumerate the patient-focused concepts discussed in each chapter. These strategies can help healthcare executives improve their satisfaction efforts, especially in today's highly competitive environment and with highly informed consumers. Both patients and employees know who is doing a good job and who is not.

I hope you enjoy this new edition. The authors worked hard to provide new takeaways. Although the authors have won awards from the American Academy of Medical Administrators, they should be recognized as well for making a difference in the healthcare field. As George Bailey ultimately learned in "It's a Wonderful Life," we all should never underestimate the difference we can make.

Preface

Like the first edition, *Achieving Service Excellence: Strategies for Healthcare*, second edition, presents and organizes the available best practices and information related to the provision of a superb total healthcare experience. Current trends, research, and examples are included throughout, offering readers a foundation for understanding the concepts discussed.

The book is designed to help executives and managers implement a customer-focused service strategy in today's customer-driven market. The book may also be used, as we have used it, as a primary text in both academic and executive education programs, as it covers the theories, methods, and techniques behind multiple aspects of customer service excellence.

Each chapter of this book is anchored on a service principle that has proven to work inside and outside the healthcare industry; see the inside cover for a complete list of these principles. These principles are the key strategies followed by benchmark organizations that use service as a competitive advantage and distinguish themselves from competitors that are merely good.

BOOK CONTENT

The book is divided into three parts—Service Strategy, Service Staff, and Service Systems. Each component is an important contributor to the ultimate goal of meeting and exceeding the needs, wants, and expectations of internal and external customers.

Strategy (Part I) is the set of plans for fulfilling the organization's mission and vision, engendering its values and culture, and achieving its goals. All service efforts are based on this strategy. Part I comprises chapters 1 through 5 and covers many topics, including the following:

- The current market reality, including more informed and more demanding patients, and the practice of "guestology"

- The three components of the total healthcare experience: service product, service setting, and service delivery system
- The strategic planning process as it relates to the service strategy
- Environmental assessment, alignment audit, and action plans
- Quantitative and qualitative forecasting tools
- Evidence-based design and the healing environment
- The customer-focused culture

Staffing (Part II) represents the human resources activities that yield the personnel who develop, implement, improve, and monitor the strategy. Part II contains chapters 6 through 9 and addresses issues such as the following:

- Job analysis and person–organization fit
- Recruitment, selection, and retention
- Leader and staff development and training
- Employee empowerment, motivation, and rewards
- Coproduction of healthcare services

Systems (Part III) refer to the processes, policies, standards, and other practices that support the strategy and the staff. Part III includes chapters 10 through 15 and explores various concepts, including the following:

- Health information systems
- Blueprinting, fishbone analysis, Program Evaluation Review Technique/ Critical Path Method (PERT/CPM), and simulations
- Wait times and the psychology of waiting (perception versus reality)
- Measurement and feedback methods
- Recovering from and preventing service failures
- Service excellence model

Finally, all chapters end with Service Strategies—key points to remember from the chapter discussion as well as our recommendations for action. In this edition, sidebars that pertain to a concept have been included in most chapters, and all references have been moved to the back of the book to facilitate reading.

CONCLUSION

Often, the total healthcare experience in many facilities is less than ideal, causing dissatisfaction of all stakeholders and driving patients to defect to competing providers. Patients and their families no longer just need, want, and expect a positive clinical outcome; they also need, want, and expect great quality and great value from the service experience. These customers are taking advantage of Web-based information and tools to make all kinds of healthcare decisions. They know who does what well and who is falling behind. All other stakeholders, including clinicians and employees, are similarly informed.

This book is a comprehensive guidebook for delivering an excellent total healthcare experience.

Myron D. Fottler, PhD
Robert C. Ford, PhD
Cherrill P. Heaton, PhD

Acknowledgments

WE THANK MANY people for reading our manuscript and offering suggestions for inclusion in the second edition. Their insightful comments added great value to this book.

Myron Fottler thanks his wife, Carol, for her patience during the approximately 18-month period of manuscript preparation. He also thanks his students in the Master's in Health Services Administration program at the University of Central Florida (UCF) who contributed ideas for this book and suggested improvements; specifically, he thanks Megan McLendon, whose assistance was crucial in the preparation of the final manuscript. Last, he thanks Dr. Aaron Liberman, chair of the Department of Healthcare Management and Informatics at UCF, for his support of this project.

Robert Ford thanks his wife, Barbara, for her patient support throughout this project. Her tolerance, understanding, and help during the production of this book are greatly appreciated. Also, he acknowledges and thanks his "guestology" mentor Bruce Laval, former senior vice president of planning and operations at The Walt Disney Company, for his willingness to share his incredible knowledge on managing outstanding guest service organizations.

Cherrill Heaton thanks his wife Marieta for her help and support. He also thanks Dr. Allen Tilley for his support and encouragement.

The authors thank the acquisitions staff at Health Administration Press (HAP)—Janet Davis, Eileen Lynch, and Audrey Kaufman (former acquisitions manager at HAP)—for their encouragement, support, and patience. We also thank Jane Calayag, editor at HAP, for her editorial assistance in shortening and focusing the manuscript.

We also extend our gratitude to Quint Studer. He inspired us to put together our collective knowledge of and experience in excellent customer service and to share them with the healthcare management field. Finally, we thank readers who have sent us comments and suggestions. We appreciate all of these ideas and have included those that fit the framework of this second edition.

PART I

The Service Strategy

Whatever your discipline, become a student of excellence in all things. Take every opportunity to observe people who manifest the qualities of mastery. These models of excellence will inspire you and guide you toward the fulfillment of your highest potential.
—Michael Gelb and Tony Buzan

CHAPTER 1

Customer Satisfaction as Competitive Advantage

Service Principle:
Identify and manage all aspects of the healthcare experience

IN THIS CHAPTER, we address the following:

- The rise of the informed, empowered healthcare customer
- The needs, wants, and expectations of today's patients
- The healthcare market trends driven by knowledgeable customers
- The state of customer service in healthcare
- The ways by which benchmark service companies and cutting-edge healthcare organizations are responding to the current market reality.

Also, we enumerate and describe the three concepts—focus on the customer, treat the customer like a guest, and manage the total healthcare experience—that serve as the foundation for the 15 principles of achieving service excellence. Each chapter in this book explores one of these principles.

A WORD ABOUT TERMINOLOGY

Both the traditional healthcare term *patient* and the general term *customer* are used throughout the book. But these words are not interchangeable because all patients are customers, but not all customers are patients.

For our purposes, we define these terms as follows:

- Patients are those who directly receive either clinical services from healthcare providers or processing services from third-party payers.
- Customers refer to anyone with whom the organization conducts a transaction. In healthcare, patients are the primary customers. The secondary customers include physicians and other clinicians, family members of patients, visitors, third-party payers, vendors, and support and ancillary staff.

Throughout this book, we use "patients" to refer to the actual recipients of healthcare services and "customers" to indicate all categories of healthcare consumers.

Although the word *guest* is introduced in Chapter 2, it is typically associated with the hospitality industry. However, the most successful healthcare organizations treat their customers like guests. Regardless of the term used, the idea is to exceed the expectations of all customers by treating each of them as an honored guest.

THE RISE OF THE HEALTHCARE CUSTOMER

The healthcare industry is made up of organizations that (1) provide healthcare and related services and (2) pay for and regulate the delivery of those services. This diverse industry includes hospitals, health systems, outpatient and retail clinics, medical practices, nursing homes, public and private regulatory agencies, managed care companies, and other third-party payers.

Because the principles and practices presented in this book apply to a wide range of settings, this expanded concept of the healthcare industry is our framework throughout the book.

A Shift in Stakeholder Focus

Historically, healthcare organizations have concentrated on meeting the expectations of their key stakeholders—medical staffs and third-party payers (Blair and Fottler 1990; Fottler et al. 1989). Because most physicians are affiliated with more than one hospital, they have the power to decide where their patients receive healthcare services. Thus, healthcare organizations go to great lengths to make their medical staffs and other physicians in the community happy. Because third-party payers, rather than patients, pay most of the bills, organizations expend considerable effort in satisfying them as well. To retain the approval of third-party payers, healthcare managers focus on increasing market share, restructuring, decreasing costs, and increasing revenues; to please their medical staffs, managers provide sophisticated technology and in-house amenities.

Patients are also key stakeholders and hence need to be satisfied. Traditionally, however, managers have focused on meeting patients' clinical needs, not their wants, needs, and expectations as customers. In a traditional healthcare environment that caters primarily to physicians' needs, many clinicians offer minimal medical consultations with patients and their families. Such treatments lead to increasingly unhappy and vocal patients who express their unhappiness by filing lawsuits and by seeking service alternatives.

Healthcare managers are expanding their aim, providing patients with service that ensures not only positive clinical outcomes but also positive total healthcare experiences (Ford, Bach, and Fottler 1997; Fottler et al. 2000). In the current healthcare marketplace, customer service is the new competitive advantage.

The Voice of Patients

A survey commissioned by the Voluntary Hospitals of America in the 1990s reported that public trust in healthcare institutions markedly declined, with health plans losing more ground than physicians or hospitals (*Alliance* 1998). This decline in trust was especially pronounced among survey respondents aged 40–59; those with higher income and education levels; and those who had recently changed, added, or selected a physician or hospital. These respondents gave hospitals only a 67 percent satisfaction rating. Among 31 other industries, hospitals ranked 27th, which placed them just above the Internal Revenue Service and only 10 percentage points below the tobacco industry.

More recently, findings from a survey by the National Coalition on Health Care (2008) indicate a lack of consumer confidence in the quality, cost, and accessibility of healthcare services and in the U.S. healthcare system as a whole. Eight out of ten survey respondents believed that something is seriously wrong with the healthcare system, and six out of ten were not optimistic about its sustainability in the future. Also, seven out of ten respondents agreed that healthcare quality is often compromised to save money, while eight out of ten stated that high-quality services are not affordable for the average person. In general, respondents who were 65 or older were more satisfied with quality and coverage than those who were in their 30s and 40s.

These results are not surprising. Services paid for by private or government insurance are not as likely to fulfill patients' preferences for convenience and personal control as those services that are paid for by the consumers.

The National Partnership for Women and Families (1998) undertook a research project to examine women's mind-sets regarding health and healthcare in the United States. DYG, Inc., a social and market research company, conducted six focus groups for the project. Focus group members (composed entirely of women) perceived the following flaws of the U.S. healthcare system:

1. It promotes an emphasis on money rather than care.
2. The greed of insurance companies and providers represents a real threat to quality.
3. Costs to consumers are high and rising.
4. Average people are treated poorly by uncommunicative and arrogant healthcare providers and insurers.
5. Access is often constrained or denied, even for those with employer-provided insurance coverage.

According to most focus group participants, the healthcare process increases their stress levels because it is insensitive to patients' time, inefficient, and needlessly complex. For example, requiring a female patient to obtain a referral from a primary care physician before she can see a gynecologist is unnecessary, is offensive, shows a lack of respect, and wastes her time. In response to such conditions, female healthcare consumers have demanded improvements to or have become activists for women's healthcare (National Partnership for Women and Families 1998).

Although this study is more than a decade old, its conclusions are still relevant today. Americans value personal control in all areas of life, including healthcare. This value is evident among members of the focus groups, who reported that they had confronted the individual healthcare system, provider, or insurance plan to personally resolve their healthcare concerns. These women, and other patients like them, demand one critical aspect of the rise of customer-driven healthcare: respect.

PATIENT NEEDS, WANTS, AND EXPECTATIONS

The unique and multilayered players (e.g., third-party payers, physicians, regulatory agencies) in the healthcare industry have caused healthcare organizations to pay less attention to their primary customers—the patients. However, various trends in the healthcare environment, along with the hypercompetitiveness of the market, have motivated healthcare organizations to be more responsive to this customer group. Although the organization must continue to maintain good partnerships with physicians and third-party payers, it has to forge relationships with patients as well. When the patient has healthcare choices, competing at a reasonable price is no longer enough. The organization must convince the patient that it is also the most capable of delivering a satisfying total healthcare experience.

For the organization, identifying and then meeting the needs, wants, and expectations of patients—regarding participation and control, convenient access, cultural competence, caring interaction, and information and value—can make the difference between success and failure in the future. Today's consumers demand and have grown accustomed to getting a lot of respect from the businesses they patronize.

Healthcare organizations must meet all of these expectations to become their patients' first choice. Healthcare executives, therefore, must spend more time and energy on being responsive to customers, providing excellent service, and marketing their institution's strengths.

Participation and Control

Today's healthcare consumers use the Internet, among other sources, to find information on a wide range of healthcare issues—from a provider's quality data to treatment and medication alternatives to clinical protocols and innovations. Consequently, these patients are more empowered and get involved in decisions about how their dollars are spent (Green and Himmelstein 1998; *Orlando Sentinel* 2001). Vocal consumer groups also encourage healthcare consumers to change their attitudes about healthcare, which transforms them from patients to active participants. Regina Herzlinger (1997) characterized healthcare consumers as "well-informed, overworked, and overburdened with child and eldercare responsibilities, whose demands for convenience and control have caused many American businesses to greatly enhance their quality and control their costs."

Convenient Access

A study by PricewaterhouseCoopers's Health Research Institute (2007) revealed that patients want healthcare facilities that are geographically nearby, are open long hours, and have a process that ensures short doctor visits. When asked what factors they considered in deciding where to go for nonurgent care, 90 percent of survey respondents said "proximity," which rated higher than "prior experience" and slightly lower than "confidence in the quality of medical staff." Following are the main lessons from this study (Lutz 2008):

- Retail clinics will prompt payers to rethink primary care. Because healthcare consumers want convenient access, they expect healthcare providers to function like stores, banks, and hotels.
- The public holds the healthcare industry to a higher standard than it reserves for other service industries. As a result, healthcare needs more regulation and more social responsibility. Consumers are not afraid to contact the elected government representatives in their areas to right perceived wrongs.
- Not only do consumers want to obtain healthcare services close to their homes, they also want to be able to conduct business transactions online, to customize services according to their own needs, and to *not* be treated as merely a number.
- Survey respondents believe that healthcare executives have been less involved and provided less leadership (than advocacy groups, physicians and nurses, and individual citizens) in improving the healthcare system.

Cultural Competence

Customizing healthcare services is a consumer desire that is at odds with the standardization goal of regulatory agencies and third-party payers, among others. These groups view standardized care as more cost effective, more efficient, and safer than customized services. Customization, however, enhances customer satisfaction.

One positive aspect of customization that has been documented in the literature is culturally competent care delivery—that is, healthcare that is responsive and sensitive to the unique needs of ethnically and culturally diverse patients. Educational institutions that prepare students (including administrators, physicians, and other caregivers) in the healthcare field are urged to offer cultural competence training or courses that help these future professionals understand and better communicate with various diverse patients and other customers. Research indicates that clinical and customer satisfaction of ethnically/culturally diverse patients tends to improve when clinicians have received training in cultural competence (Beach et al. 2005; Romana 2006).

Caring Interaction

Caring interaction can enhance customer satisfaction and loyalty. According to one study, three attributes have the most impact on patient satisfaction in primary care practices: physician care, staff care, and access, in this order (Otani, Kurz, and Harris 2005). Under the physician care attribute, a major contributor to satisfaction is the length of time a clinician spends with the patient. Under staff care, the most desirable traits are willingness to listen, compassionate behavior, and prompt service. Under access, survey respondents cited caring interaction with appointment personnel as a satisfier.

Findings of this study present several lessons for healthcare organizations: physicians should allocate time for patient questions or concerns about their medical conditions; nursing and ancillary staff should recognize the anxiety felt by patients and their families and interact with them in a sensitive manner; waiting times for all processes should be reduced; and support personnel should efficiently manage the process for scheduling appointments.

Information and Value

A patient chooses a provider on the basis of published outcomes and word-of-mouth information. After a provider is selected and the service/procedure is received, the patient then determines the value and quality of the healthcare experience on the basis of multiple factors. The patient's holistic perception begins before admission and ends after discharge and bill payment, and the provider must deliver an excellent clinical and customer service experience throughout. Each component of this experience contributes to the value perceived by the patient.

To sustain the relationship, the organization must continually remind the patient, through various communication means, that it is a high-quality provider that can meet and exceed his needs, wants, and expectations.

CUSTOMER SATISFACTION LEADS TO CUSTOMER LOYALTY

Why should healthcare executives and health administration students be concerned whether patients are satisfied or dissatisfied with their total healthcare experience? The answer is simple: Customer satisfaction leads to a variety of positive outcomes; conversely, dissatisfaction results in negative consequences.

High levels (extremely and highly satisfied ratings) of customer satisfaction increase market share, improve financial outcomes, enhance the public's perception of the institution and its leaders, encourage former patients to return to the facility when needed, and bolster recommendations by patients to friends or family to use the services offered at the facility. Conversely, low levels of customer satisfaction undermine the long-term viability of the organization.

Customer satisfaction is a short-term product of one excellent encounter, while customer loyalty is a long-term outcome of an ongoing satisfying experience (O'Malley 2004a). Customer loyalty is dependent on the consistent delivery of a memorable service experience that leaves the patient with a constant favorable impression of the provider. Loyal customers generate word-of-mouth advertising, avoid litigation, refer the organization to friends and family, make financial donations, and volunteer their time and talents. Also, as patients, they are more likely to follow the prescribed treatment regimen and thus achieve the desired medical outcomes.

In an environment of cost containment, satisfying customers and building customer loyalty make sense because doing so generates revenue, reduces expense, and saves time (Dube 2003; O'Malley 2004a).

True Customer Loyalty

Smith (2009) notes that *loyalty* is a misused term. Most organizations think that loyalty is about customers being devoted to patronizing their business, but it should be the other way around. The organization should show its loyalty to repeat customers by offering an added value—that is, a service or product not generally experienced in the mass market.

True loyalty happens when a customer experiences an emotional engagement with the organization or product. This engagement comes from experiencing the brand or organization in a unique way that creates value for the customer. This emotional engagement matters because companies that successfully created both functional and emotional bonding had higher customer retention ratios and higher ratios of "cross-selling" and "up-selling" than those that did not. True loyalty requires you to know who your most profitable customers are and to consistently deliver an outstanding customer experience so as to create a high degree of trust in your brand. These loyal and highly profitable customers are then prepared to recommend your organization to others (Smith 2009).

True loyalty is a long-term commitment that depends on the organization's ability to consistently deliver a memorable customer experience that leaves customers with an ongoing favorable image, feeling, and union with the provider. A memorable customer experience is not a single event, but includes many differentiating service encounters that are delivered over a wide spectrum of employee–customer encounters. These customer experiences are more than the sum of the individual service encounter parts (O'Malley 2004a).

Loyal customers generate positive word-of-mouth advertising; are less likely to sue; and are more apt to volunteer, refer others, and donate time and money. Greater customer loyalty also encourages greater customer cooperation, which may lead to better clinical outcomes because the customers conform to treatment plans and may be more likely to purchase other service offerings. Thus, loyal customers may enable the organization to achieve greater revenue growth. They also reduce costs for the provider because they do not require an investment in marketing and do not bring lawsuits. Unfortunately, most healthcare organizations do not have a customer loyalty program in place.

Any deviation from total satisfaction erodes loyalty. Customers who are not totally satisfied tend to change providers after they complete a particular course of treatment. Reducing such defections by 10 percent to 15 percent can double profits. Similar benefits could also accrue to healthcare organizations that work to bring out their customers' true loyalty.

In many healthcare organizations, however, customer service is given lip service and not the resources for selecting, training, and rewarding employees who possess or can develop customer-service skills (Mayer et al. 1998). This is particularly true in an economy that is in recession, where consequent financial pressures cause healthcare executives to cut staffing and staff support in ways that may negatively affect customer service.

MARKET TRENDS

Gaining a competitive advantage in today's healthcare environment is increasingly difficult, so examining today's trends is important. A healthcare organization will sustain a competitive advantage only so long as the attributes of the service it delivers correspond to the key buying criteria of a substantial number of customers in its target market. Sustained competitive advantage is the direct result of the *value differential*—a marked difference in clinical quality, service quality, or price between two competing services—that customers believe one organization has over another. Benchmark healthcare organizations know that the quality and value of their services are largely, if not entirely, determined in the mind of the customer.

One way to achieve a competitive advantage is to develop capabilities that are difficult for competitors to duplicate in the short run or, even better, in the long run. Such capabilities enable the organization to deploy competencies and tangible and intangible resources that produce desired services. Implementing appropriate principles and practices that have been proven effective by the best service organizations strengthens organizational capabilities.

Five major market trends affect healthcare organizations. Each of these trends is discussed in this section.

Trend 1: Awareness of Customer Expectations

Exhibit 1.1 lists eight major customers of healthcare organizations, their customer type (i.e., primary or secondary, external or internal), and their service expectations beyond clinical excellence. As the exhibit shows, the expectations of these eight customers overlap. Although the patient is the primary customer, secondary customers (e.g., families, vendors, physicians) are not unimportant. As mentioned earlier, the organization has to maintain good relationships with its internal and external stakeholders, including the medical staff and unaffiliated community physicians.

Understanding the expectations and key drivers of all customers helps the organization formulate the strategies, staffing, and processes necessary to deliver an excellent total healthcare experience. Because the patient is the principal customer and the ultimate reason that the organization exists, benchmark healthcare organizations focus their attention on the patient's needs, wants, and expectations. Certainly, the service principles and practices applied to patients also work to satisfy other customer groups.

Trend 2: Quality Improvement from the Patient's Perspective

In the past, efforts to improve the quality of healthcare have centered on the provider's needs rather than those of the patient. For example, in 1991 The Joint Commission (formerly the Joint Commission on Accreditation of Healthcare Organizations) made the adoption of continuous quality improvement (CQI) methods a criterion for accreditation. The Joint Commission proposed that healthcare organizations set expectations, develop plans, and implement procedures to assess and improve their governance, management, clinical services, and support services. The goal here was to improve organizational structures and processes (The Joint Commission 1991). Although worthy, this CQI pursuit had mixed results at best (Bigelow and Arndt 1995). Further, the proposals were aimed at improving caregiving from the viewpoint of providers, not patients. Specifically, the recommendations did not require obtaining consumer input or benchmarking against the best practices of service organizations outside of healthcare.

Today, healthcare organizations can use ORYX in their quality pursuit. In 1997, The Joint Commission introduced ORYX, a system hospitals can use to gather and report their performance data. ORYX provides a list of the core and noncore measures that should be collected and submitted to The Joint Commission as part of the hospital accreditation process.

Following are clinical measure sets that may be selected by hospitals (The Joint Commission 2008):

Exhibit 1.1 Customers of Healthcare Organizations, by Type and Service Expectations

Customer	Customer Type	Service Expectations Beyond Clinical Excellence
1. Patients	External/primary	Personalized care, prompt attention, professionalism, communication, respect, privacy, and clear information
2. Families	External/secondary	Professionalism, communication, respect, privacy, and clear information
3. Visitors	External/secondary	Professionalism, respect, and clear information
4. Third-party payers	External/secondary	Prompt attention, professionalism, privacy, and clear information
5. Vendors	External/secondary	Prompt attention, professionalism, and clear communication
6. Clergy	Internal or external/secondary	Professionalism, communication, privacy, and clear information
7. Physicians	Internal or external/secondary	Respect, conflict resolution, teamwork, communication, privacy, and clear information
8. Staff	Internal/secondary	Professionalism, conflict resolution, communication, respect, privacy, teamwork, and clear information

- Acute myocardial infarction
- Heart failure
- Pneumonia
- Pregnancy and related conditions
- Hospital-based inpatient psychiatric services
- Children's asthma care
- Surgical care improvement project
- Hospital outpatient measures

Reporting and collection of measurement data must follow the framework of a Joint Commission–endorsed system.

The report card movement embodies an attempt by the healthcare industry to improve quality and present information that helps consumers make better decisions about health plans and providers. The Healthcare Effectiveness Data and

Information Set (HEDIS), developed by the National Committee for Quality Assurance (NCQA), is a performance measurement system designed specifically for health plans. Using HEDIS, health plans can measure and compare their own performance on numerous health metrics, including management of high blood pressure and smoking cessation, against the performance of other insurers. HEDIS measures are updated annually (NCQA 2009).

Consumer Reports (1996) noted that HEDIS data on health plans were uncorrelated with its own surveys of patient satisfaction. Some dimensions of the customer experience were generally ignored in providers' measures of quality, including patient comfort, convenience, satisfaction, and service quality. Increasingly, however, data requirements—by The Joint Commission and NCQA, for example—are beginning to incorporate select measures of consumer satisfaction.

Today, one of the most consumer oriented of all the available measurement systems is the CAHPS (Consumer Assessment of Healthcare Providers and Systems), developed by the Agency for Healthcare Research and Quality. CAHPS creates and makes available surveys for healthcare customers. Because they are customer centered, the surveys include items and questions that address all aspects of the healthcare experience, including staff's interpersonal and customer service skills. Patients, families, potential customers, providers, and health plans are among those who read the survey results to guide their decision making on buying, switching, dropping, or keeping services. The outcomes are also used in quality improvement efforts (CAHPS 2009).

Because the customer perspective is now represented in report cards and other performance measurement instruments, more healthcare organizations are redesigning their systems to better respond to patients. Here are several ways that clinical and customer service data are collected and distributed within the industry:

- Hospital Compare is a website (see www.hospitalcompare.hhs.gov) that contains information on how hospitals provide care to patients who suffer from medical conditions such as heart disease and diabetes. The website also includes patient ratings of attributes such as cleanliness of the hospital room and bathroom and the customer's intention to recommend the hospital to others (Geggis 2008). The goal of Hospital Compare is to make healthcare practices more transparent and to aid consumers in making informed decisions. Thus far, it is unclear whether the information on Hospital Compare sways consumers to shift their healthcare spending toward hospitals that exhibit the highest quality ratings.
- Consumers Union, a consumer advocacy group and the publisher of *Consumer Reports*, launched a hospital ratings service, adding to the growing providers of consumer information on the Internet (Mathews 2008). On its

website (see www.consumersunion.org), Consumers Union offers assessments of health insurance plans, drugs, and some medical treatments.

- Athenahealth, Inc. (see www.athenahealth.com) is a Web-based medical practice management company that ranks health insurers on the basis of clients' assessments of the insurers' level of responsiveness. Among the attributes these clients evaluate are delays in payment and dropped insurance plans, both of which reduce plan members' access to care.

- The American Customer Satisfaction Index (ACSI), an indicator created by the University of Michigan's Ross School of Business, tracks customer satisfaction scores in various industries. In 2008, ACSI reported that hospitals ranked 28th among 45 other service industries, while health insurance was ranked 36th out of 45. In 2006, ACSI found that health insurers ranked near the bottom in consumer satisfaction, just above airlines and wireless phone providers (Hindo 2006). A major factor in consumer dissatisfaction is cost cutting—that is, companies minimize their overhead by eliminating services, products, or extras that consumers have grown to expect.

- J.D. Power and Associates conducted a customer satisfaction study for *Business Week.* Although this study included only companies with at least $1.5 billion in annual revenue (hence excluding any healthcare organization), its findings have implications in the healthcare industry. The top 25 companies (including Marriott, Publix, UPS, Lexus, and USAA) exceeded customers' expectations through a variety of means. They took advantage of technological innovations, provided employee training and incentives, centered their corporate strategies on customer service, regularly evaluated their service performance, selected employees on the basis of their service orientation, and offered concierge services and customer guarantees. Most of these successful companies involve their top executives in customer service initiatives, and a few of them even developed a "chief customer officer" position (McGregor 2007).

Trend 3: Formal and Informal Reporting of Performance Results

In the United States, the performance data of healthcare organizations and providers are widely and easily accessible. National magazines, such as *U.S. News & World Report*, publish an annual list of "best hospitals," while local news outlets (print, television, and Internet) occasionally feature the best-rated providers in the community. For example, each year *Pittsburgh Magazine* and *New York Magazine* run a list of their respective region's best physicians and hospitals. In addition, statistics and studies on physician malpractice or nursing home performance can be searched on the Internet with a few keywords. Every 9–15 months, the Massachusetts Department of Public Health inspects the quality and compliance with standards of all nursing care facilities across the state. The inspections are not scheduled, and the results are publicized (MassLongTermCare.org 2009). Publicizing performance data and ratings emphasizes the impact of consumers on the organization's overall outcomes and thus the importance of treating customers well.

More and more consumers opt out of company-prescribed channels, such as call centers, to voice their grievances. Instead, they turn to technology to share and spread their opinions (McGregor 2008). Consumer blogs, some of which contain persuasive videos, detail the customer's transactions and eventual disappointment with a product, service, or provider. After getting no help or satisfying response from customer service representatives and supervisors, some consumers send out "e-mail carpet bombs" to the company's executives or top-level personnel. Here, the idea is not only to reach a full resolution to the problem but also to call attention to the inadequacies of the company's customer service function.

Dissatisfied customers are willing to express their dissatisfaction to a worldwide audience—that is, it does not take long for one disgruntled person to spread the word to his or her contacts on a social networking site, such as Facebook.

Trend 4: Consumer-Driven Movement

Historically, in the United States, healthcare services have been provided on a wholesale basis. The government, employers, and insurance companies have been the primary purchasers of these services, leaving the direct consumer (the patient) out of the pricing and purchasing decisions. Often, doctors have dictated what services are needed and where and how these services should be delivered. Today, consumers are taking control of their own healthcare for several reasons, including new tax laws, high insurance deductibles and copayments, health savings accounts, the wide availability of medical information, and the emergence of retail health clinics (see Malvey and Fottler 2006; Hanaman 2006) and other outpatient centers.

Giving employees the responsibility for managing their own healthcare benefits (just as they do their retirement savings) adds momentum to the patient-involvement movement in healthcare. Many employers have created websites to help employees make health-benefit decisions and sign up for plans. Entrepreneurs, in turn, offer online services that greatly reduce the need for employers to manage this type of employee information. Such online services offer employees tools and information that facilitate health-related decision making.

Dysfunctional insurance-related incentives prevent healthcare organizations from developing entrepreneurial consumer-oriented services. The solution to the lack of healthcare entrepreneurship, according to some healthcare insiders, may be consumer participation (Cannon and Tanner 2005; Porter and Teisberg 2006; Kapp 2007). The assumption with such websites is that individual consumers (rather than health plans) are best able to allocate their own resources and determine their own healthcare needs. One experimental model entails a high-deductible health insurance policy, a health savings account, and gap coverage. Under this model, the individual consumer is empowered—that is, he or she exercises a high degree of personal choice, direction, and control regarding healthcare (Cannon and Tanner 2005; Porter and Teisberg 2006; Kapp 2007).

Corporations are self-insuring in increasing numbers. This means that healthcare services are increasingly paid for and managed by employers rather than by insurance companies. One significant advantage of self-insurance is that the health plans offered to employees are more flexible and allow employees to have a voice in how these plans work and what they provide.

Trend 5: Globalization of Healthcare

Employers, insurance companies, and patients have discovered that in some other countries the costs of some healthcare services are lower and their quality and outcomes comparable to those achieved in the United States. The result is medical tourism—the practice of U.S. patients traveling outside the country to obtain surgical services (Connell 2006). Medical tourism has grown rapidly in the last decade because of high healthcare costs, long waits for some surgical procedures, new technology and skills in destination countries, lower transportation fares, Internet marketing of such services, and the globalization of the world economy.

Countries in Southeast Asia, particularly India, have been the primary destinations of medical tourists. In many of these foreign-run facilities, language barriers are not an issue and the standards of care are similar to those followed in the United States. In some instances, U.S. patients achieve equal clinical outcomes and receive higher service quality, although follow-up care may be difficult to maintain.

International migration of healthcare professionals is a major part of globalization and can present challenges for U.S. healthcare executives. Foreign-born/trained physicians and nurses need support in multiple areas, such as visa applications, healthcare system training, acculturation and adaptation, credentialing and continuing education, and interpersonal relations (Masselink 2008). Healthcare organizations that recruit foreign professionals must be aware of the ethical implications on these workers' native countries—that is, by hiring these people to practice in the United States, are U.S. employers depriving the native countries of healthcare knowledge and resources?

LESSONS FROM BENCHMARK SERVICE ORGANIZATIONS

The modern economy is dominated by service organizations. According to Rust (1998), even businesses that deal primarily in physical goods "view themselves primarily as services, with the offered good being an important part of the service (rather than the service being an augmentation of the physical good)." These businesses have adopted traditional service terms such as customer satisfaction, customer retention, and customer relationships.

Throughout this book, we present lessons learned from benchmark healthcare and service organizations to show how today's healthcare organizations can use their strategy, staff, and systems to provide each patient with a seamless healthcare experience. To do so, healthcare organizations must pay close attention to the three components of the total healthcare experience—service product, service setting, and service delivery system. Providing the standards in each component alone will meet the patient's basic expectations, but excellence in all components will make a patient say or think, "They did their best for me. What a superb healthcare experience!"

The principles of managing the total healthcare experience are the same for all organizations, from a neighborhood clinic to a national managed care organization to a rural community hospital to an urban academic medical center. These principles stress service in a way not often done by academic programs and healthcare management seminars. That is, in this book, we argue that excellent practices in other service industries, such as airlines, amusement parks, and hotels, are equally applicable to healthcare enterprises. The most successful healthcare organizations treat their customers like guests and offer not only positive clinical outcomes but also superb total healthcare experiences.

Most organizations that treat customers like guests and provide memorable experiences do not come from the healthcare industry. This is why many of the examples in this book are about other fields. For example, The Walt Disney Company, which refers to its customers as "guests," is considered one of the best at service excellence. It was the first to think in terms of delivering experiences rather than goods or services. As such, Disney is a worthwhile customer service model for any organization, in and out of healthcare.

Ford and Bowen (2008) point out that other service businesses have the following customer service fundamentals:

- Producing a memorable customer service experience is the ultimate goal.
- The customer coproduces or cocreates the value of the experience.
- Employee and customer attitudes and relationships are key to customer satisfaction.
- All tangible (visible to the customer) aspects of the service are managed.
- The customer determines how organizational effectiveness is measured.
- Culture is viewed as a mechanism for control and inspiration.
- Service errors are sought and fixed.

Judging by these fundamentals, the healthcare industry indeed has much to learn from benchmark organizations in other service fields. The improvements that result will carry over to the bottom line, a welcome change in these financially uncertain times.

THE CHALLENGES OF PROVIDING SERVICE EXCELLENCE IN HEALTHCARE

Healthcare executives face multiple challenges to their efforts to provide superb customer service.

First, primary care physicians are in short supply in the United States. Unlike in other countries, this country values its specialists more than its primary care physicians (Pho 2008). As a result, the odds are stacked against primary care, causing a disincentive for these physicians. Primary care demands too much work for too little pay. Insurance companies dictate the price for each service, and telephone and e-mail communications between doctors and patients are not reimbursed. The only way for primary care physicians to raise their income is to see more patients, which is antithetical to service excellence. Because of the shortage of primary care physicians, U.S. patients have to wait longer for appointments than do patients in other countries (Arnst 2007). This is one reason for the rapid rise of retail and other walk-in clinics (Malvey and Fottler 2006).

Second, healthcare's unique reimbursement system acts as a barrier to great customer service. In manufacturing, for example, the customer receives a product or service and then pays the producer or distributor directly. In contrast, in healthcare, the parties that pay for the product or service—such as a managed care company, Medicare, or Medicaid—are not always the ones who receive that product or service. These third-party payers impose rules, regulations, guidelines, clinical protocols, and incentives on providers that constrain the services provided to the patients. If the provider fails to comply with these requirements, the third-party payer may deny reimbursement for the services already provided. Although being customer focused is important from a strategic and competitive perspective, it has to fit within the political and economic framework set by the third-party payers, a constraint that most other service industries do not have to grapple with.

Third, healthcare does not hand out monetary rewards for excellence nor penalties for mediocrity (Goodman 2007). Service excellence, then, tends to be the result of the energy and enthusiasm of a few individuals who receive (or expect) no financial bonus for their efforts. The reason for this is that health insurance reimburses for the number (volume) of procedures performed, not the clinical or service quality. Under this reasoning, hospitals and doctors can make more money providing inefficient, mediocre care to many patients. Healthcare settings in which third-party payment is rare or nonexistent (e.g., walk-in clinics or laser surgery) are vibrant, entrepreneurial, innovative, and competitive. Herzlinger (2007a) makes a similar point when she decries the lack of innovation in healthcare and ties it to the inflexible regulatory and reimbursement system.

Only recently have healthcare researchers and management scholars begun to consider the management of the total healthcare experience as part of the healthcare manager's responsibility. Therefore, much of what is known in this area is based on anecdotal information and case study examples, which makes perfect sense. In the early stages of inquiry into any field of business, the logical approach is to find the best organizations and study them to discover the principles that drive what they do. A review of the service management literature quickly reveals several benchmark organizations; these include Southwest Airlines, Marriott, Ritz-Carlton, Nordstrom, USAA Insurance Company, and The Walt Disney Company.

Some healthcare organizations, such as Shouldice Hospital, SSM Health Care, Sharp HealthCare, and Baptist Health Care, have learned the importance of understanding what their customers expect from all parts of their service experience, and they manage their businesses to enable them to exceed expectations. Because they have studied their customers long and hard, they know what their customers want, what they are willing to pay for it, and how to give it to them. Outstanding healthcare organizations meet customer expectations at a minimum and then go beyond them. As a result, customers, clients, patrons, and patients return, again and again.

THREE FUNDAMENTAL CONCEPTS

Three fundamental concepts of service excellence underlie the "service principle" and "service strategies" in each chapter:

1. Focus on the customer.
2. Treat the customer like a guest.
3. Manage the total healthcare experience.

Focus on the Customer

Everything the healthcare organization does should revolve around the customer—usually the patient. Too many healthcare managers think first about reimbursement procedures, clinical standards, and physician needs. Most major processes—such as designing a service product, creating the climate in which the patient interacts with the organization, and setting up the service delivery system—start with executives, third-party payers, or physicians. This is management from the inside out.

Focusing on the customer, however, requires managing from the outside in. Start with the customers. Study them endlessly to find out what they need, want, value, and expect and what they actually do. Then, focus everyone in the organization on doing a better job of meeting and exceeding their expectations in a way that allows the organization to achieve its financial goals.

Another way of pursuing customer focus in healthcare is to "think retail" or follow the retail model. This means taking on the perspective of the consumer when developing service features and attributes; this effort, in turn, will prompt the consumer to "buy" from your organization (Goldman and Corrigan 1998). Retailers employ three basic strategies to maximize customer satisfaction and create customer loyalty:

1. Enhance the customer experience.
2. Capture a greater share of the consumer's spending for related needs.
3. Create new sources of revenue by discovering unmet or unacknowledged needs.

The recent growth of independent primary care practices that do not accept health insurance exemplifies the value of practicing the principles of customer focus. Known as *concierge medicine,* these facilities only accept a limited number of patients, provide quick appointments, and dedicate an above-average amount of time to each patient. Such facilities are growing fastest in affluent cities and suburbs (Beck 2009) where the average consumer can afford "boutique" services. These doctors lobby Congress to create more financial incentives for employers to offer workers medical savings accounts, which let people put aside pretax earnings for healthcare expenses. Proponents of medical savings accounts argue that people who allocate money specifically for healthcare purposes will spend the funds on independent doctors who provide excellent customer service.

Successful healthcare organizations are those managed by leadership teams who are committed to customer service and instill a service philosophy in their cultures (Girard-DiCarlo 1999; Studer 2008). These leaders continually enhance their core competencies and set and sustain standards that enable their organizations to satisfy the needs of customers at all times in all service locations. They know that each interaction with a customer or potential customer represents a "moment of truth" that needs to be endowed with caring and courtesy.

In a consolidated health system, the service excellence philosophy must be followed by all leaders at all facilities so that the customer service focus prevails across the organization (Girard-DiCarlo 1999; Studer 2008). This philosophy must be embraced by the system's outsourcing partners as well to ensure that high-quality customer service is provided consistently.

As the Baldrige Award winners have shown, focusing on the customer is an ongoing effort. It should begin with selecting customer-oriented employees and providing service training and should continue on to measuring results and rewarding employees for customer service accomplishments.

Treat the Customer Like a Guest

In the last decade, healthcare has undergone a positive paradigm shift. Increasingly, patients are treated as guests, healing (which addresses the whole body) is preferable to curing (which focuses only on the illness), and patients are viewed as active participants or collaborators. Willis (2000) has argued that this paradigm shift is a return to the original purpose of hospitals: to provide hospitable accommodation to strangers. Today, healthcare has become a business; the treatment of a particular disease, a product line; and the hospital, a cost center. As mentioned earlier, consumer surveys suggest that many healthcare facilities do not provide the little things that make patients feel like honored guests.

Implementing the concept of treating the customer (especially the patient, as the primary customer) as a guest requires a change of attitude, not merely a switch in terminology from "customer" to "guest." Many outstanding service companies constantly remind their employees to think of their customers as guests. Disney even coined the term *guestology*—the scientific study of guest behavior—to better understand the needs, wants, and expectations of its customers. As discussed earlier, in this book, we generally refer to healthcare consumers as "patients" and "customers," but regardless of the terminology used, our message is the same: Healthcare organizations must instill the mind-set among their staff that customers are guests.

This mind-set changes the way the organization (through its employees) performs its responsibilities. For example, if a patient comes to the emergency department with a broken arm, the organization is obligated to have the following available: the physician and other support staff, bed or space, and equipment and supplies. If the organization appropriately meets the basic requirements for attending to and setting the broken arm, then the patient leaves satisfied with the service.

With a guest mind-set, however, the organization does more than what it is obligated to deliver. It adds extra touches throughout the entire care experience, such as acknowledging and apologizing for the long wait; giving status updates; or offering water, coffee, or reading material. As a result, the patient goes home impressed with how he or she was respected and treated as a customer. Feeling like a guest is a welcome change for healthcare customers. It is pleasantly unexpected and thus exceeds the expectations of the typical healthcare experience. Moreover, it encourages patients to return and refer others to the facility. Repeat business and referrals are critical to the organization's long-term viability and profitability.

Apply this concept to your own experiences as a customer. Will you patronize a business again if it made you feel central to its operation rather than merely a component of a commercial transaction? Your patients and other customers think the same way.

Manage the Total Healthcare Experience

In healthcare, the primary goal is to achieve a positive clinical outcome. The rest of the patient experience, however, often receives much less attention, to the detriment of all concerned. Managing the total healthcare experience means ensuring that every component of care—the physical environment, organizational culture, clinician and staff behavior, interpersonal relations, communication system, administrative policies, clinical protocols, and standards of operation, to name a few—is efficient, consistent, and responsive to the needs, wants, and expectations of all customers, especially patients.

In the current "experience economy," a term coined by Pine and Gilmore (1998), well-rendered clinical care may no longer be enough. Today's patients are seeking more from their healthcare providers, and they expect it each time they come for any service. In Chapter 2, we discuss the three parts of the total healthcare experience: service product, service setting, and service delivery system. We also show how benchmark healthcare and service organizations use their strategy, staff, and systems to provide each patient (viewed as a guest) with an excellent service experience.

CONCLUSION

Focusing on the customer, treating customers like guests, and managing the total healthcare experience seem to be simple concepts. In reality, however, they are huge managerial challenges on which innovators in healthcare spend considerable time and energy. Healthcare organizations that follow these concepts not only raise the bar but also take business away from competitors that have only a vague understanding of these principles.

Service Strategies

1. Identify the needs, wants, and expectations of your healthcare customers (both primary and secondary).
2. Create a plan to overcome and reverse negative customer perceptions about healthcare delivery systems in general and your healthcare organization in particular.
3. Ensure that your organization's website provides links to healthcare resources and related information.
4. Research what the best healthcare and other service organizations are doing to serve their customers, and then adopt those techniques that make sense in your environment. In other words, benchmark against the best.
5. "Think retail" when developing product/service features and attributes to convince the customer to "buy" from your organization.
6. Implement the three fundamental concepts of customer service: (a) focus on the customer, (b) treat the customer like a guest, and (c) manage the total healthcare experience.

Hail guest! We ask not what thou art: If friend, we greet thee,
hand and heart; if stranger, such no longer be. . . .
—Arthur Guiterman

CHAPTER 2

The Customer as Guest

Service Principle:
Meet or exceed the quality and value that customers expect

SERVING PATIENTS AND making products are so dissimilar that each requires different management principles and concepts. Catching a defective tire or a paint blemish at the final inspection stage is one thing; it is quite another to listen to an irate patient complain that the hospital, clinic, group practice, or managed care company failed to live up to its promise of quality and value. In the first instance, the quality inspector—one of many intermediaries between the maker of the product and the final customer—can send the defect back so that the customer never sees the faulty product. In the second situation, the poor service has been delivered, and the quality inspector is the customer. The administrator or manager can only apologize for the failure, offer options to fix it, and assure the patient that such an unsatisfactory experience will be evaluated.

The challenge for healthcare organizations is that patients want and expect not only outstanding clinical interventions but also excellent customer service—every single time. Compounding this challenge is that service quality and value are judged not only by administrators, third-party payers, and governmental oversight agencies but also by patients and their family and friends. *Consumer Reports* occasionally reviews managed care plans and *U.S. News & World Report* annually rates hospitals, but patients evaluate their healthcare experience each time.

Therefore, on any given day, a patient (who may have been happy with a previous experience) could deem a given service to be of poor quality, a particular doctor to be inept, or the entire hospital to be a major disappointment. Just one unfortunate incident can negatively influence the opinion of the patient *and* anyone with whom the patient comes in contact, either directly through talking or indirectly through a blog entry. Many organizations have discovered that being "average" or "good" is not good enough when one angry or dissatisfied customer decides to seek revenge for a bad experience. Google any organization followed by the word "sucks" and be amazed at the number of hits.

In this chapter, we address the following:

- The meaning of "guestology"
- The nature of service and service product
- The three components of the total healthcare experience: service product, service setting, and service delivery system
- The relationship among quality, value, and cost.

WHAT IS GUESTOLOGY?

Guestology, a term coined by Bruce Laval, former senior vice president of planning and operations at The Walt Disney Company (see Ford and Dickson 2008), is the scientific study of guests' demographic characteristics, needs, wants, expectations, and actual behaviors. Guestology turns traditional management thinking on its head because it forces the organization to systematically examine the service experience through its customers' points of view. The goal of guestology is to create and sustain a customer-centered experience that effectively responds to guests' expectations and actual behaviors and, at the same time, meets financial and clinical objectives.

For a healthcare organization, guestology means studying patients' needs, wants, and expectations as well as observing their behavior while they are in the facility. Findings of such a study then guide healthcare managers in changing or developing services and practices that meet *and* exceed patient expectations of the organization's service product, service setting (also called environment), and service delivery system. Guestology aligns the organization's strategy, staff, and systems with the interests of the patient by starting with a study of the customer and her key drivers of satisfaction.

With guestology, the saying, "It all starts with the customer" becomes the truth (or mind-set) that everyone in the organization accepts and uses to guide everything they do, say, and write.

Desired Qualities of Guest-Service Providers

In the Judeo-Christian tradition, the concept of kindness to strangers traces back to the Israelites' days of slavery in Egypt. In the Torah, the following is written:

> When a stranger sojourns with you in your land, you will do him no wrong. The stranger who sojourns with you should be to you as a native among you, and you should love him as yourself; for you were strangers in the land of Israel. (Leviticus 19:33–34)

Early Christians believed that what separated the "sheep" from the "goats" on Judgment Day was whether they "took strangers in" (Matthew 25). Early Christians built houses that served as lodging (where food was served) for travelers and other strangers. Eventually, they added sections to these houses where sick travelers could stay to get care and treatment for infectious diseases. After many centuries, these houses for strangers were renamed "hospitals"—from the Latin *hospitas,* meaning "guest" or "host." Only much later did hospitals come to specialize in caring for the sick and injured (Willis 2000).

Today's healthcare consumers are looking for the same type of hospitality from their providers. Healthcare organizations must have *functional service quality characteristics*—attributes of caregivers that please (and are easily evaluated by) patients. Research has identified the five most important service quality characteristics (Mittal and Lassar 1998; Parasuraman, Zeithaml, and Berry 1988):

- *Responsiveness:* willingness to help and provide services
- *Assurance:* knowledge and courtesy of staff
- *Empathy:* caring and individualized attention
- *Tangibles:* availability of equipment and appearance of physical environment
- *Reliability:* ability to perform the promised service dependably and accurately

Possessing these characteristics sets the stage for a superb guest experience and turns customers into loyal patrons or repeat guests. Treating customers as guests may seem simple, but it is a major undertaking that healthcare organizations must master to compete successfully in a customer-driven marketplace (Ford, Heaton, and Brown 2001).

THE CUSTOMER SERVICE CHAIN

Exhibit 2.1 shows how customer service begins and ends for a healthcare organization. The external environment (top left corner of the exhibit) influences customers' expectations (bottom left corner), and vice versa (which is illustrated by the two-way arrow). For example, some incentives within the industry may not be supportive of the provision of high levels of customer service. If physicians are pressured by managed care organizations to limit the time spent with each patient so that they can see more patients, the physicians and patient will not be satisfied.

Consumer expectations reflect both the present benefits of the healthcare service received and the anticipated benefits of future services (MacStravic 2005). If consumers are frustrated by elements of the external healthcare environment, they may pressure the system to change. For example, several years ago consumers rallied their political representatives to ease managed care's tight controls over access to certain services and specialists. The managed care industry responded to customers by loosening its grip. A high level of consumer satisfaction with a recent service is a good predictor that the customer will use the service in the future.

Both the external environment and customer expectations have an impact on the organization's strategies, staffing, and systems. For example, if the health insurance plan does not reimburse e-mail communications between patients and physicians but does pay for brief office visits, then face-to-face interaction becomes the preferred medium of contact. The customer's perception of the total healthcare experience (second box from the right of the exhibit) is, in our opinion, the true determinant of satisfaction with a service (which is short term) and loyalty to the organization (which is long term), although many healthcare organizations may argue that their superb performance on clinical measures alone drives their success.

If a customer thinks the experience exceeded his expectations, he is delighted or thrilled. If a customer perceives that the experience met her expectations, she is likely to be satisfied; but if she deems that the service fell below standards, she is not only unhappy but also not likely to come back to the facility. While customer satisfaction may be the result of an excellent, one-time encounter, customer loyalty results from repeated positive transactions over an extended period (O'Malley 2004a). Over the long run, levels of customer satisfaction and loyalty can have a tremendous impact on a business's customer relationship and revenue stream (Peltier, Schibowsky, and Cochran 2002). One bad encounter represents a lost opportunity for the organization to gain a loyal customer (and loyalty means not only repeat service but also a referral).

Exhibit 2.1 Satisfaction–Loyalty–Outcomes Chain

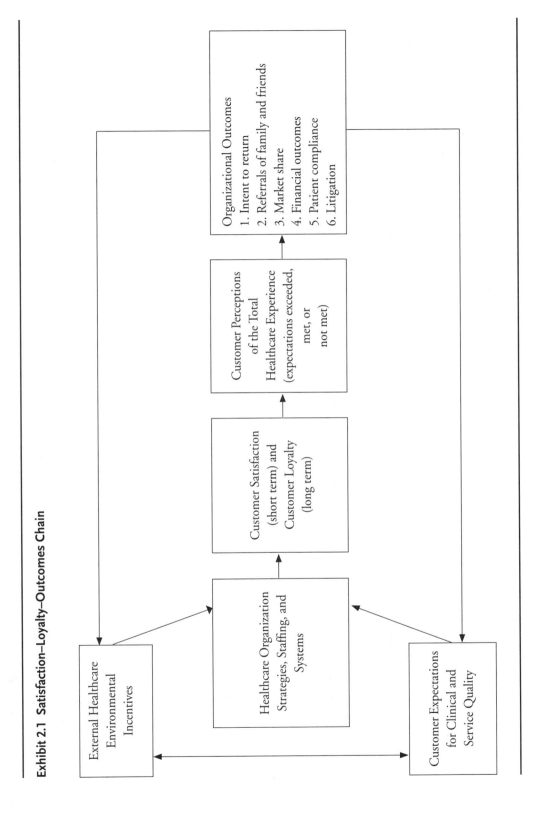

One study of adult medical patients found an empirical link between customer satisfaction and customer loyalty (Garman, Garcia, and Hargreaves 2004). The results revealed that how well physicians and nurses attended to and provided information to patients and their families significantly influenced patients' intention to return to the institution. The financial implications of this finding were substantial.

This customer service chain ends with outcomes (last box on the right of the exhibit). High and low levels of customer satisfaction and customer loyalty yield different results. On the positive end, the organization may see an increase in patients' intent to return, a greater likelihood that patients will refer the facility to their friends and family, a growth in the market share, an improvement of the bottom line, higher rates of patient compliance with treatment, and less litigation (Dube 2003; Harkey and Vraciu 1992; Nelson et al. 1992; Pink and Murray 2003). Conversely, low levels of satisfaction and loyalty are associated with negative outcomes in all variables.

EXTERNAL OR PRIMARY CUSTOMERS' EXPECTATIONS

Discovering the Key Drivers of Satisfaction

Excellent service organizations intensively study the key drivers of people who use their products. Key drivers are the needs, wants, and expectations that are most important to customers, and they should be part of the organization's knowledge base. The best way to learn these key drivers is to continually and carefully study customers.

Many healthcare managers think they understand the factors that contribute to customer satisfaction and intent to return. Most times, however, management's perception does not represent the customers' point of view, creating a disconnect between what managers think consumers prefer and what consumers actually want.

As mentioned earlier, Disney created and developed the concept of guestology to learn about its customers' expectations. Other superb service organizations train their direct-contact employees to regularly ask guests about their customer experience. For example, the Ritz-Carlton has identified 18 key drivers through the use of customer surveys. Ritz-Carlton realized that these key drivers are so important that it designated one employee in every one of its hotels to be in charge of ensuring the delivery of each of the 18 key drivers (Ford and Heaton 2000).

Customer Relationship Management

Benchmark service organizations live by the old sayings "the only constant is change" and "success is never final." That is, they exert much effort into identifying and responding to changes in customer expectations and demographics. Indeed, this is the underlying principle of *customer relationship management,* the organizational practice of focusing all activities on the needs, wants, and behaviors of its customers (Dickson, Ford, and Laval 2005).

According to Berkowitz (2006, 195), customer relationship management (CRM) is "the organization's attempt to develop a long-term, cost-effective link with the customer for the benefit of both the customer and the organization." Simply, CRM shifts the service thinking from the individual transaction to relationship building. Thomas (2005, 309) states that CRM involves

> the creation of a centralized body of knowledge that interfaces internal customer data with external market data. This integrated data set can be analyzed to determine patterns relevant for the task at hand. More specifically, it involves identifying customers and their past purchase behaviors for the purpose of guiding future marketing decisions. It involves building a comprehensive data base of customer profiles and initiating direct marketing based on these profiles.

Well-designed and well-implemented CRM programs yield substantial returns, and new technologies only expand this opportunity. Common goals for a CRM program include the following (Thomas 2005):

- Improve customer service and satisfaction
- Increase profitability
- Reduce negative customer experiences
- Allocate resources more efficiently
- Lower the cost of customer interaction
- Attract and retain customers and prospects
- Build stronger customer relationships
- Improve clinical outcomes

Most organizations use customer satisfaction to define CRM success. Given that most hospitals already use patient satisfaction as a key performance indicator, adopting CRM strategies should not feel like a big leap. However, healthcare organizations seem to have a difficult time switching from being inside-out driven to being outside-in driven. Kaiser Permanente, Celebration Health, and Mayo Clinic all have made significant strides in becoming customer (outside-in) driven. However, they are the exception, not the rule.

CRM is ideal to apply to managing customers in the following areas or activities (Thomas 2005, 313):

- Disease management for the chronically ill
- Employee assistance program
- Physician-to-physician marketing
- Community health screening and prevention
- Frequent-customer program

Managing Expectations

Among the crucial influences on expectations include the individual's needs, values, previous experiences, information from others, intentions, attributes, moods/emotions, perceived consequences of outcomes, social/demographic background, social norms, group pressures, and perceptions of equity (Thompson and Sunol 1995). Because benchmark healthcare organizations dig deep to discover the key factors behind patient expectations, they are able to personalize (as much as possible) each patient's service experience using the information at hand.

Some organizations even document patients' expectations, along with their clinical record, to ensure that the expectations are met on the patients' next visit. Other organizations manage patient expectations by providing accurate information about their services ahead of time. That is, before the patient arrives, she would have already read material or spoken to a staff member regarding the procedure or care she will receive. This type of information may be conveyed through advertisements, preadmission calls, brochures, and website postings. The more accurate the patient expectations are, the more likely the organization can meet or exceed those expectations.

Superb hospitality and other guest-service organizations are also acutely aware of the importance of setting expectations and living up to them. For example, Wendy's defines its offerings well: its food is high quality, its restaurants are open late, and its restrooms are clean. Wendy's customers, then, notice and get disappointed if the food is subpar, the restaurants are closed early, or the restrooms are dirty.

Another example is the way Disney anticipates and meets expectations even before customers enter its amusement parks. Disney's guestology studies revealed that when confronted with a choice in direction, people who are indifferent to where they are going tend to go toward the dominant handedness. Because most guests are right-handed, Disney built the road from the Magic Kingdom's Main Street square to Tomorrowland (which leads right) wider than the road to Frontierland (which leads left). This is guestology in practice, and any organization can benefit from a similar study of its customer needs, wants, behaviors, and expectations.

In healthcare, however, managing patient expectations is challenging because patients' needs and wants are ambiguous and variable. This is especially true if the organization has infrequent or no previous contact with its patients. Unlike visitors to a theme park, many patients are sick, are reluctant to get care, value privacy, need "whole person" service, and are at medical risk (Berry and Bendapudi 2007).

First-time patients may have generalized expectations, such as a clean room and environment, knowledgeable and helpful staff, and a positive clinical outcome. Repeat patients, on the other hand, are likely to have specific expectations that reflect their previous experience with the healthcare provider. This variability is more reason for healthcare organizations to study the key satisfaction drivers for all customers.

Furthermore, patients have high expectations of large healthcare organizations with a well-known brand—Mayo Clinic, for example. Potential customers know of Mayo Clinic's superior reputation: They have read articles, have heard Mayo's name for years, and have possibly been referred to it by their primary care physician. When these first-time patients arrive at Mayo Clinic, they are definitely expecting outstanding services at all levels.

If the organization realizes that it cannot meet the identified patient expectations, it must say so right away before the patient is disappointed. The institution must assess its own capabilities and competencies so that it knows which patient expectations it can meet, thus avoiding the pitfall of overpromising and underdelivering. In addition, healthcare managers must communicate any problems so that patients do not develop unrealistic expectations at any point in the service experience.

Welcoming Complaints

Today's unhappy patients are no longer restricted to talking with friends and neighbors over the backyard fence or the phone. They are also equipped with the Internet, which can quickly spread their message of dissatisfaction to the whole world. Websites that are dedicated to bashing non–customer friendly providers and organizations have proliferated. Enough negative write-ups or mentions on these websites will severely affect an organization's reputation and put its business model at risk. Furthermore, recruiting new customers is much more costly than retaining an existing customer base (Mittal and Lassar 1998), a research finding that was as true in the late 1990s as it is today.

Surveys and interviews are not required to determine that most patients expect a positive experience from a healthcare provider. Patients complain when they encounter factors or situations they do not expect. These complaints are a good source of information, however. Examining what customers do not want can provide insight into what they do want. In his book *Discovering the Soul of Service*, service expert Len Berry (1999, 31) lists the ten most common customer complaints, which are still valid in today's healthcare marketplace. A common thread in these complaints is that healthcare customers feel disrespected:

- Complaint: lying, dishonesty, and unfairness by the organization and employees
  Patient expectation: to be told the truth and treated fairly
- Complaint: harsh, disrespectful treatment by employees
  Patient expectation: to be treated with respect
- Complaint: carelessness, mistakes, and broken promises
  Patient expectation: to receive careful, reliable healthcare and the promised clinical outcome
- Complaint: employees without the desire or authority to solve problems
  Patient expectation: to receive prompt solutions to clinical and nonclinical problems
- Complaint: waiting in line because some service lanes or counters are closed
  Patient expectation: to wait as short a time as possible
- Complaint: impersonal service
  Patient expectation: to receive personal attention and genuine interest from employees
- Complaint: inadequate communication after problems arise
  Patient expectation: to be kept informed of problem-solving efforts after reporting or encountering problems or service failures
- Complaint: employees who are unwilling to make extra effort or who seem annoyed by requests for assistance
  Patient expectation: to receive assistance rendered willingly by employees
- Complaint: employees who do not know what is happening
  Patient expectation: to receive accurate answers to common questions from informed employees
- Complaint: employees who put their own interests first, conduct personal business, or chat with each other while the customers wait
- Patient expectation: to have customer interests come first

Using Customer Service as the Competitive Edge

When patients are unable to readily distinguish the difference in clinical quality between one healthcare provider and another, the organization's excellent customer service reputation can become its competitive advantage. This reputation is a product of the organization's ability to combine its service product, service setting, and service delivery system in a way that meets or exceeds the needs, wants, and expectations of its customers. In a competitive market, customer service is the competitive edge.

INTERNAL CUSTOMERS' EXPECTATIONS

As mentioned in Chapter 1, internal customers include persons (all employees and clinicians) and departments or units that depend on and serve each other. The principles of an outstanding service experience apply not only to external customers but also to internal stakeholders.

For example, when a physician requests a patient's x-ray film from the radiology department, a radiology technician should treat the request as if it were coming from the patient himself—that is, fulfill the request in a pleasant, friendly, and timely manner; provide the correct film; ask clarifying questions if needed; and offer to help in any way possible. If the radiology department does not meet the physician's basic expectation (to acquire the patient's x-ray quickly or by a certain date), then the physician comes away from this transaction dissatisfied with radiology's service. Although the physician cannot stop using the organization's radiology services (as an upset patient might), she can spread the word that the department and its technicians are slow, incompetent, or inefficient. Furthermore, she might become so frustrated that she refuses to practice at the hospital in the future, causing the hospital to lose any future revenues this physician may generate.

This same logic applies to the relationship between administrators and employees. All employees expect their employers to treat them fairly, with care and consideration, and with respect for their dignity and abilities. This is the same basic treatment that benchmark healthcare organizations ask their employees to extend to their patients and other external and internal customers. Viewing employees as guests, thereby motivating and empowering them, is critical to organizational success. (See Chapter 8 for a complete discussion of motivating and empowering staff.)

THE NATURE OF SERVICE AND SERVICE PRODUCTS

By nature, service occurs between two (or more) parties—the consumer and the provider. Usually but not always, service involves both a tangible and an intangible component.

In healthcare, the intangibles are those that patients cannot take home, such as the friendliness and responsiveness of the staff or the promptness and efficiency of the service. The tangibles, on the other hand, are those that patients can physically hold or feel, such as a stethoscope or a thermometer. Sometimes, the intangibles include a tangible part, and vice versa. This bundle or combination of the tangible and the intangible makes up the *service product*.

Both the healthcare organization and the patient define the service product, but each party may define it differently. For example, the organization may think the service product is the positive clinical outcome of a heart transplant. Meanwhile, the patient may perceive the service product as the sum of the whole experience—that is, it includes the successful operation as well as the clean room, caring and informative physicians, supportive and cheerful staff, and outstanding follow-up care. To the patient, the warmth displayed by the caregivers and the bedside manner of the surgeon may be more memorable than the clinical reason for the hospital stay.

For this reason, the organization should define its service product in terms of not only its own interests but also the needs, wants, and expectations of its primary customers. Long ago, Charles Revson, former head of Revlon, Inc., drew this important distinction between what the company makes and what its clientele buys: "In the factory we make cosmetics, in the store we sell hope" (Levitt 1972). This distinction is even more important today as patients seek positive experiences and outcomes.

Tangible Versus Intangible

Manufactured products are different from healthcare service products because manufactured products tend to be exclusively tangible. They are produced, shipped, and purchased now for consumption later, and their producers (manufacturers) have minimal, if any, interaction with the consumer. In contrast, service products are often intangible and demand consumer contact and even customer participation. The tangible item—eyeglasses, a prosthetic device, or prescription drugs, for example—accompanies the intangible service. The combination of the service product, setting, and delivery system defines the total healthcare experience.

Purely intangible services can also be called "service products" if they are the only "product" an organization offers. Think of it this way: A service product is a general term that does not necessarily include a tangible item. For example, the diagnosis of a disease is the service product. The service product consists of information given by the doctor; the nurse's ability to gather health information and explain the doctor's instructions; the promptness with which the front desk signed the patient in and processed the payment; and the availability of the nurse to answer questions before, during, and after the visit.

Interaction Between Customer and Provider

A study by Berry and Bendapudi (2007) enumerates the similarities between services in healthcare and those in other industries. Like others, healthcare services require intense labor and skill, offer intangible and tangible benefits, are usually provided in the presence of the customer, are often perishable, and are not readily clear or understandable to the recipients. Interactions between the customer and the provider are at the heart of healthcare service.

Exhibit 2.2 is a matrix of the types of interactions between the customer and the service provider; it also lists common examples of services that fit each type. As the exhibit shows, different services call for different interactions. For example, vending machines and ATMs (automated teller machines) do not require the provider to be present. Because the provider is not there when a customer uses these machines, the provider must ensure that the system is foolproof for all types of customers who encounter it. Take ATM services, for example. Not only are more and more ATMs equipped with multilingual options, they have also become more customer friendly, allowing users to conduct most of their banking needs without

Exhibit 2.2 Interaction Between Customers and Service Providers

	Customer Is Present	**Customer Is Not Present**
Service Provider Is Not Present	Electric/gas utilities, ATM, vending machine	Answering services, TV security services
Service Provider Is Present	Healthcare, hospitality, other professional services	Lawn service, watch repair

the help of bankers and tellers (Online Search Authority 2009). This functionality is another way banks can forge relationships with their busy customers and hence add value to the experience.

In healthcare and hospitality industries, the provider must almost always be present when the customer is present. Here, the service interaction is the major means for the provider to add value to the customer's experience. For example, in a medical office, the receptionist or front-desk staff is responsible for not only greeting the patient and ensuring that the clinician (physician or nurse) is aware that the patient is waiting to be seen but also for processing payments and making follow-up appointments later in the process. During this (hopefully) brief interaction with the front desk, the receptionist represents the provider. As such, the receptionist can add value to the encounter by exceeding the patient's basic expectations for that part of the visit.

In healthcare, the only services that do not require provider–customer interaction are those performed "back of the house," such as lab work, insurance claims processing, and plant maintenance. Advances in medical technology, however, are widening the possibility of less direct contact between providers and patients. Remote patient monitoring—mostly geared toward patients with chronic illnesses and the elderly—has experienced tremendous growth. Two industry giants—GE and Intel—recently announced a joint venture that will enable physicians to "remotely monitor, diagnose and consult with patients in their homes or assisted-living residences" (Lohr 2009). Telehealth and robotic surgery are among the main practices that allow clinicians and other caregivers to interact remotely and provide care outside of the traditional care setting. As long as these innovations are designed with patient capabilities in mind, they can enhance the service experience.

Implications of Service Intangibility

Service intangibility has several implications for healthcare managers:

1. *Accurately and objectively assessing the intangible service's quality or value is impossible.* The only way to measure its quality or value is through subjective techniques, the most basic of which is to ask the customer. But even using this technique is problematic because each healthcare customer has unique needs and wants, so no two patient experiences are exactly alike. Every patient judges a service on the basis of his or her own views and mind-set. Thus, the less tangible a service, the more patient experiences will vary, regardless of the similarity in what services they received and how they were treated.

2. *Intangible services cannot be stockpiled or stored in an inventory.* For example, a 10:00 a.m. doctor's appointment or an empty hospital bed on Monday cannot be held for use on Tuesday. This temporal aspect of the service can cause patient dissatisfaction, as patients think the healthcare organization has capacity problems. Whether that perception is true or not, managers must manage capacity. They must ensure that the facility can meet expected volumes so that no patient has to wait a long time or go to another provider. However, managers must also be careful about having too much capacity, because if it exceeds demand, then the facility's human and physical resources will sit idle.

3. *Intangible services are difficult to articulate in marketing efforts and to comprehend by customers who have not experienced these services.* Including affirming photographs in advertising pieces, posting quotes and testimonials by satisfied patients and families on the organization's website, publicizing customer service and clinical quality awards, and seeking genuine endorsements from respected community and civic leaders can go a long way toward spreading the organization's good work. Such efforts make the intangible tangible, help potential customers form a mental image of what to expect, and guide employees in what to provide.

4. *Intangible services require human interaction and coproduction.* These interactions can be face to face; over the phone; or by mail, e-mail, or text, and they can be brief or lengthy. Regardless of the format, contact between providers and customers shapes the customer's perception of the organization.

Empowering the Service Provider

To understand and meet customer needs, wants, and expectations, healthcare organizations must work from the patient backward, which follows the concept of guestology. Working backward entails training and empowering the people who provide the services.

Benchmark organizations empower their employees, instead of tightening managerial control systems (which is the practice of bureaucratic organizations), to ensure consistency and predictability of service and employee behavior. They know that no manager can watch every patient–employee interaction and that the staff can make or break the healthcare experience.

Therefore, they place their trust on the capabilities of service providers, to whom they provide ample guidance on and training in customer service principles and organizational mission. Furthermore, these organizations help their employees understand that the organizational mission must be aligned with employee behavior—that is, everything they say must be in concert with everything they do.

Rather than review employees' performance only on an annual basis or after a negative event, healthcare managers should provide ongoing coaching, feedback, resources or tools, and education on a broad set of topics, including customer service. Well-trained and mission-driven staff will provide excellent service.

From Service Economy to Experience Economy

Too few organizations in all industries yet understand that, for many consumers, well-made goods or well-rendered services are no longer sufficient. More and more customers want and expect a memorable experience from the service or product for which they paid. Of course, in healthcare, hospitals are still expected to provide high-quality care at a fair price, doctors are still obligated to prescribe appropriate medications and treatments, and insurance companies and other payers are still relied on to pay the bills on time. However, patient expectations have gone beyond those basics.

In their publications, authors Pine and Gilmore (1998; 1999) argue that society has moved from an industrial to a service to an experience economy. In an *experience economy*, businesses must offer products and services that are memorable and personal for the customers. As a response to this shift, some healthcare organizations (e.g., North Hawaii Community Hospital, Baptist Health Care, and Mid-Columbia Medical Center) have incorporated innovative patient experiences into their practice, such as offering a total healing environment, installing a "wow" team, and making the facility feel more like a cozy inn than a rigid hospital (Pine and Gilmore 1999).

The underlying lesson here is that patients should not be viewed as statistics or as abstract representations of society's healthcare recipients. Each patient is unique, and each presents to the facility with varying emotions and levels of need. They can arrive calm but may be in need of pain medication and serious medical intervention, or they may show up frustrated and afraid but may only need a confirmation that they will be okay. The key to appreciating these differences is learning about the patients, as discussed earlier and as illustrated by guestology. A healthcare organization would want to know not only what ails the patient physically but also what drives the patient mentally and emotionally (e.g., attitudes, beliefs, values). From there, the organization can create a memorable healthcare experience that is tailor made for the patient's needs, wants, and expectations.

The caveat is that meeting the needs, wants, and expectations of a patient who arrives already agitated can be challenging. For example, most dental patients neither enter nor leave the dentist's office filled with joy. If the clinical outcome turns out to be negative (a botched root canal, for example), the challenge to satisfy the patient intensifies. However, healthcare literature shows even if the clinical outcome is less than satisfying (but not too negative), a provider can stem or minimize lawsuits or poor evaluations by attending to the nonclinical aspects of the healthcare experience (Studdert, Melo, and Brennen 2004). Several studies have shown that up to 80 percent of all medical malpractice suits have nothing to do with the clinical quality of the medical services delivered (Berkowitz 2006). A major reason for lawsuits is that the patient or loved ones were angered by the way in which service was delivered, independent of whether the care was injurious.

As Exhibit 2.3 shows, a relationship exists between a patient's medical status and the importance of the total healthcare experience to that patient and his family. Generally, the sicker the patient, the less concerned she is about the service experience. For example, a patient who has lung cancer is focused on getting appropriate and exceptional clinical treatment, not the cleanliness of the bathroom or the cheerfulness of the staff. Conversely, a patient who just received a clean bill of health from a physician tends to notice how welcoming the front desk and the receptionists were or how long the appointment delay was. Regardless of a patient's health status, however, the healthcare organization should provide the best possible

Exhibit 2.3 Relationship Between Probable Clinical Outcome and the Importance of Service Quality

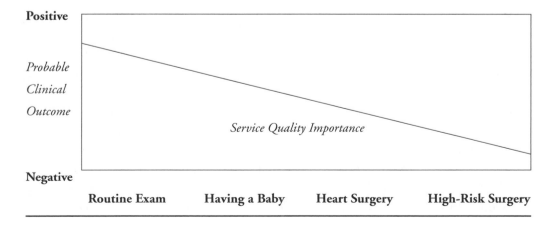

healthcare experience for all its patients because, many times, the positive can off-set the negative.

THE TOTAL HEALTHCARE EXPERIENCE

The total healthcare experience is the sum of all the activities that fall within the three main components of service—product, setting, and delivery system.

As mentioned earlier, no two healthcare experiences are exactly alike because each patient has unique needs, wants, and expectations. This uniqueness becomes the primary challenge for healthcare organizations, but it should not prevent providers from at least trying to enhance the healthcare experience. Benchmark healthcare organizations spend considerable time, effort, and money to ensure that each part of the total healthcare experience adds positive value. They look for and correct service mistakes, and they use probability models to predict how their customers will react or respond to services. O'Malley (2004b) argues that healthcare administrators can improve the total healthcare experience by performing a service inventory of all critical customer-contact points. Armed with an inventory list, managers can identify areas of weakness and address the needs of each area, thereby improving them.

Service Product

The service product is the primary reason that a patient comes to a healthcare provider. In fact, the name of many healthcare businesses reflects their service product—for example, Orlando Regional Medical Center, Orthopedic Associates, CVS Pharmacy, Jones Chiropractic Clinic, Millhopper Family Dentistry, and Vi-sionCare.

Most service products consist of both tangible and intangible elements, and the rest are solely dependent on the intangible, such as the expertise of the provider. Almost always, patients primarily seek the intangible product, and a tangible item may or may not accompany the service. For example, when an elderly patient consults with an orthopedic doctor regarding the pain in his hip, the patient is there to get expert advice and opinion, not to buy an artificial hip. If the orthopedic surgeon deems that a hip replacement is necessary, the patient will receive the artificial hip. In this case, the combination of the intangible (including the orthopedist's knowledge and experience) and the tangible (including the artificial hip) composes the service product. Sometimes, however, the service product does not include a tangible item, which makes paying attention to the intangible aspects even more important for the provider.

Service Setting

The term *servicescape* or *healthscape* refers to the physical environment in which the service product is provided.

The service setting includes the layout of the unit/department, rooms, receiving and waiting areas, cafeterias, and other private and public spaces; employee dress code; the background or ambient music and noise; the lighting, signs, wall hangings, and other decorative elements; and equipment and supplies. Every aspect of the service setting communicates to patients and other customers whether the organization is orderly, clean, and capable and ready to render services. Most important, the setting articulates whether the organization understands the needs, wants, and expectations of its customers.

A service setting that is spotless, has good air and traffic flow, and is pleasant to the customers' senses can promote patient healing and satisfaction, among many other benefits.

Service Delivery System

The service delivery system has by three organizational components:

1. *Clinicians and employees.* This component includes not only physicians and nurses but also orderlies, receptionists, billing clerks, and other personnel.
2. *Physical production tools.* This component includes the technology, equipment, supplies, and space used in the course of producing and delivering a service.
3. *Organizational processes and information systems.* This component includes admission, discharge, accounting, patient records, clinical information, operations management, communications, housekeeping, and food services.

The healthcare delivery system is unlike the manufacturing assembly line. Generally, a factory's product is created behind closed doors, is always tangible, and is often delivered through an intermediary. In healthcare, on the other hand, the product is on demand, intangible, and delivered directly, thus making it an experience rather than an object.

All aspects of the delivery system are equally important and must be managed well, separately and together. The most challenging of these three is the people component. Many patients and other customers gauge the value of their service experience on the basis of the staff's or the clinicians' attitude, concern, and help-fulness. At the moment of the encounter, the patient views that one clinician or employee as the representative for the entire department, the entire organization, or even the entire healthcare industry. Thus, if that one clinician or employee be-haves unprofessionally, gives inaccurate information, fails to meet basic expecta-tions, or disregards the patient's viewpoint and preferences, the patient can regard the entire service experience as dissatisfying. This one event can set off an avalanche of negative consequences for the organization, as the patient proceeds to tell others about the experience.

Moment of Truth

The term *service encounter* refers to the time in which an interaction or a series of interactions (which is usually face to face) takes place between the customer and the service provider. In healthcare, the length of a typical service encounter varies depending on the service sought. For example, a chest x-ray is considered a brief procedure that lasts less than 30 minutes, while a meeting between a patient and a billing clerk could take more than an hour. One hospitalization involves dozens of service encounters.

Any service encounter can make or break the total healthcare experience. Jan Carlzon (1987), the former president of Scandinavian Airline Services (SAS) who reenergized the stagnant company by adopting a customer service focus, termed the "first fifteen golden seconds" of service encounters as *moments of truth*. Every service encounter a customer has with a provider has the potential to make or break customer satisfaction and customer loyalty.

In healthcare, the moment of truth can extend beyond the first 15 seconds and involves more than personal interactions. The healthcare moment of truth refers to any patient encounter with the three components of the service delivery system—with a nurse assistant, with an ATM on the premises, or with a discharge system. Management's responsibility is to ensure that its staff and systems are capable of handling these moments of truth.

Following are recommendations from customer service experts that can enable employees to shine at the moment of truth (Zibriskie 2009):

* [Do not] act as though patients are dead.
* Ask patients for information at the time they arrive.
* Be mindful of others who can hear what you are saying.
* For many people, the issue of weight is sensitive and [should not] be

broadcast. Just write it down, and [do not] argue with patients who insist the scales are wrong.

- Unless otherwise directed, call adult patients Mr., Ms., or Mrs.
- Know the difference between being pleasant and friendly and being too personal.
- Clean up your act to establish credibility.
- Never talk about patients within earshot of other patients.
- Let the patient know what you are getting ready to do and the degree of discomfort she will likely experience as a result.
- Slow down, and speak in plain English (or get a translator, if necessary).

The Beryl Institute (2007) studied one particular moment of truth in hospitals: when a customer or potential customer calls the hospital switchboard. Findings from this research indicate that the interaction between the customer and the switchboard operator has the potential to enhance or detract from customer service success. Specifically, the study found that

- more than 12 percent of switchboard operators incorrectly told customers that the hospital had no referral system;
- more than 40 percent of callers were given another number to call for physician referral, rather than being transferred to the referral hotline, and only 40 percent of callers were transferred to the hotline; and
- nearly 8 percent of callers were transferred to the wrong number.

In light of these findings, the Beryl Institute recommends the following strategies for improving customer contact:

- Start at the top.
- View each call as a potential (or repeat) customer.
- Implement technology.
- Communicate, communicate, communicate.
- Train for results.
- Provide benchmarks.
- Staff appropriately.
- Hire outside support to make assessments and recommendations.

Although these recommendations are specific to enhancing the patient's switchboard experience, they may also apply to other customer-contact areas. To see the complete list and explanations of these strategies, go to www.theberylinstitute.net/publications.asp.

Critical Incident

In general, a critical incident is an event so unusual that it can cause a change in mind-set, behavior, or plans. These incidents may or may not be adverse and, as such, may be classified as customer satisfiers or dissatisfiers. In healthcare, however, a critical incident refers to negative occurrences, such as the following:

- Multiple complaints about the long wait for a routine doctor's appointment
- Miscommunication between the pharmacy and the nursing staff about a physician's order
- A patient's refusal to comply to prescribed medication or treatment
- An employee action that undermines the organization's ethical policy
- A clinician's failure to get patient consent or approval for a delicate procedure

These critical incidents can lead to dire consequences, from confusion to loss of the customer's business to litigation to death. To minimize these eventualities and encourage a trusting environment, one healthcare organization established a policy to disclose all critical and sentinel events to its patients. Created in 2006, this policy includes "a list of items that must be documented to show disclosure of a critical incident has taken place" (Thompson 2009). According to this organization, patients and their families find this transparency valuable.

QUALITY, COST, AND VALUE

In healthcare and other service businesses, "quality," "cost," and "value" have special meanings. Two equations (discussed later) can clarify these meanings and show how quality and value are determined, not in an absolute sense but by the customer (Heskett, Sasser, and Hart 1990, 2).

Because healthcare service is mostly intangible and patient expectations are variable, no objective determination of quality level (and therefore of value) can be made. In manufacturing, a quality inspector can define and determine the quality of a product before a customer even sees or receives it. But in healthcare, that is not possible. Physicians, other clinicians, and medical experts do their part: They develop the standards and protocols for delivering and achieving the best possible health outcomes, and they assess the effectiveness and quality of those methods. However, as mentioned, healthcare consumers today are more involved. They are making their own determination of a service's quality and value, and their perspective is not solely focused on clinical success.

In this consumer-driven environment, healthcare managers must make the patient believe that he is always right. Even when the patient is wrong, the manager must allow that patient to be wrong with dignity. For example, if the patient is accusing the clinic of selling his medical records to pharmaceutical companies, the clinic's manager cannot simply deny the allegation and quote HIPAA rules. The manager must provide the patient with evidence that supports the clinic's privacy policy and must calmly address the patient's concerns. This way, the discussion remains professional but friendly, and the patient does not feel disrespected.

Quality

The quality of the total healthcare experience is evaluated by comparing the quality the customer expects against the quality the customer gets. If no difference exists between the expectation and the actual, quality can be rated as average or normal—that is, the patient received what she expected and is thus satisfied. If the actual exceeds the expectation, then quality can be rated as positive. Conversely, if the actual fails short of the expectation, then quality is viewed as negative.

The quality of two distinct organizations can be assessed this way also. A patient will perceive that a neighborhood health clinic's quality is more superior than that of an academic medical center if the services he received at the clinic exceed his (somewhat lower) expectations, while the services at the medical center did not live up to his (somewhat higher) standards.

This method of determining quality can be expressed with this equation:

$$Q_e = Q_{ed} - Q_{ee}.$$

Here, Q_e is the customer-perceived quality of the healthcare experience, Q_{ed} is the quality of the actual or delivered experience, and Q_{ee} is the quality expected. If Q_{ed} and Q_{ee} are equal or about the same, the Q_e is average or normal. If the Q_{ed} is higher than the Q_{ee}, the Q_e is above average. If the Q_{ed} is lower than the Q_{ee}, the Q_e is below average. Ideally, the Q_{ed} should be higher than the Q_{ee} in all aspects of the total healthcare experience.

Quality under this definition is not necessarily dependent on cost or value, but they may be related. Quality is determined by the difference between what was expected and what the patient experienced. A healthcare consumer may be dissatisfied with the value (because of high costs), but he may view the quality positively. High quality, as perceived by the consumer, will enhance the consumer's perception of value and will lower costs.

Cost

Cost is the sum of all the tangible and intangible expenses associated with a given healthcare experience.

For example, the monetary costs of eye care include the exam, the glasses or contact lenses, the optometrist's fee, and the necessary supplies for the glasses or contact lenses. If the patient has vision insurance, a health savings account, or other coverage and discount plans, these costs are minimized. Opportunity costs are also incurred—that is, if the patient opted to go to another eye center or forgo the doctor appointment altogether, would she have saved money?

Assigning a dollar figure to the patient's time is difficult, but time cost must be considered. The patient is devoting a significant amount of time to the entire care process. She has to make an appointment, commute to the eye clinic, wait to be seen by the optometrist, get measured or fitted for the glasses or contact lenses, and pick up the final product. Finally, a risk cost exists. The patient faces a risk, slim but real, that the clinic's staff or system will damage her vision.

Value

The value (Ve) of the total healthcare experience is determined by comparing the quality delivered (Qed) against all costs (monetary and nonmonetary). This relationship is expressed in this equation:

$$Ve = Qed \div Costs.$$

Patients expect quality to match with cost. That is, if they receive poor quality, they expect low cost; on the other hand, if they receive excellent quality, they expect high cost. If quality is proportionate to the monetary cost, then patients will deem the healthcare experience a fair value but will not necessarily be impressed; after all, they are still paying. Many healthcare organizations "add value" to the experience by offering amenities or extras without increasing the price of the service.

The cost of quality is an important concept in the service industry, including healthcare. These organizations want their customers to realize that although the monetary cost of providing quality service is high, the economic and risk costs of performing poorly are even higher. Fixing errors, compensating customers for those errors, turning around low employee morale, convincing patients to return, and combating negative word of mouth are just some of the inevitable expenses of poor service quality.

Preventing and recovering from errors are so critical that Chapter 13 is devoted to this topic.

CONCLUSION

Guestology is helpful in organizing consumer knowledge in the hospitality and service industries. But the concept can also be applied to healthcare organizations. In this environment of global economic crisis, the idea of treating all customers (internal or external, primary or secondary) as guests can benefit any healthcare enterprise and give it a competitive edge.

Why should leaders think of staff and physicians as guests as well? The answer lies in a leader's answer to this question: Which organization would you prefer to patronize or work for—an organization that treats everybody well or an organization that considers people an interruption and a nuisance?

The answer should be obvious. The healthcare organization that patients and staff prefer invests time, money, and energy to determine their needs, wants, and expectations and their opinion of quality and value. Then, that facility offers this type of experience and expresses its sincere appreciation for customers' patronage. This organization cares about not just the clinical service it provides but also the total healthcare experience. The ultimate goal is to exceed expectations and in so doing make customers return and spread positive word of mouth.

When matters of life and death are involved, the clinical side becomes front and center, of course. The patient, family, physicians, and other caregivers are focused on improving the health condition, not the attitudes of the staff or the flow of the waiting room. But in other situations, the nonclinical aspects of healthcare are important and can determine the success or failure of a healthcare enterprise.

Service Strategies

1. Treat each patient like a guest.
2. Study your customers (be a guestologist). This effort will reveal, among other things, the customers' definition of quality and value, which is likely different from the organization's definition.
3. Recognize that we live in an experience economy by designing services that provide memorable moments.
4. Manage the three components of the total healthcare experience—service product, service environment, and service delivery system.
5. Calculate the tangible and intangible costs of services. Remember that the costs of providing high-quality care are low when compared with the costs of errors and all the consequences.
6. Underpromise but overdeliver. Expect that customers have high expectations, and strive to deliver the best outcome.

Those who fail to plan, plan to fail.
Leaders who are not planners are simply caretakers and gatekeepers.
—Major General Perry Smith, U.S. Air Force

CHAPTER 3

Enhancing Customer Service Through Planning

Service Principle:
Identify and focus on the key drivers of customer satisfaction
in strategic planning

THE SERVICE STRATEGY is an outcome of the comprehensive effort to align the organization's mission with all other activities specified in the strategic plan. An effective plan requires managers to analyze internal strengths and weaknesses and to forecast external opportunities and threats. These analyses and forecasts are used to systematically align all organizational activities and actions with the mission.

Developing and implementing a strategic plan are simple to talk about but are difficult to do. In theory, the basic steps are straightforward: identify or review the mission, vision, and values statements; conduct an environmental and internal assessment to determine threats, weaknesses, opportunities, and strengths; develop a strategic plan and specific actions that are aligned with the mission, vision, and values and resources; and monitor the plan and results regularly.

Unfortunately, patient expectations change often and quickly, competitors duplicate and even take away the organization's competitive advantages, governments pass new laws and regulations, and technological advances make current systems obsolete. When the only constant is change, strategic planning is challenging. The healthcare organization must change to stay competitive and viable.

In this chapter, we address the following:

- The strategic planning process as it relates to the service strategy
- Environmental assessments

- Action plans
- The alignment audit
- Methods for enhancing a service strategy, with examples from benchmark organizations along the way

THE STRATEGIC PLANNING PROCESS

Benchmark organizations work hard to discover the kinds of experiences that customers view as meeting or exceeding their expectations, and they plan ways to deliver them. In healthcare, many exemplary organizations have identified strategies and tactics to meet these expectations. Examples include boutique medicine, medical homes, patient information systems, health savings accounts, and healing environments. All of these will be discussed in this book.

The strategic planning process not only aligns the efforts and activities of the organization but may also spark innovative thinking because it requires organizations to understand, anticipate, and even create the future needs of their customers. Although a detailed explanation of the healthcare strategic planning process is beyond the scope of this book, we offer an overview of the main components of strategic planning as a framework for customer service and patient satisfaction:

- *Mission, vision, and values.* The mission articulates the organization's purpose—the reason it was founded and the reason it exists. It defines the path to the vision and ensures the values are incorporated into organizational actions. It guides the overall organization in how it delivers its product or service and should incorporate its commitment to service excellence. The mission, vision, and values drive the design of the service product, setting, and delivery system. The vision clearly communicates the organization's desired state in the future. Because it communicates a goal or an aspiration, the vision can inspire and unite employees to achieve the common ideal. Values represent the priorities of the organization and its stakeholders, including its employees and its customers; examples of values include excellent customer service and clinical excellence.
- *Environmental assessment.* This component ("the long look around") evaluates the surrounding environment to identify external opportunities and threats, which in turn enables the organization to generate strategic premises. These premises are educated guesses concerning how the future external environment may change depending on recent and current data and experience. The premises then form the basis of the service strategy.

- *Internal assessment.* This examination (searching within) aims to determine the organization's own strengths and weaknesses. An internal assessment leads to an adjustment, a definition, or an affirmation of core competencies, which enable the institution to compete in the future.
- *Alignment audit.* Just as a financial audit ensures that the funds are used properly, a strategic plan audit ensures that the proposed activities, plans, tactics, and policies are aligned with the established mission, vision, and values.

Each of these components is explored in later sections. As shown in Exhibit 3.1, healthcare strategic planning begins with the mission and vision and ends with specific action plans for management, employees, capacity, budget allocations, and marketing. Typically done annually, strategic planning should follow a predictable time frame—for example, every August—to keep everyone focused. No plan should be set in concrete. As things change, the plan must change. The plan must

Exhibit 3.1 The Healthcare Strategic Planning Process

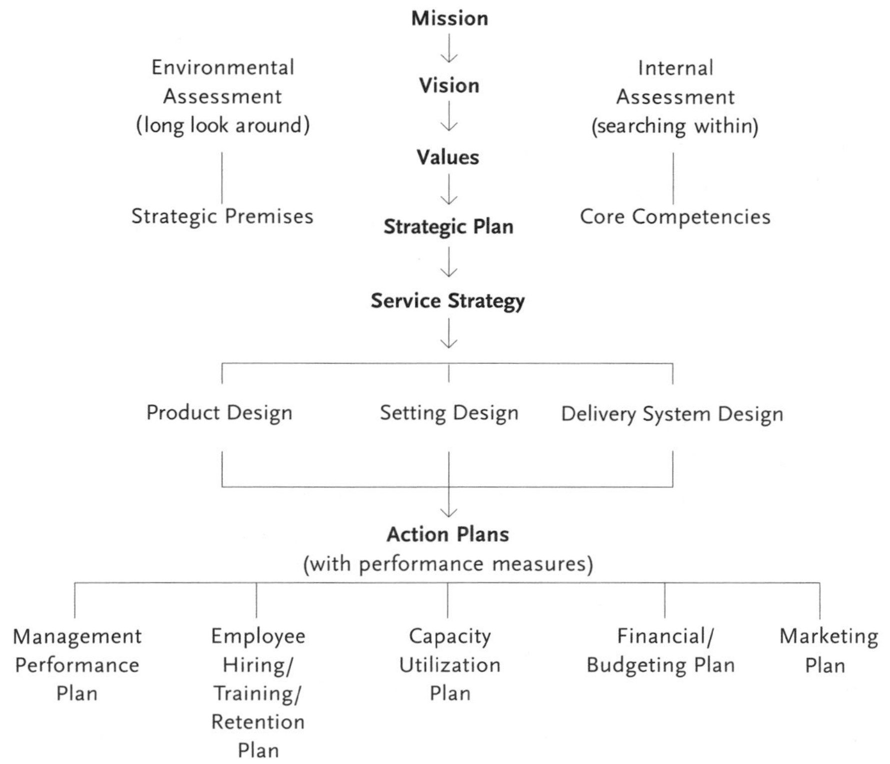

be flexible enough to allow for changes in the environment, the organization, and the customers' expectations.

Strategic planning is a systematic effort to apply rationality and predictability to an irrational and unpredictable world. Thus, it will inevitably lead to missed opportunities, mistakes, wasted time, and frustration. Nevertheless, the process is worthwhile. Although no one knows exactly what the future will bring, everybody has to anticipate and prepare for it.

Strategic planning provides the organization with a method not only for making the best possible decisions today to operate in the future but also for communicating the desired direction to all stakeholders. Once the mission, vision, and values are articulated and the internal and external assessments are completed, the organization can develop and implement the service strategy that will best meet the future needs, wants, and expectations of its customers.

FORECASTING TOOLS FOR EXTERNAL ASSESSMENTS

Many forecasting tools are available, ranging from quantitative or objective methods to qualitative or subjective techniques. Quantitative methods include statistical forecasting, design day, and yield management. Qualitative methods include brainstorming, the Delphi technique, focus groups, scenario planning, and creative thinking.

The principle behind most forecasting tools is that the future is connected in some predictable way to the past. For example, if in the last 30 years a hospital's patient growth rate has been about 5 percent per year, the assumption that the growth rate in the coming ten years will stay the same is reasonable. Similarly, if a clinic's records for the last two years show that a certain percentage of all patients scheduled for the day do not show up, use of physician time can be improved by allowing for "no shows" when scheduling patient appointments.

Unfortunately, using past data to predict future outcomes can be misleading. Innovation (technological or otherwise) can disrupt statistical trends. For example, when the telephone first became widely used, a fixed number of operators were needed for each telephone system. If population growth were used exclusively back then to predict the number of operators needed today, without accounting for factors such as improved technology, the number of operators forecasted for today would be in the millions. Of course, telephone operators are now obsolete. The point is that predictions based only on past and limited experiences and information can be invalidated by advances in technology, work productivity, and other societal changes that may not be foreseeable.

Over the years, lifestyle trends have been the basis of many astute business predictions. For example, the availability of the automobile led to the forecasting of related needs or services: More motorists signaled interstate highways, while more highways signaled roadside hotels, eating accommodations, and rest stops. One of Walt Disney's astute calculations was that the growth of the interstate highway system would result in the development of the theme-park industry. In the 1970s, amid rising healthcare costs, several entrepreneurs predicted that employers and governments (local, state, and federal) would be looking for ways to manage costs. One result of this forecast was the establishment and subsequent growth of for-profit healthcare providers and managed care organizations.

Forecasting techniques are useful in determining the impact of past experiences and trends on future business. However, they are but one part of the external assessment process, which requires thoughtful consideration of other sources and a creative ability to see the connections between today's and tomorrow's customer needs, wants, and expectations.

Quantitative Techniques

An accurate forecast of future demand enables the healthcare organization to make adequate capacity available. This is true for both clinical and nonclinical capacity. Ensuring appropriate coverage is a basic patient expectation in today's marketplace.

Statistical Forecasting
Econometric, regression, time series, and trend analysis are major types of statistical tools. Each type shows that a definable and reliable relationship exists between or among variables.

Econometric models are elaborate mathematical descriptions of multiple and complex relationships that are statistically assembled as systems of multiple regression equations (Pearce and Robinson 2005). An econometric analysis can show the impact of population growth, income changes, and changing demographics on projected demand for a particular health service. In regression analysis, variations in dependent variables are explained by variations in one or more independent variables. Time series and trend analyses extrapolate past data into the future. A time-series forecast will project the future rates in total demand, patient waits, and occupancy rates, for example, on the basis of growth rates in the past (say, the last ten years). These numbers may also be adjusted to account for changes in the economy.

Design Day

Building a new facility (e.g., hospital, clinic, life care community) entails capacity planning—that is, determining how big it should be and how many patients it can serve at one time. A facility cannot be designed to accommodate extreme levels of demand (such as after or during a natural or man-made disaster or a pandemic) because doing so is too expensive. Conversely, a facility's capacity should not be so limited that it is unable to meet normal anticipated demand.

The design-day method is helpful in planning capacity before a facility opens and even afterward, when capacity is already fixed but has to be expanded. Based on information derived from past experiences and knowledge of the demand patterns in similar facilities, the design-day capacity decision can allow the facility to be built to accommodate the demand that is likely to fit the service mission. If the decision is to build to accommodate demand half the time, the facility will be unable to handle demand the other half. Patients will be unhappy, and other stakeholders will be upset. On the other hand, if the design day is set at 100 percent of the time, the facility will be underutilized whenever the highest level of patient demand isn't reached.

To illustrate this concept, consider a clinic that wants to expand capacity. The clinic uses past and predicted patient volume figures to tentatively set the design day at the 50th percentile. This means demand will exceed capacity 50 percent of the year, and capacity will exceed demand 50 percent of the time. Because the clinic is customer focused, however, and does not want patients to experience excessive wait times (when demand exceeds capacity) at any time, it changes the design-day percentile to a higher percentile. The higher the percentile, the lower the number of days that patients have to experience long wait times. For example, if the design day is set at the 75th percentile, the clinic's wait-time standards are exceeded on only about 90 days of the year. If set at the 90th percentile, the standards are exceeded on only about 36 days of the year.

A high percentile design day means an increase in capacity and hence requires additional investment in capital and human resources. A low percentile design day, on the other hand, costs less initially, but because it means a decreased capacity, it tends to result in patient dissatisfaction. This dissatisfaction could discourage repeat visitation, lead to negative word-of-mouth recommendations, stunt revenue growth, and increase the risk of litigation. Management must balance the trade-offs when establishing the design-day percentile: A high level is expensive but meets customer expectations, while a low level is cheaper but may result in dissatisfaction.

Yield Management

Yield management is the process of maximizing the profitability and use of existing capacity. Pioneered by the airline industry, yield management relies on timely information about available capacity and customer demand so that the right capacity (such as airline seats) can be sold to the right customer at the right price. This method is advantageous to organizations that have limited capacity and perishable products or services. Because capacity planners must have accurate and up-to-the-minute data, they cannot properly apply yield management without computers and links to Web-based information systems.

Yield management allows a healthcare organization to quote different rates to different people or groups. For example, HMO patients may be charged prices lower than those given to patients who are under a different or no insurance plan, or different rates could be offered to elective surgery patients to fill in gaps in a medical facility's schedule. A yield management approach encourages the organization to base its pricing structure on three factors:

1. Bargaining power of a group and its importance to the organization
2. Demand patterns by customers
3. Capacity projected to be available at any given time

Qualitative Techniques

Among the qualitative or subjective tools that an organization may use are brainstorming, the Delphi technique, focus group, and scenario building or war gaming.

Brainstorming

Brainstorming is a strategy that entails having members of a group generate as many ideas as possible about a certain topic without stopping to evaluate the details or the usefulness of the ideas. The goals of brainstorming are to spark creativity, generate many possible alternatives, promote participation, and encourage teamwork. In a forecasting discussion, brainstorming opens up the minds of the participants to yield creative and novel insights into trends, perspectives, and other information that may not have been revealed had the discussion not been opened to team participation or if criticism or evaluation had been allowed during the brainstorming session.

Of course, brainstorming does not work for everybody. According to a survey by BNET and Harris Interactive, 37 percent of respondents dislike their team's brainstorming process; specific complaints are that opinions are not heard and participants are unclear about goals (Palfini 2008). Neverthless, brainstorming has the potential to bring about innovative ideas and informed forecasts.

Delphi Technique

The Delphi technique is a structured, multistep method that draws on expert knowledge to forecast an unknowable future. Let's say a hospital wants to know what percentage of overall surgical capacity will be filled at this time next year. The hospital calls on a panel of industry experts to make individual estimates on the basis of their knowledge about past patterns and current trends. Then the hospital compiles and averages the estimates. The hospital then shows the experts the summary, along with the reasoning behind each expert's estimate (without the expert's names, however), and ask them for a second round of estimates. The process is repeated until the variance of the experts' estimates is narrowed down.

The Delphi technique cannot guarantee a precise forecast of the future, such as how many elderly people will need hip replacements. However, this method relies on the best information available from experts and thus can yield a reasonable estimate.

Focus Group

A focus group is a discussion facilitated by a trained leader about a specific issue. Often, focus groups are held to assess the quality of a product or service already received or rendered, but they can be conducted also to determine customers' preferences or wishes for a future offering or innovation. In this case, the organization forms a focus group that is demographically and psychographically (e.g., values, attitudes, interests) representative of its target market. For example, senior citizens are frequently asked to discuss their opinions and expectations related to healthcare services for the elderly. Findings from these focus groups are used to forecast future needs of aging patients.

Scenario Building or War Gaming

With this technique, a certain future situation or scenario is imagined, and its implications for the organization's operations are assessed. For example, a diagnostic clinic's future scenario may be the rapid rise of online diagnostic services. Under this scenario, people will be able to schedule appointments, find related clinical information, pose questions to a physician, receive test results, and get a second opinion if needed. The downside of this innovation is that people may no longer opt to travel to a physical diagnostic clinic if they can get full service on the Internet. If this scenario becomes a reality, how will the clinic entice its patients back? The answer may be some form of organizational redesign.

Although scenario building stimulates creative thinking, it should be based on realistic situations, not on conditions so imaginative that they yield even unlikelier implications and solutions and thus render the exercise futile.

Predicting Other External Factors

The environmental assessment also examines trends and changes in the wider society, including demographics, technology, market expectations, politics, policy, economics, competition, foreign trade, workforce, and sources of capital. All of these factors will affect the way the organization strategizes today and develops innovative services and initiatives in the future.

Some factors are both simple and easy to predict because hard data already exist. For example, estimating the number of people who will be eligible to join the workforce in ten years is a straightforward calculation based on current birth and immigration rates. On the other hand, some factors are simple but unpredictable because they entail multiple variables. For example, estimating the number of skilled and trained people who will join the workforce in a certain geographic area in ten years is complicated to calculate because of many unknown variables, such as population growth, education variability, and migration into and out of a location. Migration is influenced largely by location of jobs, and job location is stimulated by the ups and downs of technology. If technology advances to the point that most healthcare services can be performed remotely, some jobs at local facilities may be filled by people at a distant location.

A complete environmental assessment uses both quantitative and qualitative tools to consider all external factors, regardless of how complicated the factors are to predict, measure, or categorize. The assessment leads the way to the strategic premise or informed predictions for the future. Even if the predictions are not wholly accurate, a strategic plan prevents the organization from reacting day to day without focus or direction.

INTERNAL ASSESSMENT

An organization cannot create a strategy until it discovers its weaknesses (e.g., undeveloped potential, lack of resources) and identifies its strengths (e.g., core competencies, competitive advantages). By conducting an internal assessment, the organization will identify the areas that need to be improved, eliminated, or capitalized on.

Core Competencies

In *Competing for the Future,* authors Gary Hamel and C. K. Prahalad (1994, 221–22) define core competencies as follows:

> Core competencies are the collective learning in the organisation, especially how to co-ordinate diverse production skills and integrate multiple streams of technologies.... Core competence is communication, involvement and a deep commitment to working across organisational boundaries.... Core competence does not diminish with use. Unlike physical assets, which do deteriorate over time, competencies are enhanced as they are applied and shared.

Simply, an organization's competencies are what it does well (through its strategy, staff, and systems) and how it sets itself apart from the competition. For example, HealthSouth's core competence revolves around physical rehabilitation of people who have undergone surgery or suffered injuries. Some healthcare organizations develop core competencies to "help define performance expectations to achieve.... goals and objectives," as is the case with Washington State Hospital Association (WSHA 2009). WSHA's competencies include a service commitment to its member hospitals, ability to deliver results, personal integrity, and cultural competency (WSHA 2009).

Core competencies should be embodied in the organization's mission statement (see, for example, Exhibit 3.2). Understanding what it does (or strives to do) enables the organization to know what it should not do. When an organization strays from its established core competence, it exposes its weaknesses to competitors. For example, in the late 1980s and into the 1990s, many health systems invested in physician practices, real estate, health insurance companies, laundry and cleaning services, and other businesses in an effort to diversify and grow. Most of these new ventures failed primarily because the health systems, although capable in delivering inpatient care, were not equipped to manage an expanded business model that included noncore businesses. The problem was not expansion per se; the problem was expanding into areas beyond core competencies.

An internal assessment will also inform the organization of competencies it does not currently possess, but which would allow it to take advantage of opportunities in the marketplace. For example, a surgery clinic learns that it does not have the capability of handling elective surgery, but the external environmental analysis reveals that, in the foreseeable future, the aging of the population will create a robust market for elective surgery. Based on this evaluation, the clinic should develop the capability for performing elective surgery as an added core competence.

Managerial Competencies

A factory manager and a hospital manager may have many of the same managerial skills, but the two professionals are not likely to be successful if they switch jobs. Each industry requires its leaders and managers to have competencies that enable them to handle the unique issues encountered in that industry. In healthcare, many managerial competency models have been developed by various professional associations and partnerships, such as The Healthcare Leadership Alliance (HLA). The HLA's model is comprehensive and evidence-based, emphasizing five domains that are relevant in healthcare management practice (Stefl 2008, 364):

1. Communication and relationship management
2. Leadership
3. Professionalism
4. Knowledge of the healthcare environment
5. Business skills and knowledge

Other than "knowledge of the healthcare environment," the HLA competencies are not exclusive to healthcare. These competencies are necessary in all other industries. In healthcare, a leader or manager must be able to apply these competencies to the unique internal and external environments of the organization. As Stefl argues, "today's healthcare executives and leaders must have management talent sophisticated enough to match the increased complexity of the healthcare environment." We cannot agree more.

Assets

Internal assets help define the organization's core competencies. These assets include reputation; human capital (employees); managerial capabilities; resources; and competitive advantage brought on by the organization's technology, patent, brand, and customer loyalty. For example, Baptist Health Care in Pensacola, Florida, reported a $2.6 million savings and improved patient outcomes as a result of installing a hospitalist program (Free Library 2004). Undoubtedly, the decision to start a hospitalist program followed an evaluation of internal assets. Back in 1997, Baptist embarked on a "turnaround" journey, seeking to develop programs and strategies that promote patient satisfaction, employee empowerment, and physician support (Nathan 2000). In 2007, Baptist was selected by *Fortune* as one of the "100 Best Companies to Work For," a recognition that has been bestowed on the organization repeatedly (Baptist Health Care 2009). All of these assets allow Baptist to deliver its core competency of customer service excellence.

VISION AND MISSION STATEMENTS

Most organizations spend a great deal of time formulating their vision and mission statements, and for good reason: If you do not know what you want to do (vision), you cannot know how you will do it (mission). Vision and mission statements vary from the simple to the complex, and the simpler the better. Exhibit 3.2 provides examples of vision and mission statements of top-ranked healthcare organizations.

To a certain extent, vision and mission statements contain overlapping goals, and sometimes the terms are used interchangeably. However, these concepts have distinct purposes. While the vision represents an overarching goal, the mission identifies the principles behind that goal. For example, a customer-focused mission states who the customers are, what customers need, and how the organization can meet those needs. Simply, the mission expresses how the organization achieves its vision (Pearce and Robinson 2005).

Vision

The vision articulates the organization's aspirations or ideal state in the future. Hamel and Prahalad (1994) refer to the process of achieving the vision as the "quest for industry foresight," wherein the organization is doing everything possible today to gain a deep understanding of the trends and opportunities to be able to lead in tomorrow's marketplace. Simply, visioning is the task of visualizing what does not yet exist (Hamel and Prahalad 1994).

According to Hamel and Prahalad (1994, 221–22), a vision statement should have the following traits:

1. Imaginable: paints a picture of the future
2. Desirable: appeals to all stakeholders

Exhibit 3.2 Example of Mission and Vision Statements

Waynesboro Hospital (Waynesboro, Pennsylvania)

Mission: The mission of Waynesboro Hospital is to provide quality health care to, and improve the health and well-being of, the people of the Hospital's service area. We will strive to offer these services at a cost that provides the greatest value to the community.

Vision: Waynesboro Hospital will be the dominant force for promoting healthy communities by serving as the provider of choice in our area for hospital sponsored care and by leading the coordination of high quality individual and community health services.

Values: We believe that the delivery of quality health care can best be achieved by caring for both our community and coworkers with the regard for the dignity of the individual that we would wish for ourselves.

King's Daughters Medical Center (Ashland, Kentucky)

Mission: To Care. To Serve. To Heal.

Vision: World-Class Care In Our Communities

Baptist Health South Florida (Coral Gables, Florida)

Mission: The mission of Baptist Health is to improve the health and well-being of individuals, and to promote the sanctity and preservation of life, in the communities we serve.

Vision: Baptist Health will be the preeminent healthcare provider in the communities we serve, the organization that people instinctively turn to for their healthcare needs. Baptist Health will offer a broad range of clinical services that are evidence-based and compassionately provided to assure patient safety, superior clinical outcomes and the highest levels of satisfaction. Baptist Health will be a national and international leader in healthcare innovation.

Indiana Regional Medical Center (Indiana, Pennsylvania)

Mission: Indiana Regional Medical Center, in partnership with its communities, strives to be the center for quality, accessible, cost-effective healthcare. We are dedicated to promoting health and wellness through education and compassionate, caring services.

Vision: To be the best community hospital in Pennsylvania.

Values: We value people, health and exceptional performance.

Source: This information was retrieved from the organizations' websites.

3. Feasible: is realistic and attainable
4. Focused: provides clear guidance
5. Flexible: allows individual adaptations
6. Communicable: can be explained in five minutes

For the vision to gain stakeholder support and following, it must be clear and well communicated. In addition, it must incorporate organizational values (Mittal 2009), which in turn define the corporate culture (Atchison and Carlson 2009). Sometimes an organization is created to fulfill a personal vision, as former Chili's CEO Norman Brinker has said: "I have a vision, then I create an atmosphere that involves the people in that vision" (Brinker and Phillips 1996, 191).

Mission

The mission statement defines three organizational truths:

1. Why it exists
2. What it does and how
3. Who it serves

The mission guides leaders and managers in developing strategies, allocating resources, creating initiatives, and establishing employee standards for dealing with patients and other customers. In this sense, the mission represents the organization's core values.

Customer service is almost always an integral part of a mission statement. When Southwest Airlines began operating in 1971, its customer-focused message to employees was, "Get your passengers to their destinations when they want to get there, on time, at the lowest possible fares, and make darn sure they have a good time doing it." Today, Southwest's mission has stayed the same: "Dedicated to the highest quality of Customer Service delivered with a sense of warmth, friendliness, individual pride, and Company Spirit." Also, Southwest is "committed to providing Employees a stable work environment with equal opportunity for learning and personal growth" (Gittell 2003).

Results of one study of hospital mission statements are presented here to illustrate the link between mission and customer orientation. The study found that the components most common among missions were purpose (76 percent), specific customers served (62 percent), one clear compelling goal (56 percent), values and beliefs (56 percent), products and services offered (52 percent), concern with satisfying customers (50 percent), and concern for employees (41 percent) (Barr 1999). In addition, the survey also found that top management satisfaction with financial performance was significantly and positively correlated with a mission statement that contains three types of information: customers served, concern with satisfying customers, and products/services offered. Moreover, top management satisfaction with financial performance was also higher if management was satisfied with how well each of the following mission statement components was written: specific customers served, concern with satisfying customers, and concern for employees.

Once the mission has been established and communicated to all stakeholders, it should be used as a guide for all internal and external initiatives. In this way, the organization (including its governance board) and the community at large are assured that every activity, practice, and policy is aligned with the mission.

THE SERVICE STRATEGY

The service strategy is the detailed plan for meeting and exceeding the customers' expectations of a healthcare experience. The service strategy should be based on informed judgment and should involve structured studies (environmental assessment) and consumer surveys. Led by the mission and vision, the service strategy guides the development of the service product, service setting, and service delivery system. That is, based on the why, what, and who defined in the mission, the organization can craft the service product, its setting, and its delivery system. For example, if the mission is to provide elective cosmetic surgery to an upscale, educated group in a specific geographic area, then the strategy should be to provide high-touch and high-tech services in an elegant environment.

The needs, opinions, preferences, and expectations of the targeted consumer group should be incorporated into the service strategy. Assessing the external and internal environment is not enough to gain insight into the key drivers of customer satisfaction. The organization must also ask its customers. Only customers can voice what they really think about the quality and value of a product or the role the organization's core competencies play in service delivery.

As discussed in Chapter 2, The Walt Disney Company surveys its guests constantly. On one such survey, the company asked guests at Disney World to rate their experiences with various aspects of their visit in relation to their intention to return and their overall satisfaction (Lee 2004). The fast food and transportation system received low ratings; however, analysis of the data revealed only a weak statistical relationship between the low ratings and the customer's intention to return and overall satisfaction. In other words, the customer-perceived quality of the food and the transportation did not matter much in determining return visits. After all, people do not fly from across the world to eat or ride basic transport.

What did matter (key drivers) to customers were the hours of operation, employee friendliness, and the fireworks display. Ratings in these two areas were strongly correlated to both intention to return and overall satisfaction. As a response to these survey findings, Disney invested available funds in extending park hours, hiring friendly employees, and expanding the fireworks displays. Disney made an improvement decision based on information provided by its guests: It allocated its scarce resources to enhancing the services that were perceived most valuable by its customers and that were the key drivers of their behavior and attitudes toward the Disney experience. Healthcare organizations can learn a lot by identifying its patients' key drivers and, like Disney, by making decisions based on what the patients declare as important.

Service expert Len Berry (1999, 65–68) suggests that an excellent service strategy commits the organization to four key factors: quality, value, service, and achievement. Press (2003) found that three key drivers were correlated with overall patient satisfaction based on data derived from 992,000 outpatients at 516 outpatient facilities in 2001: "Staff sensitivity to your needs," "How well staff worked together to provide care," and "Response to concerns/complaints made during your visit."

Quality and Value

An excellent service strategy emphasizes quality and value. A healthcare organization truly committed to customer service will make a commitment to providing both high quality and high value. A commitment means that the organization invests the necessary resources (money, time, and labor) to identify and measure patients' perception of quality and value. It is perception that matters in determining quality and value and not the actual cost or engineered quality. Patients must perceive that the total healthcare experience was worth the price—that is, offered a good value.

Previous research has shown that many healthcare managers do not know what really matters to patients (Duffy, Duffy, and Kilbourne 2001). The main reason for this gap in knowledge is that, typically, managers do not ask patients, preferring instead to assume they know what patients think. Quint Studer (2008, 270–72) recommends an easy method for finding out and remembering customer needs, wants, and expectations: A manager fills out a preference card for customers (patients and physicians) on the unit. The patient preference card may include personal information such as favorite foods, sleeping habits, and a visitor list. The physician preference card may include professional requests such as the appropriate time to call the physician about a patient's condition. These convenient cards allow managers to customize the service product, setting, and delivery, which increases the customer's perception of quality and value.

Service and Achievement

An excellent strategy must emphasize service and achievement of goals, not just quality and value. Again, organizational commitment to service excellence, not just lip service through the mission statement, is imperative. Commitment to service (and, by extension, achievement of service goals) requires the following:

- Recruitment and retention of physicians and employees who believe in the merits and efficacy of customer service
- Allocation of appropriate resources to employee-training programs, service product development and evaluation, and service performance and reward systems, among others
- Action plans that support the service mission
- Regular and clear communication about service initiatives to all stakeholders

A culture of service can foster a sense of genuine achievement among employees and clinicians. It can stretch people's service abilities and, in so doing, expand the capabilities of the entire organization, resulting in performance that exceeds everyone's expectations. At one time, 90 percent of Taco Bell restaurants operated properly without full-time managers (Berry 1999). That is an impressive scenario that is possible when people are committed to service and achievement of service goals.

ACTION PLANS

Action plans lay out the specific tactics of the service strategy—that is, how the organization will operate, what each department or employee group will be expected to do, and what time frame will be followed. (Exhibit 3.3 shows how a service strategy can be converted into action plans.)

Exhibit 3.3 From Service Strategy to Action Plans

Service Strategy

- Study similar organizations that excel in customer service and benchmark against them.

- Use a service audit to survey customers based on quality, value, service, and achievement.

- Develop a strategy to reduce the gaps between desired and actual customer service expectations.

Action Plans

- Use cross-functional teams to create tactical plans that focus all parts of the organization on customer service.

- Use cross-functional teams to integrate all of the tactical plans.

- Use various techniques, such as brainstorming, to create customer service initiatives in each tactical area.

- Carefully select one or two customer service priority areas for intense focus.

- Empower employees to meet customer expectations.

- Include customer outcome measures in assessment strategies.

- Ensure that key stakeholders support new strategic customer service initiatives through continued communication of benefits of change and risk of the status quo.

- Involve staff in identifying ways to implement strategy.

- Use social norms and opinion leaders to create support for strategic initiatives.

- Audit the alignment of customer service plans with mission, vision, values, strategies, staffing, and systems.

Action plans should be established in five key areas:

1. Management performance
2. Staffing (hiring, training, retention)
3. Capacity utilization
4. Finance/budget
5. Marketing

Performance criteria in each of these areas must be established and measured. Measurement ensures that the right steps are taken, the right people are involved, the right time line is followed, and the right goals are pursued. More important, measurement allows the stakeholders to see their progress and contributions toward the overarching strategy.

The action plan in each area must be created with careful consideration of the action plans in other areas. For example, when establishing the marketing plan, the capacity utilization plan must be consulted to prevent conflicts in priorities. What if the marketing plan is designed to draw thousands of new patients to the hospital but the capacity plan is intended to drastically reduce services on the weekends? Similarly, what if the management performance plan demands managerial innovation but the finance plan provides no budget for accomplishing this innovation goal? Action plans need to integrate the activities of the organization. Action plans make little sense if they are not supported by other organizational components or if no money has been allocated to execute the activities.

Action plans provide a road map and put the responsibility for achieving the service strategy into the hands of employees (managers and frontline staff alike). In this sense, everyone knows how his contribution helps the organization reach its mission, and everyone is held accountable for meeting and exceeding patient expectations. The most obvious and the biggest opportunity for delivering customer satisfaction is direct patient contact. Exhibit 3.4 lists the ideal behaviors to display during service delivery, while Exhibit 3.5 recommends protocols (what you do) and scripts (what you say) for selected drivers of patient satisfaction.

THE ALIGNMENT AUDIT

Strategy scholar Michael Porter (1996) suggests that the best way for an organization to achieve a sustainable competitive advantage is to reinforce its strategic plan by aligning functional policies, staffing decisions, structure, and all other activities with the established mission. In addition, Nadler and Tushman (1997, 34) argue that "The degree to which the strategy, work, people, structure, and culture are smoothly aligned will determine the organization's ability to compete and succeed." Quint Studer (2008) organizes an entire book around the benefits of alignment.

Empirical research has found that when internal organizational factors (i.e., mission, vision, values, and communication methods) are aligned with the strategic plan, employees feel higher levels of commitment and satisfaction (Ford et al. 2006). In turn, staff commitment and satisfaction lead to positive financial returns, competitive advantage, and customer satisfaction (Atkins, Marshall, and Javalgi 1996; Fottler et al. 2006; Schneider, White, and Paul 1998). A study by

Exhibit 3.4 Employee Behaviors That Deliver Patient Satisfaction

1. Make people feel welcomed. Smile, make eye contact, introduce yourself, use customer last names, and offer help.

2. Protect privacy and confidentiality. Knock before entering patient rooms, cover patients, and watch what you say to whom.

3. Show courtesy and respect. Say "please" and "thank you," be sensitive to cultural differences, and find out what customers want and need.

4. Explain what you are doing. Let customers know what to expect, speak in ways customers can understand, check to see if the message is understood, and keep the staff informed.

5. Handle with care. Slow down and handle patients gently when moving or touching them, and listen and respond to what they are saying.

6. Maintain a customer-friendly atmosphere. Reduce noise and keep the environment clean and clutter-free.

7. Follow-up and follow through. Work to solve problems and complaints, let customers know what you can and cannot do, and find out who can help and then follow-up and "close the loop."

Source: Used with permission from *Journal of Healthcare Management* 46 (3): 153. (Chicago: Health Administration Press, 2001).

Exhibit 3.5 Protocols and Scripts for Key Drivers of Patient Satisfaction

Key Driver	Protocol (What you do)	Script (What you say)
1. Respect for privacy and dignity	Knock on patient's door and say patient's name	"Mrs. ____? My name is ____. I am here to _____. Is this a good time?"
2. Feel listened to	Ask if patient has any special needs or requests	"Is there anything else I can do for you?"
3. Experience responsiveness to concerns and complaints	Ask if the previous concern (e.g., low room temperature) has been resolved	"Is the room temperature still uncomfortable? Can I get you another blanket?"

Source: Adapted with permission from *Journal of Healthcare Management* 46 (3): 154. (Chicago: Health Administration Press, 2001).

Goldstein and Schweikhardt (2002) reveals that organizations that focus on the 19 dimensions of the Malcolm Baldrige National Quality Award provide high levels of customer service and satisfaction. This finding rings true for Sharp HealthCare (see sidebar), a recipient of the Baldrige Award and a proponent for aligning mission with all organizational components and activities.

Although healthcare organizations routinely audit their financial plans and operations, they are doing so to monitor financial progress, not to check if the plans are consistent with the mission; plus, most organizations do not audit their patient services and management processes. In light of the advantages that an alignment brings, an organization should conduct an alignment audit to ensure that all of its undertakings are in sync with its mission (Crotts, Dickson, and Ford 2005). Such an audit (Exhibit 3.6) may be conducted annually, much like a financial audit is performed.

If what gets measured gets managed, then measuring alignment will guarantee that the mission is managed (Laborwitz 2005). More important, conducting an audit communicates a powerful message: The organization is serious about its service mission.

Cues

Managers communicate organizational needs, wants, and expectations to employees by sending various *cues*. Cues can be explicit (such as the written mission statement) or implicit (such as a verbal story about an exemplary employee). Human resource policies (such as requirements in a job description or system procedures for handling customer calls) also serve as cues. From these cues, employees learn what the organization (and their superiors) deems important and desirable regarding employee performance and behavior.

When cues are aligned with the mission, they send a message that the mission is more than just a theory; it is applicable to everyday practice. An alignment audit systematically measures how well each cue supports the mission. Because aligning each cue with the mission does not by itself achieve mission excellence, an alignment audit reveals whether all cues (verbal, written, behavioral) are sending a consistent message.

For example, when managers say customer service is important, do they reward those who go above and beyond their duties to please customers, or are reward programs in place to recognize an employee's customer orientation? Similarly, when a mission statement claims that the organization is a leader in medical innovation, do top executives strive to recruit and retain staff who have expertise, experience,

SIDEBAR: SHARP HEALTHCARE

In 2007, Sharp HealthCare, the largest integrated delivery system in San Diego, California, received the Malcolm Baldrige National Quality Award.

Sharp's quality journey began in 2001 with the launch of the Sharp Experience, a performance improvement initiative aimed at making the organization the best place to work, the best place to practice medicine, and the best place to receive care. Guided by its mission, vision, and values, Sharp conducts a strategic planning process with an eye toward the satisfaction of patients, staff, physicians, employees, third-party payers, and community representatives (Sharp HealthCare 2007). Moreover, Sharp reinforces its mission, vision, and values by constantly communicating them to stakeholders. In addition, Sharp pursues (and then measures) a wide range of short- and long-term objectives that increase customer satisfaction, customer loyalty, and market share. Everything at Sharp—from strategic plans to meeting agendas—is aligned with the Six Pillars of Excellence, which are "the foundation for its vision to transform the health care experience" (Sharp HealthCare 2009). Following are the award-winning principles behind Sharp HealthCare's success.

MISSION STATEMENT

To improve the health of those we serve with a commitment to excellence in all we do. Offer quality care and service that set community standards, exceed patient's expectations, and are provided in a caring, convenient, cost effective, and accessible manner.

VISION STATEMENT

Redefine the healthcare experience through a culture of caring quality, service, innovation, and excellence. Recognition as the best place to work, practice medicine and receive care . . . become the best healthcare system in the universe.

VALUES

- Integrity
- Caring
- Innovation
- Excellence

SIX PILLARS OF EXCELLENCE

1. Quality
2. Service
3. People
4. Finance
5. Growth
6. Community

EMPLOYEE BEHAVIOR STANDARDS

Confidentiality; Manners; Diversity; Skills and competence; Lasting impression; Talk, Listen, and Teamwork; Service recovery; Safety; Appearance; Ease waiting times; Smile; Take people to destination; Scripting; Attitude of gratitude; Round with reason; Acknowledge; Introduce yourself; Explain; Thank you

CRITICAL SUCCESS FACTORS

- Define, measure, and communicate climate and service excellence
- Increase patient and community loyalty
- Attract, motivate, maintain, and promote the best healthcare workforce in the area

COMMUNICATION PLAN

Use multiple communication processes to convey vision, values, and goals annually (all staff assembly, employee satisfaction survey, and physician satisfaction survey), quarterly (leader development seminar and employee forums), monthly (departmental meetings, action teams, operations meetings, board meetings, and newsletters), and day-to-day (CEO letters, global emails, intranet, and thank you notes).

PLANNING HORIZONS

- Long-term (five years)
- Short-term (one year)

Long-Term Service Strategies (2007–2012)

- Focus on top patient satisfiers (key drivers) as identified by Press Ganey Patient Surveys
- Hospitals, medical groups, and physician satisfaction
- Physician leadership development and satisfaction
- Extensive education and tools for leaders and staff

CUSTOMER/PARTNER-DRIVEN ENVIRONMENTAL ANALYSIS

During the strategic planning process, a customer-partner driven analysis is produced. Sharp continually assesses key customer groups, competitor activities, market share, demographic data, customer group feedback, and industry trends data.

CUSTOMER SERVICE METRICS

Patient satisfaction surveys (Press Ganey); Physician and staff satisfaction surveys; Focus groups; Mystery shopping; Interviews; Encounter data online; Nurse connector web center; Call center; "Rounding with Reason" logs; Comment cards; Interdepartmental surveys; Complaint system; Health plan surveys; Customer contact centers; Web page; and Annual meeting for payers and medical groups.

Source: Reprinted with permission from Sharp HealthCare, San Diego, California.

---

and training in advanced clinical technology? In other words, an alignment audit enables managers to discover the inconsistencies between their words and actions. Management's hope that physicians and employees do what they are told is folly if management does not behave in accordance to its own cues or offer rewards to those who abide by those cues.

Well-aligned cues guide internal stakeholders' (managers, employees, and clinicians alike) performance and behavior in every patient or customer encounter.

Framework

The deeper the audit delves into the organization's policies, procedures, and practices, the more likely the audit will reveal misalignment, but the greater the opportunity for improvement will be. In this section, we discuss the framework of an alignment audit.

Core Elements

The audit should focus on three main areas: (1) strategic and tactical practices, (2) staffing policies and processes, and (3) system procedures and design. Using other categories of focus may be equally useful, but these three areas comprehensively address the elements most critical to organizational functions. Exhibit 3.6 presents sample audit questions for each core element that may be used as a starting point or a template for an alignment audit. Managers may expand or revise these questions according to their organizational needs or preferred areas of focus.

Steps for Conducting an Audit
The audit should be structured as follows:

1. Define the goals of the mission in measurable terms (e.g., scores on customer satisfaction surveys).
2. Identify key policies, procedures, practices, and communications that cue employee performance and behavior (e.g., job descriptions).
3. Formulate questions that evaluate if the mission is reflected in each key policy, procedure, practice, and communication (e.g., see Exhibit 3.6)
4. Answer the questions honestly.
5. Develop a list of misaligned items for immediate or future corrections and improvements.
6. Compare the audit results (step 5) with the mission goals (step 1).

The purpose of step 6 is to audit the audit—that is, to affirm that the items audited are the ones that matter according to the mission goals or outcomes desired. In addition, step 6 establishes a measure of the organizational benefit gained by undertaking an alignment audit—that is, the gap between the desired versus the actual behavior is determined. Lastly, step 6 documents the alignment process, which serves as proof that the organization has put in effort toward alignment.

Research by Caldwell and colleagues (2008) indicates that successful implementation of strategies (step 6) requires a change in employee behavior. Changing that behavior calls not only for the relentless communication of customer needs and expectations but also for the involvement of staff in identifying the action steps.

CONCLUSION

Healthcare service planning lays out the necessary path and identifies the mileposts that the organization must follow to fulfill its mission, to achieve its vision, and to serve its customers. Whether the organization is a large medical complex, a managed care company, or a physician's office, it can lose its competitive stature if it foresees the wrong future, misdiagnoses its core competencies, poorly defines its mission, or chooses the wrong service strategy. Of course, unforeseen developments may disrupt or overturn even the best-laid plans.

Exhibit 3.6 Mission Alignment Elements with Audit Questions

Strategic and Tactical Practices

1. Departmental goals are aligned with mission.

   - Does management specifically reward unit/department managers on how well they score on mission related measures?

   - Does management specifically reward managers on how well their unit/department provides excellent service to other units/departments?

2. Environmental setting and physical design communicate mission.

   - Is our physical facility/room layout designed to communicate our mission?

   - Are our temperature, lighting, and environmental conditions designed to be customer friendly?

3. Stories relate and successes celebrate excellence in mission achievement.

   - Does management formally celebrate the performance of employees who help achieve mission objectives?

   - Is the achievement of mission outcomes formally recognized and rewarded in our reward system?

4. Top management walks the mission talk.

   - Does management shows its commitment to our mission by visibly walking the mission talk?

5. Performance standards are aligned with mission.

   - Is achievement of mission outcomes incorporated in each manager/supervisor's annual plan/ goals/objectives?

   - Has management established standards of service quality for all aspects of the achievement of mission outcomes that are important to our customers and us?

6. Budget allocations are aligned with mission.

   - Do our departmental/unit supervisors have the financial resources to train employees how to achieve mission outcomes?

   - Are employees reminded that achievement of all mission outcomes is no less important than achievement of financial goals?

Staffing Policies and Processes Factors

7. Job descriptions include mission.

   - Does every key job description include responsibility for achievement of mission outcomes?

8. Job ads include mission.

   - Does our recruitment literature mention our commitment to achievement of mission outcomes?

9. Interviews include questions about commitment to mission.

   - Do we routinely ask applicants about their commitment to achieve mission outcomes in employment interviews?

   - Do we use commitment to our mission as a criterion in selecting who we hire?

continued

Exhibit 3.6 Mission Alignment Elements with Audit Questions (continued)

10. Orientation programs emphasize mission.

- Do we routinely explain our commitment to mission achievement in our orientation of new employees?

11. Performance appraisals include and reward mission.

- Is commitment to achievement of mission outcomes part of everyone's annual performance evaluation?
- Can specific failures in achievement of mission outcomes lead to employee discipline including discharge?

12. Training programs include retraining in mission.

- Does management routinely schedule time to remind staff members of their commitment to achievement of mission outcomes in regular staff meetings?

System Procedures and Design Factors

13. Mission achievement elements are systematically measured.

- Do we follow a set plan for consistently collecting information about achievement of mission outcomes?
- Do we follow a set plan to consistently fix customer service problems that interfere with achievement of mission outcomes?

14. Measurement of mission outcome achievement is systematically provided to all.

- Do we follow a set plan to consistently share feedback about achievement of mission outcomes with our employees?
- Are unit/department comparisons of achievement of mission outcomes performance scores systematically measured and publicly shared across units/departments?

15. Service quality systematically measured.

- Do we consistently measure the degree to which our service experience meets or exceeds our customers' quality expectations for reliability, responsiveness, expressions of empathy, and the tangibles of the destination?

16. Service delivery system design reflects mission.

- Do we follow a set plan to consistently record how long customers wait for service?
- Do we follow a set plan to consistently keep our customers informed about all aspects of their experience?

Source: Reprinted with permission from Crotts, J., D. Dickson, and R. C. Ford. 2005. "Aligning Organizational Processes with Mission: The Case of Service Excellence." *The Academy of Management Executive* 19 (3): 57.

Good plans (strategic, service, and others) attempt to bring rationality and stability to an organization's operations and efforts, despite the unpredictability of governments, the market, the economy, technology, customers, and the future. Thus, managers should not ignore the trends and changes in the marketplace, which may render any plan irrelevant and noncompetitive. The process of planning should be tied to a yearly calendar and placed on everyone's time-management screen.

Note that plans laid out in August may be turned upside down by September because of external events such as competitors' innovations; new laws and regulations; technological developments; changes in customer preferences; organizational disruptions such as the illness or death of a CEO, a massive lawsuit, or a labor strike; or societal upheavals such as an economic recession, a natural disaster, or a terrorist attack. In the face of such events, plans have to be revised immediately. In this sense, plans must be designed to be flexible, allowing the organization to respond to any unforeseen variables. Many organizations create contingency plans or alternative strategies because the future is unpredictable.

Increasingly, organizations are involving frontline employees in the planning process for several reasons. First, employees know more than anyone else about the key drivers of patient satisfaction (Fottler et al. 2006), and as such they have heard and thought about many ideas about products or services that could be added, redesigned, or eliminated in an effort to increase customer satisfaction and perceptions of quality and value as well as to reduce costs. Second, smooth implementation of any plan necessitates gaining employee buy-in. Employees will resist the plan if they do not understand the logic and reasoning behind it. The organization must make every effort to communicate and educate all internal stakeholders about its strategies. If employees are aware of how important the plan is to achieving a mission they believe in, they are more likely to support it and work hard toward its achievement. The more they know about how the plan affects their daily work and functioning, the more apt they are to offer support and help the implementation.

Service Strategies

1. Engage in service strategy planning to design a customer-focused product, setting, and delivery system.
2. Base all plans and subsequent activities on the vision, mission, and values of the organization.

3. Use appropriate tools to forecast future needs and demands, but do not let them replace managerial judgment.
4. Perform an internal and external environmental assessment to discover strengths, weaknesses, opportunities, and threats. Core competencies, internal assets, and market trends are just some of the many products of such an assessment.
5. Consider the customer's perception of quality and value when creating a service or product and establishing the setting and delivery system.
6. Develop action plans to implement the service strategy, and communicate those plans to all internal stakeholders.
7. Conduct an alignment audit to ensure that all critical activities are in sync with the mission and that written cues are consistent with verbal and behavioral cues.
8. Involve employees in the planning process to gain buy-in and ensure a smooth plan implementation.

The hospital, grey, quiet, old,
Where Life and Death like friendly chafferers meet.
—William Ernest Henley

CHAPTER 4

Creating a Healing Environment

Service Principle:
Exceed customer expectations regarding the healthcare setting
in both reception and patient care areas

IN A CONSUMER-DRIVEN, experience economy, a healthcare service is no longer just an economic transaction. Patients and their families expect more, including comfort, convenience, safety, information, and even entertainment in the physical setting in which the service is delivered. As such, the environment or setting is not merely a background to the service experience; it is an important contributor to patients' well-being, mood and attitude, and perception of value and quality. The physical setting—including layout, décor and furnishing, lighting, signage, odor, and cleanliness—is part of the total healthcare experience.

Any provider—from a 500-bed university hospital to a small rural clinic—should create an environment that enhances and complements the total healthcare experience, although each provider's approach will differ depending on its available space, capabilities, resources, and customers' expectations.

For example, a state-of-the-art medical complex may communicate its commitment to patient care and satisfaction through its sprawling size, modern architecture, wide use of advanced technology, and carefully laid-out public and private areas. A small rural clinic, on the other hand, may convey the same message, but through colorful and fragrant plants and flowers in and around the facility; clean, well-lit, and functional spaces; a prominently placed registration/information desk; and pleasing artwork in rooms and hallways.

In other words, the physical environment is a tool for adding value to the experience. A clean, safe, well-appointed, and attractive setting alleviates the stress of the healthcare service for patients, families, and staff.

In its landmark report, *Crossing the Quality Chasm*, the Institute of Medicine (2001) identifies several problems with the U.S. healthcare system: It is unsafe, ineffective, inefficient, untimely, inequitable, and lacking patient-centeredness. Since publication of that report, a patient-safety-and-quality revolution has swept the country, leading to numerous initiatives and research. Even before the IOM report, however, studies were underway regarding the effects of the physical healthcare space on various areas, including quality, delivery, and stress and fatigue of both patients and staff (Geboy 2007). And studies have contined: Sadler, DuBose, and Zimring (2008), for example, found that the environment may unintentionally contribute to negative outcomes, such as those listed in the IOM report.

In this chapter, we address the following:

- The many dimensions of the service setting, including its importance to the healthcare experience and its effects on the healing process
- Evidence-based design
- Healing environment
- Environmental trends and strategies that engender customer loyalty
- Four environmental dimensions
- Servicescape

Throughout the chapter, we provide examples of healthcare organizations that have enhanced their environments to achieve better outcomes.

THE IMPORTANCE OF THE SERVICE SETTING

In healthcare, the service setting serves multiple purposes. First, it is the stage on which the organization's staff can please or disappoint its customers. Second, it creates and conveys a tacit message about the organization. For example, if clean and orderly, the organization is saying that it cares about safety and quality; if dilapidated, the organization is communicating that it is in serious financial trouble and hence cannot appropriately provide care. Third, it is viewed as part of the experience, especially when coordinated with the service product. For example, a well-tended garden on the cancer center's grounds sends a message about the healing services provided inside. Fourth, it adds to or takes away value from other clinical functions.

Simply, the setting influences patient satisfaction, intention to return, willingness to recommend to others, and even the rate of healing. Research supports this argument: One study indicates that an appealing hospital room leads to positive patient evaluations of doctors, nurses, and the overall service experience (Swan, Richardson, and Hutton 2003). Furthermore, a patient can form judgments and expectations about a healthcare organization's capability and service quality the first time he or she sees the facility and even before he or she receives any medical intervention. Thus, the organization should take care to ensure that the environment makes an outstanding, positive first impression.

Perception is almost always more important than reality. That is, even if the quality of care at an old hospital is equal to or comparable with that provided at a modern facility, the perception (among patients and employees alike) is that the old hospital provides substandard care. For example, before undertaking a significant renovation, a public teaching hospital in Atlanta, Georgia, had a poor public image despite the fact it consistently provided high-quality healthcare. After the renovation and improvements, the hospital's reputation soared, even though its service quality remained about the same (Fottler et al. 2000).

Previous Mind-Set

In the past, most healthcare organizations focused their efforts almost exclusively on the medical needs of patients. As patient satisfaction surveys became more widely used in the 1990s, however, organizations began to learn that patients and their families considered the service environment more important than was previously understood. Findings from research, surveys, and focus groups indicated the following:

- Members of a hospital focus group stated that physical features, more than any other service attributes, are a determinant of their satisfaction and perception of service quality (Singh 1990).
- Patients want privacy, cleanliness, quiet, closet space, and the ability to control temperature (Malloch 1999).
- Environments at most facilities fail to meet patient expectations (Lawson and Phiri 2000).
- One hospital's physical appearance was rated at the bottom of all service attributes, leading some patients to switch healthcare providers (Bowers, Swan, and Koehler 1994).
- The healthcare setting is a major determinant of perceived quality and customer satisfaction and can lead to sustainable competitive advantage (Taylor 1994).

- Atmospherics or environmental factors have been shown to lead to customer satisfaction, continued patronage, positive word-of-mouth advertising, and an improved image for the organization (Bitner, Booms, and Stanfield Tetreault 1990).

More recently, a focus group of patients revealed the following environmental factors as important determinants of their perceptions of quality of care (Gupta 2008):

- Modern, state-of-the-art equipment
- Comfortable, clean, and visually appealing facilities
- Neatly and appropriately dressed physicians and staff
- Convenient location
- Good housekeeping and laundry services

EVIDENCE-BASED DESIGN

Evidence-based design is more than the beautification of the facility. It is founded on the idea that the facility's construction and design should incorporate the principles and research findings from healthcare architecture and design, environmental psychology, human factors, and industrial engineering (Henricksen et al. 2007). Evidence-based design strives to improve air quality and lighting, reduce noise, encourage hand hygiene, reduce walking distances, improve wayfinding, incorporate nature, and accommodate family needs.

Recent research has demonstrated the positive impact of environmental factors on clinical outcomes, patient satisfaction, and providers' work/life quality (Ulrich et al. 2004; Marberry 2006; Joseph 2006). Because it is outcomes focused, evidence-based design constructs single or private rooms, not only to satisfy the patient's need for quiet and privacy but also to lower the likelihood that the patient will contract an infection.

Kroll (2005) enumerates several principles of evidence-based design:

1. The change has to bring about measurable, positive outcomes, not just serve as an attractive feature.
2. The design has to target significant healthcare delivery or patient care concerns, not just stress. Reducing the rate of medication errors and shortening the hospital stay are good clinical aims for evidence-based design.

3. No two designs can be exactly alike, because every organization is unique. Findings from research must be adapted and applied to the reality and circumstances of the facility.

Cost

Unless you are building a new facility, one of the challenges of using evidence-based design in healthcare facilities is its expense. Major environmental renovations or design alterations can be costly. Tight budgets make justifying these design investments difficult. Thus far, one study shows that the initial investment can be offset by the positive outcomes and savings from those improvements (Kroll 2005), but much work still needs to be done in providing the cost–benefit justification for using evidence-based design principles.

HEALING ENVIRONMENT

Evidence-based design is part of the healing environment concept. Numerous studies show that a healing environment has therapeutic effects on both patients and staff. Research by Ulrich and colleagues (2004) found that a healing environment leads to faster recoveries, higher levels of patient satisfaction, reduced pain, fewer cases of infection, and lower stress levels in visitors and staff. Similarly, Zborowsky and Kreitzer (2008) argue that "these changes also can help prevent medical errors and hospital-acquired infections, while improving staff morale and efficiency."

Initially, the redesign of the service setting focused on public spaces (e.g., lobby, reception areas, grounds) but overlooked the private areas (e.g., patient rooms, exam rooms). Organizations were installing spa-like features, harnessing natural lighting, and planting gardens. Bigger redesigns included new building facades, soaring atriums, water features, and marble lobbies—all of which project an impressive image. Although such designs contribute to a welcoming, soothing setting, they do not affect the areas in which patients undergo or wait for treatment (Landro 2008).

Thanks in part to the growing evidence-based design movement, more organizations are paying closer attention to how both public and private spaces contribute to patient health and satisfaction. Following are examples of this design trend:

- Orange City Area Health System, Orange City, Iowa: Private patient rooms are situated in the back of the building and have a view of the prairie, a pond, and a healing garden. Each room also has a "family seating area" (HGA 2006).

- Alta Bates Summit Medical Center, Oakland, California: The entry hall to the new breast health center is circular and covered with mosaic tiles. Benches line the hall, and sounds of flowing water and birds chirping can be heard. The waiting room has a tree-like hanging sculpture and colored glass vases (Landro 2008).
- Seattle Cancer Care Alliance, Seattle, Washington: The waiting area for patients who have breast or gynecologic cancer is a light-filled room with views of Lake Union (Landro 2008).
- The University Medical Center North, Tucson, Arizona: The American Institute of Architects honored the medical center with a Healthcare Design Award. The building itself has three courtyards and has views of the surrounding mountains. The Institute said this about the design: "It invokes the power of the desert landscape to define a place of inspiration and healing" (Landro 2008).
- St. John's Heart Hospital, St. Louis, Missouri: Artwork that conveys "feeling of hope and light" is strategically placed throughout the interior of the hospital. Pottery, sculptures, paintings, prints, and other pieces are displayed in all patient rooms, care units, and waiting and reception areas. In the emergency department, the ceiling is painted with a sky mural and the walls are covered with oversized nature prints (Brady Spellman and Franke 2007).

According to Jain Malkin (1992), a world leader in healthcare design and healing environments, facility design should not just fulfill an aesthetic purpose; it should also reduce stress and lessen anxiety for all those who enter the facility and the treatment areas. The use of color enriches the environment and generates the same response as nature does (Beckwith 2008). Also, staff surveys conducted by Parrish Medical Center revealed that design that brings in natural light, mimics home comforts, and improves air flow have a positive effect on patient care and staff's work life (Stenz 2008).

The Center for Health Design recommends seven elements conducive to healing environments (Parrish Medical Center 2008):

1. Nature
2. Color
3. Healthy building
4. Healthy lighting
5. Physical security

6. Wayfinding
7. Cultural responsiveness

These elements are explored throughout the chapter.

Exhibit 4.1 provides a comprehensive, step-by-step approach to creating a healing environment. Such an environment can serve as the organization's competitive edge in a consumer-driven market.

Family-Friendly, Homelike Design

Consider the psychological and social benefits in a nursing home designed by healthcare architect Lloyd Landow. Landow lessened the typical monotonous effect of long hallways by placing small, angled alcoves at the entrances to patient rooms. Landow calls this technique "neighborhooding," as the design resembles a neighborhood street (Montague 1995). Neighborhooding makes the hallway feel and look like a row of front porches, where residents and visitors can sit to socialize or watch the goings-on on the unit without feeling intrusive or in the way. This design allows residents to get out of their rooms and take part in the life and activities of the facility.

Wood floors, soft lighting, cherry armoires that hold flat-screen TVs, back-lit nature photographs, and hidden medical equipment are just some of the homelike features being installed at many newly constructed hospitals (Carpenter 2009; *Medical News Today* 2006). This trend is not confined to the United States. A university hospital in Oslo, Norway, has been designed to mimic a small village: The main thoroughfare is colorful and curves, leading to patient care areas, labs, and other units that surround a courtyard. The Frank Gehry–designed Maggie's Centre (cancer care clinic) in Dundee, Scotland, follows the same healing principle. The interior is made to look like a cozy home with the use of large windows that open to the sky and the landscape, warm wood details, and curving stairs (Arcspace 2003).

Link to Nature

Nature can distract patients from their illness and enhance their sense of well-being. According to Stone (2009), "natural images such as flowers and trees, the sound of water, and natural materials like wood and stone resonate with us on a deep level and help us reconnect with our own basic nature." Moreover, empirical

Exhibit 4.1 Approaches to Creating a Healing Environment

Environmental Dimension	Approach
1. Ambient Conditions	
A. Objective: A feeling of physical comfort before, during, and after service delivery	A. Provide private and public spaces that are clean, odor-free, quiet, well-equipped, and temperature-controlled (i.e., not too cold, not too warm); use nonslip flooring and padded material
B. Objective: A feeling of psychological comfort before, during, and after service delivery	B. Place vibrant décor and furnishings in all rooms; incorporate natural elements and warm colors; offer soothing music, if available
2. Spatial Conditions	
A. Objective: A positive first impression	A. Present a clean, well-lit interior, manicured or well-tended exterior, abundant greenery, clear and wide hallways and pathways; well-lit and well-furnished rooms and waiting areas; well-lit parking lots with uniformed staff
B. Objective: Comfortable, well-laid-out patient room	B. Present clean rooms, easily accessible equipment, wide doorways, nonslip flooring
3. Signs, Symbols, and Artifacts	
A. Objective: Signs that are easy to use, find, and understand	A. Use simple language in big, bold letters; place signs in obvious and expected locations; make signs available in another language (e.g., Spanish); use international symbols, not obscure representations; use clear maps, arrows, or kiosks to direct foot traffic
4. Other People	
A. Objective: Staff attire that meets customer expectations	A. Survey customers about their uniform preferences (e.g., scrubs color, likes/dislikes of lab coats); implement good ideas with approval from staff

studies show that postsurgical patients who are assigned to rooms with views of nature (e.g., parks, gardens, water) give better nurse evaluations, take less medication, and have shorter hospital stays (Horburgh 1995). Even painted nature scenes have a positive impact on patient outcomes (Wiley 1999).

The award-winning rooftop garden at Schwab Rehabilitation Hospital in Chicago was built to alleviate the stress and pain of physical recovery (AHRQ 2009). Anecdotal evidence indicates that the Schwab rooftop garden yields benefits: "Patients report that the healing garden serves as a source of optimism and motivation. Therapists report that daily access to nature and the outdoors makes the rehabilitation process easier for patients, while administrators believe that the garden helps patients to gain more independence" (AHRQ 2009).

In his book *The Biophilia Hypothesis,* author E. O. Wilson introduced the term "biophilia" (which means love of life) and claimed that people are inherently drawn to and nourished by nature (Cooper 2008). This idea evolved into *biophilic design,* the concept of incorporating natural elements into living and working quarters to encourage health and well-being. Biophilic design is unlike the green movement in that its focus is on the relaxing benefits of a nature-infused setting, not on sustainability of materials, although this design certainly contributes to environmentally friendly schemes.

Indoor and outdoor gardens are elements of biophilic design, and these gardens can be found in many hospitals, such as Lucille Packard Children's Hospital in Palo Alto, California; Bronson Methodist Hospital in Kalamazoo, Michigan; and Christus St. Michael Health System in Texarkana, Texas. Various studies show that the most important benefit of hospital gardens for all users is recovery from stress (Cooper 2008). For more information on this concept, see the book *Biophilic Design: The Theory, Science, and Practice of Bringing Buildings to Life,* edited by Stephen Kellert.

A great example of bringing nature inside is Parrish Medical Center's four-story atrium that is decorated with planters and fountains that harness "light, color, texture, and sound." Located in Titusville, Florida, Parrish Medical Center (2008) was one of the first members of the Center for Health Design's Pebble Project and is considered "one of America's finest healing environments."

Use of Humor

Adding humor to the environment is another way of enhancing the moods and spirits of patients, families, and staff. INTEGRIS Baptist Medical Center in Oklahoma City established the Medical Institute for Recovery Through Humor

(M.I.R.T.H.) program (Zizzo 2008). INTEGRIS also holds an annual, weeklong "Camp Funnybone," which is "designed to teach kids to use laughter as a coping tool" (INTEGRIS 2009), Similarly, St. Luke's Episcopal Health System in Houston, Texas, has a volunteer team of "laff staff" clowns who visit patient care areas to spread fun and laughter.

Humor is also a critical component of the Healing Arts Program at El Camino Hospital in Mountain View, California. According to one of the program's supporters and creators, Dr. Joshua Sickel, a pathologist and an amateur stand-up comedian, "When people are hurting, a little humor can make a huge difference." At the hospital, "a volunteer jester . . . roams the hospital floors, connecting with patients and distracting them . . . from health problems and the hospital routine." Also, various comedy shows and stand-up routines are broadcast on the hospital's dedicated humor channel (El Camino Hospital 2009).

Importance to Employees

No one spends more time in the healthcare setting than employees do, be they clinical or nonclinical staff or full time, part time, or under contract (as in the case of most doctors). Thus, a well-designed, clean, well-lit, and safe work environment promotes employee satisfaction, which is highly correlated with patient satisfaction. A pleasant work setting enables staff to concentrate on the task at hand, communicates that management cares about staff's well-being, and instills pride and joy among staff about the workplace.

Most important, a healthcare organization that invests money, time, and energy on the details of the service setting (even those details that external customers will likely not notice) is showing its commitment to providing high value and quality. For example, an organization that cares about its positive image will not hire or tolerate people who wear unclean, ragged, or business-inappropriate clothing. It must uphold a specific dress and appearance code or policy to indicate its respect for its work, customers, and employees. Careful attention and regular enhancements to the details of the service setting result in an attractive, comfortable workplace.

Simply, just as the setting can affect the patient and family's attitude, it can also affect the employees' attitude and productivity. Employees who work in pleasant environments are more likely to provide the level of service that exceeds patient expectations, which then leads to satisfaction and loyalty (or willingness to return). In contrast, employees who work in dark, dirty, noisy, crowded, and dilapidated facilities may not be as happy to come to work or as productive as their counterparts in newly designed spaces. Research by Lin and colleagues (2008) found that a favorable perception of the physical environment is positively associated with job satisfaction and negatively related to employees' intention to leave or to reduce working hours.

ENVIRONMENTAL TRENDS AND STRATEGIES THAT ENGENDER CUSTOMER LOYALTY

When it comes to settings, empowered healthcare consumers expect more than the basics (e.g., functioning equipment, competent and helpful staff, hygienic public and private areas, easily navigable layout). They want a healthcare setting that appeals to their senses and that makes them feel comfortable, welcomed, and in capable hands. In this section, we enumerate the trends and strategies that enrich the setting and thereby promote customer loyalty.

Theming

All aspects of the physical setting—décor, size and layout, lighting, colors, signs, employee uniforms, and supplies and equipment—must complement and support each other to create the sense of an integrated design. This consistent look may be achieved through *theming*.

Theming is the process of organizing or staging the physical elements of the environment around a main idea. Receiving high-quality clinical services within an effectively themed environment adds up to a memorable experience (Pine and Gilmore 1998). This kind of experience reinforces a patient's desire to return and confirms the perception of high quality and high value.

For example, at High Point Women's Center in High Point, North Carolina, the themed design is a spa. The waiting room has Asian-style furniture, screens, and lamps as well as simple flower arrangements. A spa-themed postpartum room carries the same minimal, clean design with screen-like lighting and hidden storage for medical equipment and supplies. The spa theme works with clinical requirements and the existing space, but it "alleviates the boredom while waiting, the stress of the medical environment, and the confusion of medical procedures" (Huelat 2009). Similarly, The Windsor of Lakewood Ranch, an assisted living facility in Bradenton, Florida, has a "West Indies" theme, complete with water-resistant fabrics in bold colors and patterns (Volzer 2006).

Themes may be quite general. To create a general feeling of comfort, a hospital can use padded seating, neutral or warm paint colors, and soft lighting. To create a stimulating environment, a nursing home can use bright paint colors, lively ambient music, and action photographs. In children's and women's care units, a family-centered theme is most effective.

For example, at the new Women's Health Center of Providence Sacred Heart Medical Center in Spokane, Washington, the labor/delivery rooms are spacious and equipped with day beds, TVs and DVD players, and refrigerators. In these rooms, medical equipment is hidden from sight and the décor has a sophisticated "hotel feel," with an earth-tone palette, curved walls, and wood floors (Northwest Business Press 2005).

A themed environment may not always be appropriate in a healthcare setting, and it can present risks. The appeal of a particular theme is subjective: One group may find it attractive and consider it an enhancement, while another may be turned off by it and consider it a dissatisfier. This latter reaction could minimize the provider's competitive advantage. Healthcare executives need to be sure that whatever theme they choose does not create a negative reaction among a large segment of its customers.

Hotel-Style Amenities

A new trend in enriching the healthcare experience through improving the setting is offering hotel-style amenities, such as valet parking, spa services, and free wireless Internet access. Here are some examples of this trend:

- Dr. P. Phillips Hospital in Orlando, Florida: The emergency department is staffed with guest service representatives 24 hours a day. These employees help out-of-town patients change flights, cancel reservations, or arrange ground transportation (Sashin 2007). Similarly, Cleveland Clinic in Ohio offers a "medical concierge service" that arranges medical appointments, transportation, and hotel rooms for patients and family members from out of town.
- MD Anderson Cancer Center in Houston, Texas: The hospital owns a hotel (operated by Marriott) where patients and families who do not live in the institution's service area can stay (Petersen 2007). The hotel is connected to the medical center by a walkway.
- Celebration Health in Celebration, Florida: The waiting area in the emergency department is equipped with two computers with Internet access and two printers that are free for use by patients and families. Also, the hospital offers in-room massages and manicures, pipes in soft music to the

parking lots, and transports (on a golf cart driven by a volunteer) patients who need help getting from the front door to their cars in the parking lot (Sashin 2007).

- Sacred Heart Medical Center at RiverBend in Springfield, Oregon: Everyone who enters the hospital is greeted warmly. Fireplaces, lounges, and coffee shops can be found inside (Bush 2007).
- Henry Ford West Bloomfield Hospital in West Bloomfield, Michigan: Patients are treated as guests. This means that nurses do not come to a patient's room from 10:30 pm to 5:30 am, unless medically necessary; patients can order what they want to eat, when they want to eat; visitors are not restricted by visiting hours and may stay overnight or for an extended period; headboards are upholstered; and closets can be locked (Henry Ford 2009). In fact, the hospital's president was a hotelier, having worked for the Ritz-Carlton before his healthcare management career (Bush 2007).

Food Service

Hospital food has become fresher, tastier, and more nutritious in the last several years (Landro 2007a; McPherson 2007). Some hospitals employ trained chefs who create restaurant-quality recipes, even for patients on restrictive diets (no or limited salt, fat, and sugar). Also, dietitians are prescribing more substitutions and healthier versions of popular dishes, such as roasted instead of mashed potatoes or soy crumbles instead of ground beef. About 70 percent of U.S. hospitals are planning to roll out new menus to keep pace with evolving culinary trends in the restaurant industry. Improving hospital food service presents immediate advantages: (1) It allows hospitals to cater to each customer's unique dietary wants and needs, and (2) it offers a way to teach patients about portion control, substitution, and menu planning (Landro 2007a).

Concierge Medicine

Concierge medicine is a controversial (but growing) innovation, no matter what it is called—retainer medicine, boutique medicine, wealth care, innovative medical practice, or direct care. Under this system, patients pay an annual retainer fee to a primary care physician, who in turn provides same-day appointments, longer visits, house calls, consultations by phone or e-mail, and prevention and nutritional services (Cohen 2008; Kalogredis 2004; Zuger 2005; Fantin 2006). The retainer fee is fixed and ranges from the standard $1,500 to $25,000, depending on the services included (Sack 2009). Essentially, what the retainer pays for is the direct, no-wait, 24/7 access to the doctor, which is unattainable in the regular insurance-based system. Also, the fee allows the physician to keep the number of patients low, which in turn minimizes the demand on the physician's time. This time may then be used for longer patient visits, which increases patient satisfaction.

Concierge medicine has been criticized for exacerbating the inequities in American healthcare (Fantin 2006). However, both the concierge physicians and their patients seem quite pleased with the results (Sack 2009; Kalogredis 2004).

Green Movement

Many healthcare organizations are beginning to adopt "green" building principles as another way to respond to customers' expectations. "Green" indicates a consideration for Earth itself, and the movement intends to stem or reverse the environmental damage inflicted by human and business practices and policies. For healthcare facilities, implementing practices associated with the green movement sends a message to its employees and patients about the commitment the organization has to nature and natural things. It also can mean multiple and high costs, including new construction, restructuring old buildings, and retrofitting—all of which aim to be sustainable in the long and short terms (Guenther 2008).

Healthcare facilities are implementing sustainable approaches for a variety of reasons (Guenther and Vittori 2008):

- Many faith-based organizations consider green practices a part of their stewardship mission.
- Many nonprofit institutions count green processes toward their community benefits.
- Green buildings enhance human health and make a lot of business sense.
- Both patients and employees expect their organization to care about the natural environment and to show it in tangible ways.

Nearly every hospital that adopts green strategies reports improved worker recruitment, satisfaction, and retention (Sadler 2006), and the same improvements are true for patient satisfaction and clinical outcomes.

One lesson for hospitals considering or planning a green construction or remodeling project is to view any one-time capital costs (a major investment) in terms of long-term operational savings (Sadler 2006). While the current economic meltdown and reimbursement constraints have served as a barrier to the comprehensive implementation of green principles in some healthcare facilities, some green initiatives can be implemented for little or no cost. Vernon (2009) suggests that, despite financial realities, hospitals, health systems, clinics, and other service providers can still "green" their facilities by (1) maximizing the efficiency of mechanical, electrical, and piping systems, (2) capitalizing on incentives for sustainable practices, and (3) using lighting retrofits and other energy-saving supplies and equipment.

Reporting

The reporting of patient experiences in hospitals is now mandated by the federal government. An initiative of the Centers for Medicare & Medicaid Services and the Agency for Healthcare Research and Quality, the Hospital Consumer Assessment of Healthcare Providers and Systems (HCAHPS) is a survey that aims to do the following:

- Produce comparable data on measures important to patients or healthcare consumers.
- Create incentives for hospitals and providers to improve quality of care.
- Increase provider accountability and transparency through requiring public reporting of quality practices.

The HCAHPS (see www.hcahpsonline.org) survey is composed of 27 items, 18 of which encompass critical aspects of the hospital experience, including cleanliness, quietness, and service quality. As of this writing, no data are available that show the impact of this initiative. But it seems reasonable to predict that hospitals committed to providing safe, comfortable, and patient-centered care will be rated highly by patients.

Ultimately, HCAHPS will have a significant influence on patient provider choice and patient loyalty—both of which can boost a hospital's market share and financial bottom line.

Healthplexes

Over the last decade, healthplexes have gained rapid acceptance in the healthcare industry, generating a following among consumers who desire a one-stop-shop customer-focused experience. Healthplexes (a combination of "health" and "complexes") are hospital-based health clubs that specialize in wellness, prevention, and education. At a healthplex, members (either individually or with the whole family) can use the fully equipped gym and sports amenities, consult with a nutritionist, and attend wellness classes or presentations.

Here are some examples of a healthplex:

- *Celebration Health, Celebration, Florida.* This healthplex offers women's and men's programs, a sports medicine center, a health club with a swimming pool, a basketball court, and a day spa. Its cafeteria presents healthy meals, cooking demonstrations, and nutrition lectures. The building is connected by an impressive lobby to the hospital (Florida Hospital) and medical offices. See www.celebrationhealth.com.
- *Rush-Copley Healthplex, Aurora, Illinois.* Boxing, swimming, Pilates, tennis, and yoga are just a few of the classes taught at this healthplex. Part of the Rush-Copley Medical Center campus, the healthplex offers adults' and children's fitness activities, a fully equipped gym, consultations with personal trainers, and educational tools and information. See www.rushcopley.com/healthplex/index.aspx.

FOUR ENVIRONMENTAL DIMENSIONS

Because most patients are anxious about the healthcare experience, the service provider must demonstrate that it cares by designing a service setting that is nurturing, responsive, and active/interactive. Exhibit 4.2 shows the four dimensions of the environment: (1) ambient conditions, such as smells, lighting and colors; (2) spatial conditions, such as layout and equipment; (3) signs, symbols, and artifacts, such as signage; and (4) other people.

Exhibit 4.2 Four Dimensions of the Environment

Dimension	Sample Elements
1. Ambient conditions	Cleanliness, temperature, music, colors, odors, lighting, and textures
2. Spatial conditions	Layout, crowding, parking and drop-off areas, equipment, furnishings, functional congruence
3. Signs, symbols, and artifacts	Signage, wayfinding aids, maps
4. Other people	Employee dress code, appearance, and behavior

Consciously or unconsciously, each customer (patient or employee) responds to the environment on the basis of that person's cognitive, emotional, and physiological conditions. These reactions are internal responses that drive external behaviors. Simply, if the setting's dimensions make a patient feel bad, she will avoid it. This avoidance, in turn, has a negative effect on the ultimate results or outcomes desired by the organization. See the section on "Servicescape" for more information on these customer responses. Let's discuss these environmental dimensions.

Ambient Conditions

Ambient conditions are factors that affect the ergonomics (comfort and efficiency) of the space, such as cleanliness, air temperature, humidity, and quality; smells and sounds; and lighting. A dark, dank, and noisy room Is not consistent with the patient's ideas of calm and healing.

Noise and Music

Applied research conducted in hospitals underscores the fact that noise has detrimental effects. Noise is found to be a major cause of loss of sleep (Parthasarathy 2004) as well as psychological stress, increased blood pressure, and increased heart rates (Ulrich 2006). Strategies for reducing noise should include more than asking staff to be quiet while they perform their daily tasks. Such strategies should involve the following (Ulrich 2006):

- Seek out all sources of noise to eliminate unnecessary reverberations.
- Design a layout that minimizes the travel of sounds from one area to another.
- Use sound-absorbent materials, such as carpeting or acoustic ceiling tiles.

Environmental sounds can be controlled and should serve a purpose. Controlled sound (music) should complement the total healthcare experience and the message the organization is conveying. For example, soft music (e.g., instrumental, classical, ballads, nature sounds) is soothing and facilitates relaxation. Music can also affect behavior. For example, people tend to eat faster and drink more when fast, loud music is playing; slow music, on the other hand, encourages leisurely dining, which helps digestion. In a study of diners at the Fairfield University cafeteria, researchers found that diners chewed an average of 4.4 bites a minute to fast music and 3.83 bites a minute to slow music (Petersen 1997).

Scientific research shows that music is beneficial for the body. At Saint Agnes Medical Center in Fresno, California, a music lab gives patients and staff a chance to compose or play music on computerized pianos (Keeler 2008). This recreational activity reduces stress and promotes healing. In addition, music (along with artwork) relaxes the mind and body, which leads to a greater likelihood that the patient will respond well to treatment (Stenz 2008).

Lighting

If the lighting in a service setting is not noticeable the first time you enter, it is probably done correctly. Conversely, if the lighting calls your attention immediately, it is not appropriate. Like environmental sounds, lighting should be controlled and should have a purpose. Every area in the facility demands the right levels of light.

For example, lighting in the operating room should not be dim, and lighting in the waiting areas should not be too bright as to make patients and family members squint because of the glare. Because lighting is part of the setting, it should contribute to enhance the total healthcare experience. Things that are lit call attention to themselves, and things that are kept dark are ignored.

Natural light plays a role in lifting patient and staff moods. In one study, hospitalized patients whose rooms were situated in the path of intense sunlight experienced less stress and required fewer medicines and thus incurred lower costs than patients whose rooms were shaded from the sun (Henricksen et al. 2007). Similarly, bedridden patients who were assigned to a room with a view of nature, rather than a brick wall or a parking lot, recovered faster and needed fewer pain medications (Ulrich 1991). Unfortunately, many nurse stations and staff breakrooms are not designed with daylight-enhancing features such as tall windows (Joseph 2006), which is a disservice to those who provide direct care.

Cleanliness

Every inch of the facility must be held to rigorous sanitary standards (McCaughey 2007). The Joint Commission (2008), which emphasizes hand hygiene in its standards, conducts accreditation visits every three years to ensure hospitals' compliance with its quality standards and other regulations. This type of vigilance, however, is not enough. After all, clean hands can be recontaminated by bacteria-laden surfaces. Hand-washing should be just one among many measures that a healthcare provider takes on a daily basis. More sanitary inspections should occur in all provider settings, including physician offices.

Spatial Conditions

Spatial condition refers to the layout, size, shape, distance, and accessibility of equipment, furnishings, hallways and walkways, and doors. How the space is laid out can influence perceptions of being open and friendly or closed-in and alone. For example, wide and roomy areas are welcoming, while narrow stairways and entryways evoke crowdedness. Following are some basic principles of space design.

1. *The space must be safe and easy to use.* The space has to be designed to minimize the risk of falls and injuries, especially for elderly persons or people with physical disabilities.
2. *The space has to enable the provision of service.* For example, in a nursing home, resident rooms must be designed so that space is allocated for both personal belongings (including furniture) and required clinical equipment and supplies. Sometimes, in an attempt to achieve or replicate a homey feel, the facility will allow patients to keep too many personal items in too small a space, and this practice interferes with the provision of clinical services. A cluttered space also may depress rather than elevate the resident. The same principle applies to public areas. In this case, the challenge is balancing conflicting uses.
3. *The space should be designed to ease way-finding.* Patients, families, and visitors must be able to locate exits, entrances, restrooms, cafeterias, elevators, and other essential amenities and services without feeling disoriented or lost. Employees and other personnel must be able to traverse the facility through wide, clear, and well-connected passageways.
4. *The space must have functional congruence. Functional congruence* refers to how the equipment, design, and layout of the space fit its function. For example, in a modern birthing suite, medical equipment and supplies (the function) are hidden in wood cabinets (the general design). In this way, the suite not only serves its purpose but also appeals to the established aesthetic.
5. *The space must be adaptable to changing healthcare delivery demands.* Some hospitals are repurposing existing spaces in the emergency department (ED) to accommodate patients traditionally placed in the hallways to wait for inpatient beds (Landro 2006a). These facilities are using industrial production models to efficiently move patients from the ED to care units and then out of the hospital. Through "Adopt a Boarder" programs, EDs are sharing the

responsibility with other departments and their personnel. Nurses in other units are asked to take care of ED patients to relieve the ED staff, and special observation units are used for noncritical cases with a goal of sending them home with follow-up care from a home health aide (Landro 2006a).

Signs and Symbols

According to Carl Sewell, signs serve only three purposes: (1) to name the business (e.g., Walgreens, Humana Hospital); (2) to describe the product or service (e.g., Radiology, Hematology); and (3) to give directions (e.g., Do Not Enter, No Smoking) (Sewell and Brown 1990, 22).

Signs are explicit physical representations of information that customers want, need, and expect to find. Signs must be visible, clearly written, and located in logical places (e.g., on doors, next to a symbol, at eye level). In many clinics, signs at the entry point (e.g., reception area, lobby) direct patients where to find service areas. In a facility that serves a multilingual population, signs must be written in the languages most commonly used in the community.

The customer's point of view, rather than the organization's, must be taken into account when creating signs. For example, a "You Are Here" sign on a map of a large medical campus can be frustrating, instead of helpful, to a first-time visitor. Because such a sign is made by an insider to the organization, the sign may not consider the perspective of a customer who is oblivious to the distance between buildings or even the direction (north, south, east, west) he is headed. As a result, the proverbial "You Are Here" sign is often no better than no sign at all. A confused customer feels not only lost or disoriented but also stupid, and customers do not think kindly of organizations that cause them to feel stupid. Signs should be clear and should not be an exercise in complex terminology or subtle humor.

Circus legend P. T. Barnum set up his exhibits and signage to guide customers from start to finish. A door right after the last exhibit was labeled "This way to the egress." Circus patrons, hoping to view a rare animal or a bird (egret) on the other side, went through the door only to find themselves in an alley outside the building. Obviously, some customers were not pleased at the deception. Even though such a tongue-in-cheek sign may be appreciated by many circus patrons, it will not be welcomed at a healthcare facility. After all, much of what happens in a hospital or clinic is no laughing matter.

Signs should also ease both entry into and exit out of any treatment area. For example, a patient who just underwent a procedure that required her to take a sense-altering drug or behavior-changing intervention should be provided clear directions that enable her to navigate out of the area, especially if no one is available to assist her. In many facilities, colored tiles on the floors or colored paint strips on the walls help patients and other customers locate their destination.

Like signs, symbols convey a message or information. Sometimes symbols are made up of words, and other times the symbols are icons that represent universal ideas (e.g., symbols for recycling, no smoking, handicap, Red Cross). Universal symbols are especially important in urban healthcare settings where the patient population comes from many different nations and cultures and speaks many different languages. Colors, numbers, and shapes are used as symbols to distinguish identical areas, such as multilevel garages, vast parking lots, and elevator banks. If the patient absolutely must remember specific information, a simple symbol often aids him best.

Artifacts are physical objects that represent something beyond their functional use; as such, they are a type of symbol. Children's hospitals often use artifacts to engender warmth and hope. A little red wagon is not merely a toy, but it is also a representation of freedom to move around and play. The wagon also serves as a symbol of normalcy despite the child's ailment.

Other People

The fourth environmental dimension includes employees, other patients, and visitors. How other people look, act, and dress can have an impact on those in the healthcare setting. Tight waiting rooms, packed emergency departments, and other crowded situations make people feel as if the organization does not care about their privacy, uniqueness, or dignity. Loud, curt, or grumpy employees can negatively affect the patient's general mood. In other words, the people in the healthcare setting can influence how the patient, the staff, and family companions and visitors feel about the quality of the clinical care, the caring nature of the organization, and the perception that the organization has a strong patient focus.

Illness can also take a mental, physical, and emotional toll on patients. In such situations, they want to see that they are not the only ones with medical burdens. Studies have shown that patients tolerate pain better when they are in the company of others who suffer the same pain. Misery loves company, as the cliché goes. But patient happiness and satisfaction are also contagious.

The life-or-death trait of the healthcare setting might feel even more taxing and depressing without the presence of other people. In group therapy, for example, other people are not there as merely scenery; they exist to participate in and coproduce that treatment experience. Of course, patients do not seek out healthcare just so that they can commiserate with other people.

Other people, except for clinicians and other employees, are usually perceived as part of the environment, not as part of the service itself, but the distinction between the two is not always clear.

SERVICESCAPE

Benchmark healthcare organizations seek input from and listen to their customers (patients and employees) and use that knowledge and evidence-based principles to design a servicescape. The *servicescape* is the sum of a patient's impression on each of the four environmental dimensions—ambient conditions, spatial conditions, signs and symbols, and other people.

Because each customer experiences the environmental dimensions differently, no two servicescapes are alike. Moreover, every customer's reaction is a product of his or her personality, values, mood, prior experiences, expectations, and other moderators. Thus, a 72-year-old Asian woman's servicescape will vary from that of a 24-year-old Caucasian man, even if they received the same services from the same providers in the same environment on the same day.

Moderators

Moderators are the personal factors that influence the way a person reacts to or perceives an experience. These factors include age, cultural and socioeconomic background, physical abilities, life views and experiences, character traits, and mood on a given day. For example, Person A prefers to be alone and thus considers a waiting room crowded if it contains more than ten people. Person B, on the other hand, thrives in a group setting and thus views the same ten people as a sign that the staff are efficient in getting people in and out of the waiting room.

Cultural or ethnic background is also a major moderator. In some cultures, red is a vibrant, life-affirming color, while in others, red is offensive and threatening. A firm handshake, eye-to-eye contact, a hug, and other types of body language also communicate different meanings to different groups and could sway a person's opinion about the general environment.

A person's health status greatly affects the way he perceives the setting. For example, if he arrives in the emergency department with severe chest pains, he is not going to notice the ambient and spatial conditions of the room. A patient's disposition also plays a part—that is, if she is good-natured and is not suffering from a traumatic medical event, she is more apt to pay attention to her surroundings. She may find the music piping into the waiting room soothing or the mural on the wall comforting. Conversely, a patient in a bad mood may become irritated by the long distance he has to walk from the front door to the pharmacy or may become upset by the lack of visible signs to direct him to his destination.

People who have had no previous experience with the facility will be most influenced by environmental cues. These new patients will expect and be sensitive to the disinfectant or soapy smells of cleanliness—the kind that sends the message "This place is sanitary." In contrast, a returning patient may be immune to or familiar with the aroma in the air, but she is nonetheless expecting and wanting the same cleanliness as desired by a new patient.

Responses to the Servicescape

The servicescape brings about three types of responses: physiological, cognitive, and emotional. These responses lead the person to make one of two choices about the healthcare experience: approach or avoid. This response does not include the clinical service or its delivery; it is simply the gut-level reaction to the service environment.

Servicescape responses can affect customer satisfaction, repeat visits, employee retention, and word of mouth. Thus, healthcare managers should invest time to enhance the environmental dimensions that fit the quality and value message they want to convey to customers (both external and internal).

Physiological

A physiological response is a physical reaction to environmental stimuli. Ambient conditions, such as odor, sound, temperature, and light, almost always elicit a physiological response. Another, but less obvious, source of a physiological reaction is a person's capacity to process information.

A classic study found that the human brain can process seven (plus or minus two) random pieces of information at one time. The study was conducted for a telephone company, which wanted to know how long a telephone number should be so that people could remember it. Results led to the use of combinations of words and numbers to help people overcome their physiological limitations (Ford and Heaton 2000). Today, the method is still employed by many businesses and is reflected in toll-free numbers such as 1-800-I-FLY-SWA or 1-800-HEALTHY.

The lesson of this study for the healthcare setting is that a lot of random information coming in at the same time (e.g., too many signs, too many instructions) can overwhelm the capacity of the human mind, preventing the person from comprehending the given information and making him feel uncomfortable, confused, and uncertain. Compounding this issue is a person's illness, age, language limitation, psychological and physical stress, or unfamiliarity with the healthcare provider.

The service environment should be made rich or lean with information to accommodate a person's information-processing capability. For example, a waiting room can be layered with signs, posters, and other informational material because here the patients are only expected to sit and wait. On the other hand, if a patient is asked to find a room or go to a service, she is already preoccupied with that task, and looking at a kiosk or map that has too much information will only frustrate her and cause a physiological reaction.

Cognitive

People almost always enter a healthcare setting with expectations that are based on previous experiences. These expectations influence what actually happens.

For example, a customer who walks into a hospital cafeteria expects the place to look like all other cafeterias he has visited before, from the arrow pointing to the beginning of the line to the stack of trays to the hairnets and white overcoats worn by the servers behind the long food counter. If the visitor encounters a different cafeteria setup than the one he expected, he is not only surprised but possibly also frustrated that he has to learn how to use this unfamiliar system.

Nonverbal communication and messages also invoke a cognitive response. For example, if a patient sees a healthcare administrator typing on a manual typewriter, the patient will immediately think that the facility is not technologically sophisticated; after all, typewriters have given way to computers. Ultimately, the patient will question the overall level of technology at the organization, including the equipment used in medical procedures. This perception alone could make the patient doubt the clinical and operational capabilities of the hospital.

Healthcare organizations should consider the cues or messages that the setting (including staff and their actions) is transmitting. Customers have cognitive expectations and like to see familiar systems in place.

Emotional

Most people are not immune to an emotional response. Alumnae get choked up when they return to their alma matter for a reunion. Holiday decorations, the smell of fresh-baked bread, and an upcoming visit to the doctor or dentist can all evoke emotional responses.

Two types of emotional responses are important for the organization to balance: (1) arousal and (2) pleasure or displeasure. Arousal is the stimulation received from the environment: A noisy, chaotic department can arouse a recuperating patient. Pleasure or displeasure, on the other hand, is the reaction from the stimulus: A noisy, chaotic department can be a cause of displeasure for the recovering patient.

The organization should temper these two emotional responses by presenting a setting that offers the right amount of arousal and pleasure elements. For example, a clean and fresh-scented restroom, a picture of a colorful flower, and a smiling receptionist can all arouse and pleasure. Vibrant murals, vaulted or textured ceilings, and plush chairs can also balance arousal and pleasure.

CONCLUSION

Investments in the service setting can provide high returns in the form of patient satisfaction, reduced recovery time, improved perception of quality and value, and intention to return. The environment can influence customer satisfaction and loyalty, so its elements have to be carefully planned, designed, and implemented.

Although more study is needed to fully understand how the environment affects the health and well-being of patients, much research has been published about this relationship. In addition, a well-laid-out and maintained space reduces stress for employees and caregivers. Healthcare managers should use the setting as a tool to communicate the organization's commitment to enhance the total healthcare experience.

Service Strategies

1. Envision and create the environment from the patient's, not the organization's, point of view.
2. Pay equal attention to public (e.g., lobby, reception area, grounds) and private (e.g., treatment areas, patient waiting rooms) spaces.
3. Identify problems and improvements related to the environmental dimensions—ambient conditions, spatial conditions, signs and symbols, and other people.
4. Create an evidence-based healing environment to convey and advance the organization's patient safety, quality improvement, and customer satisfaction agenda.
5. Manage the physiological, cognitive, and emotional responses of customers.

Work together with employees to develop a "can-do" culture of
honesty, integrity, energy, and initiative.
—Norman Brinker

CHAPTER 5

Developing a Culture of Customer Service

Service Principle:
Define and build a culture committed to providing superb service
for all parts of the healthcare experience

WHEN YOU WALK into Disney World, fly on Southwest Airlines, shop at Nordstrom, stay at a Marriott hotel, or receive treatment at Baptist Health Care in Pensacola, Florida, you sense something special about the place and the people who work there. If customers of these businesses are asked about their experience, they describe it as better than expected. Employees of these companies embody their respective organization's corporate value of exceptional service. For example, Disney cast members talk about their commitment to the quality of the show they put on for park visitors.

Healthcare leaders can learn a great deal from customer service–centered organizations on how to build a culture of service excellence that both patients and staff can believe in.

Organizational culture comprises the philosophies, ideologies, values, assumptions, beliefs, attitudes, and norms shared by the internal members of the institution. Culture is the standard or guideline that the group agrees, implicitly or explicitly, to follow and support—whether in behaving, decision making, problem solving, performing a task or duty, or other group work. By nature, culture is dynamic and constantly changing. Initially, it is shaped by the founding leaders and members of the culture itself, but over time, as it is shared, it can change, as more interactions, experiences, and events occur in the environment.

In this chapter, we address the following:

- The basic elements of culture
- The critical role of leaders in defining, teaching, and communicating the culture
- The importance of adopting a customer service culture

BASIC ELEMENTS OF CULTURE

Beliefs and values, norms, folkways and mores, and subcultures are the basic elements of an organizational culture. The strength of this culture, however, is its members' commitment to it, even when subcultures emerge.

Beliefs and Values

Beliefs form the ideological core of the culture. While culture is a set of assumptions about how the organization operates, beliefs explain what those assumptions mean. Beliefs define the relationship between cause and effect. Values, on the other hand, are the organization's compass. They direct what the organization supports and accepts in terms of employee behaviors, mission focus, clinical approaches and outcomes, to name a few factors. Most institutions have a mission statement, but not as many have a separate, formal values statement. For example, a study of VA (Veterans Affairs) facilities found that the more civil the work unit, the greater the patient satisfaction with the quality of care. In addition, an emphasis on civility reduced sick leaves, absenteeism, and the number of complaints submitted to the Equal Employment Opportunity Commission (Belton and Dyrenforth 2007).

An organizational culture that values and believes in customer service has a bias for enhancing the healthcare experience for its patients, speeding up resolutions to problems and complaints, and communicating regularly with its stakeholders. Beliefs and values are integrated into every aspect of the employee/human resources management system, including recruitment, selection, performance appraisal, and rewards and compensation.

Customer-focused beliefs and values are developed and strengthened by

- actively involving employees in customer initiatives,
- applying a facilitative management (coaching) approach,

- empowering employees in decision making, and
- communicating regularly and widely with staff using all available media (e.g., intranet, internal newsletter, bulletin board).

According to service expert Len Berry (1999), "Sustained performance of quality service depends on organizational values that truly guide and inspire employees. And how does an organization get such values? It gets them from its leaders who view the infusion and cultivation of values within the organization as a primary responsibility. The responsibility of the leader in creating a culture that values customer service is perhaps the most important among his or her duties." In Chapter 3, we discussed the importance of aligning the strategic plan with values and other organizational components. Without this alignment and a strong stakeholder support for the culture created by those values, a commitment to a patient-focused mission would be impossible to achieve.

Norms

Norms are standards of behavior (e.g., what to do and say, what to wear, how to conduct oneself) expected and desired by the organization from all employees, internal associates, and even those external to the organization—customers, patients, and visitors. While some norms are immediately obvious or formally written in an employee manual, other norms are intricate, compelling a new employee to seek the advice of or closely watch a veteran employee for cues as to how one should behave while in the organization.

One norm practiced by outstanding service-focused institutions is to greet a customer warmly by smiling and making eye contact. Another norm is "the 15-foot rule," whereby an employee must make positive contact with a customer who is within a 15-foot radius. This rule applies not only to patients and their family members but also to window washers, engineers, the grounds crew, and any other visitor to the facility or unit. Positive contact includes making eye contact, asking the person if he or she needs help, or briefly engaging in conversation. These hospitality norms can enhance the healthcare experience and should be taught to all staff. For example, employees at Baptist Health Care are instructed to say, "May I take you to where you are going?" upon seeing a customer who seems lost or confused.

Cultural norms are defined and molded not only by employees and managers (including supervisors) but also by customers who make their expectations plain. Vocal customers are an advantage that healthcare has over manufacturing, in that product consumers are far removed from the organization and rarely contact the manufacturers directly to give feedback. Feedback, comments, and even nonverbal cues (e.g., glares, silence) from healthcare consumers assist managers in monitoring, reinforcing, and shaping behavior expectations. Exhibit 5.1 presents Baptist Health Care's behavioral guidelines for nurses; although these norms were created years ago, they are still useful guides to any healthcare organization seeking to shape and define customer-oriented behaviors.

Norms also apply to physical appearance, including clothing and grooming. Examples of this norm include wearing a clean and ironed uniform, maintaining a specific hair length and style, wearing gloves when handling patients, and minimizing jewelry during work hours. Although such norms can be criticized for restricting the employee's freedom of personal expression, they are not baseless. For example, wearing strong or too much perfume is often prohibited because it can trigger allergy symptoms and other uncomfortable reactions.

Similarly, looking disheveled and dirty goes against a facility's message of health, cleanliness, and well-being. Most important, customers (whether internal or external, primary or secondary) expect all workers at any healthcare facility—from the CEO to the nurse supervisor to the pharmacy technician to the orderly to the security guard—to appear friendly, caring, professional, credible, and ready to serve. Indeed, one of the frequent patient complaints is the lack of standardized staff uniforms, which can make it difficult to tell the difference between the housekeeping staff and the nursing staff. This confusion can be frustrating for anxious patients and family looking for help.

Exhibit 5.1 Behavioral Guidelines for Nurse Interactions with Patients

- Greet all patients by name and introduce yourself during the initial meeting (all three shifts).
- Provide each patient with your pager number and phone number, and invite communication as needed.
- Discuss reasons for each procedure before it is done.
- Ask patients if they need anything else before leaving a patient room.
- Explain that doors and curtains must be closed to ensure privacy.
- Respond promptly to call lights.
- Ensure that proper levels of pain medication are available for each patient.
- Never talk negatively about patients or coworkers.

Source: Reprinted with permission from Baptist Leadership Institute, Pensacola, Florida. Originally included in a presentation, "Turning Customer Satisfaction into Bottom-Line Results," by Q. Studer and G. Boylan, July 2000.

Folkways and Mores

Folkways and mores are closely related to norms. Folkways are shared practices or customs within a group. For example, shaking hands is a folkway in the business setting. Addressing physicians with "Dr." before the last name is a folkway in most societies. In a healthcare organization, regardless of size or mission, one folkway is for laboratory technicians to wear a white coat.

Mores are proper behaviors that are understood and practiced by the entire group. Examples in healthcare include wearing gloves, washing hands, and knocking before entering a patient's room. Mores, although not necessarily based on morals, can be fundamental to a code of ethics.

Subcultures

Because they are made up of distinct units and work groups, healthcare organizations are a breeding ground for many subcultures.

Categorizing staff by employment status (full time versus part time or temporary), department (laboratory versus rehabilitation), specialty (pediatrics versus intensive care unit), type (administrative versus clinical, managerial versus professional, union versus nonunion), length of service (veteran versus newcomer), or shift (weekday versus weeknight) promotes the formation of subcultures. The reason is simple: Employees bond with those who are like themselves. For example, part-time or temporary employees may form a subculture on account of the factors that tie them together—for example, limited communication with full-timers and administration, limited employment benefits, and irregular hours.

Although subcultures are not necessarily bad, they can be a managerial challenge if they conflict with the overall culture. For example, a subculture of veteran clinicians and managers may clash with the corporate customer service value because the subculture has a silo mentality, which complicates patient handoffs, impedes information exchange, and detracts from patient-focused care.

Sometimes, a subculture may be more customer oriented than the dominant culture. Take, for example, the case at the Northwest Regional Faculty Development Center of the Boise VA Medical Center in Idaho. The Center had two subcultures—the provider and the executive (Smith, Francovich, and Geiselman 2000). The values of these two cultures diverged and, as such, acted as a barrier to working together. The executives were focused on adding patients when the Center's clinical capacity was already at the maximum, while the providers were ordering expensive patient treatments and interventions that took away funds and time that could have been used to make the Center more competitive.

When data reflecting the plans and actions of each culture were presented to them in a problem-solving meeting, both groups were able to see the need to find mutually acceptable ways to bridge the gaps in their values with an eye toward providing both excellent and cost-effective service. A discussion was initiated and solutions were forwarded, including a tighter coupling between clinic capacity and patient recruitment. The result was better communication between the two cultures, higher levels of patient satisfaction, and cost savings.

Any time management confronts conflicting cultures or subcultures, it must ensure that the information that passes between the groups is not distorted, delayed, limited, or biased by the subculture's norms and values. Recognizing the existence of subcultures and knowing why they exist will allow managers to encourage collaboration among such groups. It will also help different subgroups understand how their subcultures fit into the overall organization. The ideal outcome is that the impact of differences will be diminished and collaboration will be enhanced. Subcultures may develop their own cultural values and beliefs, as long as they do not interfere with those intended to advance the mission.

Commitment

A healthcare culture requires an especially high level of commitment from its followers. Silos and subcultures are common, both of which can weaken the cultural value of service. Regardless of how ideal the beliefs, values, norms, folkways, and mores of the culture, the culture cannot be sustained if it is not fully supported by members of the group. The task of gaining commitment belongs to the leader, and that is the subject discussed in the next section.

THE ROLE OF LEADERS IN DEFINING AND TEACHING A CUSTOMER-FOCUSED CULTURE

Getting everyone—employees and contract staff alike—to commit to high levels of customer service is daunting and takes a great deal of time. This effort should start at the top with senior leaders, although all managers and supervisors play a part in translating and disseminating the established culture. Culture significantly affects employees' eagerness to serve. Thus, the culture should support employee initiatives, decisiveness, innovativeness, and rewards related to customer service (Bellou 2007).

Senior leaders, because of their high-level and high-visibility positions, must be role models within the organization. As role models, leaders set the standards of organizational behavior and influence the actions of internal stakeholders. This influence has a cascading effect. A CEO's every move is watched and imitated (even judged) by other executives in the C-suite. Vice presidents' actions set an example for managers, who in turn affect the behaviors of supervisors, who in turn guide frontline employees.

In defining and teaching the customer-focused culture, leaders must

1. make a commitment to customer service, embodying that dedication in all they say, do, and write, and
2. clearly, consistently, and regularly communicate that commitment not only with words but also through deeds.

The message itself should be intentional and explicit. For example, Marriott's founder, Bill Marriott, Sr., reportedly fired an employee on the spot for insulting a guest. After the story spread throughout the organization, employees no longer doubted that Marriott was serious about its purported culture of putting the customer first at all times.

Leaders who do what they say are viewed as consistent, participative, highly structured, considerate, and in touch with both staff and customers. They may be known as demanding, but for a reason: They are willing to do whatever it takes to develop and motivate staff to provide better service. Their expectations and insistence on results may be high, but the rewards they offer for goal achievements are equally great, if not more so. Their decisions are consistently based on the cultural values espoused by the organization (Ford et al. 2006). As a result, employees believe in the culture and its values, which in turn encourages them to stay with the organization. The more the employees accept and believe in the culture, the more likely they will uphold its values in all they do, including how they treat patients, colleagues, and other stakeholders.

Establishing a culture requires a leader who seeks to transform the organization and its members by inspiring it with a compelling vision, rather than by focusing on routine operational transactions. In the literature, vision-driven leadership is called "transformational," while routine management is termed "transactional." Transactional leaders have a place in every organization; after all, someone has to ensure that the payroll is processed on time and the bills are paid. However, real change requires transformational leaders. Kouzes and Posner (1995) identify the five roles of a transformational leader:

1. Challenge existing processes and practices to promote innovation and improvement.
2. Inspire others to share the vision by showing people how their responsibilities directly contribute to achievement of the mission.
3. Enable and empower others to act.
4. Model the way to achieve the mission.
5. Encourage the heart to give meaning to everyone's work.

Interestingly, conceptual and empirical research indicates that these strategies are commonly used by managers who are seen as "spiritual" leaders—that is, those who believe in service to others, humility, and honesty (Strack and Fottler 2002; Strack, Fottler, and Kilpatrick 2008).

Translating and Practicing the Culture

Managers at all levels are responsible for translating the culture for their direct reports. Talking about the importance of a customer service culture is not enough; managers must also "walk the talk," so to speak, by using their actions as examples, actively coaching others, and correcting inappropriate behaviors. For example, if a nurse manager witnesses a nurse's aide blatantly ignoring a patient's repeated request for an extra blanket, the manager must step in to help and then immediately speak to the aide (or even to all the staff on the unit) about the importance of providing service to the patients.

If the manager ignores the aide's behavior and assumes the incident will not happen again, the manager is communicating that such behavior is acceptable and tolerated. After a few instances of the manager looking away from an obvious disregard for the values and standards, employees will stop listening to the "talk." A major component of translating the culture is putting in place reward systems, training programs, and measures of achievement that support and reinforce the message. That is, employees who strengthen the culture are rewarded; organizational successes are celebrated; and coaching and education in customer service are an ongoing management practice.

Practicing Patient-Centered Approaches

A culture that honors patients can improve a healthcare organization's reputation and thus its competitiveness in the marketplace. Following are examples of patient-centered efforts:

- World-renowned Planetree is a nonprofit collaborative of healthcare organizations formed to promote the development and implementation of innovative healthcare models that focus on healing and nurturing the body, mind, and spirit of the patient.

  Planetree (2009) provides education and information about healing environments and patient-centered care and helps other organizations apply these principles. Planetree's success and growth demonstrate that patient-centered care is not only an empowering philosophy but also a viable, cost-effective approach to care delivery (Frampton and Charmel 2008).
- United Healthcare (2009) has partnered with IBM Corporation and selected physician practices in Arizona to develop patient-centered physician practices. The goal of this collaboration is to strengthen the patient–primary care physician relationship using the Patient-Centered Medical Home model. This model enables physicians to work closely with patients to better understand patient needs and preferences, coordinate health services, and facilitate linkages to other healthcare professionals.
- In 2004, the Picker Institute sponsored a summit to discuss patient-centered healthcare reform. Twenty-seven leaders in the patient-centered movement shared their opinions and forecasts on healthcare reform, noting that patient-centered care will be the most preferred but the least likely to be enacted. Whether this 2004 prediction will become a reality in light of the 2009 healthcare reform proposal remains to be seen.

IMPORTANCE OF A CUSTOMER-ORIENTED CULTURE

Everyone has experienced a place that feels warm, friendly, and helpful. Similarly, everyone has experienced a place that feels aloof, uncaring, and impersonal. However, few people can articulate the exact reason they perceived one place welcoming and the other cold. Fewer people may guess that the difference is the culture.

A customer-focused culture naturally leads to increased patient satisfaction, and as laid out throughout this book, happy customers are a source of many benefits, including organizational survival (Jones and Sasser 1995), increased market share (Rust, Subramanian, and Wells 1992), and profitability (Heskett et al. 1994).

First, patient satisfaction not only enhances the organization's reputation but also engenders customer loyalty (Hansemark and Albinsson 2004; Platonova, Kennedy, and Shewchuk 2008). Loyalty translates to repeat business, which in turn generates income. Second, satisfaction lowers the expenses associated with attracting new customers, including advertising, promotion, and start-up activities (Bellou 2007). Third, satisfaction drives recommendations and referrals from the patients. Fourth, satisfaction strengthens the organization's competitive edge (Gelade and Young 2005).

Employees like to work in a customer-oriented organization because they encounter less customer criticism and abuse, find their jobs more fulfilling, and perceive the company to be supportive and trustworthy.

Provides a Competitive Edge

Culture can be a significant competitive advantage if it has value to its members, is unique, and cannot be easily copied. One strategy for creating a culture that serves as a competitive advantage is to identify and then adopt successful elements in other organizational cultures. These elements can be altered to fit the realities of the organization.

Often, a unique culture exudes a fun, relaxed spirit. Patients and their families prefer this type of atmosphere as it yields many benefits, such as promoting friendly interactions among employees and between staff and patients (Ford, McLaughlin, and Newstrom 2004).

Highlights Core Competency

Culture signals the organization's core competencies. The perception is that a culture that values both high-quality healthcare and patient satisfaction will not make a move (even if it is cost-saving) that jeopardizes the quality of the service experience. Most important, this culture will ensure that operational, managerial, and clinical systems that support excellence are in place.

Bridges the Internal and External Worlds

Culture helps organizational members interact with two core groups: (1) the external environment and (2) other internal members. Ed Schein (1985) describes culture as a "pattern of basic assumptions—invented, discovered, or developed by a given group as it learns to cope with its problems of external adaptation and internal interaction—that has worked well enough to be considered valid and, therefore, to be taught to new members as the correct way to perceive, think, and feel in relation to those problems."

Culture helps its members make sense of their internal and external environments. Some organizations misinterpret the need to deal with the outside world as the need to adopt an "us versus them" mind-set. Such a closed culture approach, however, encourages people to have a negative and unreceptive attitude to ideas generated outside of their immediate setting. For example, new industry practices and innovations in other fields are downplayed or deliberately ignored, and internal methods are kept secret and protected.

On the other hand, organizations with an open culture constantly encourage growth and development by interacting with other players in the industry, benchmarking against best practices, and trying novel ideas. Members of such a culture adapt and respond more quickly to environmental and customer trends.

In addition, a customer-oriented culture establishes extensive standards or rules for behavior and performance about how to deal with the patient and other external customers. These guide the interactions among internal members and between these members and outside customers. As a whole, a customer-focused culture prepares employees to face the incredible variety of external events, patient expectations, and other situations and contingencies that can arise in delivering a healthcare experience. Ideally, these standards are written, not tacitly known. Excellent healthcare organizations, however, understand that written rules and procedures alone are not enough. Leaders and managers must invest time clarifying, disseminating, and teaching (even re-teaching) this information as well as cultural values and beliefs.

Gaps will inevitably occur between what the culture provides and espouses (e.g., values, standards, education) and what the external environment presents (e.g., industry requirements, changes in service delivery, governmental policies). In these instances, people who work in a strong patient-focused culture will adapt more readily while delivering the quality of patient experience that the cultural values promote and require.

Reinforces Values

Values are regularly reinforced in exemplary organizations, where leaders invest considerable time and money on educating the workforce about the patient-centric culture. In these organizations, values are discussed at staff meetings and are often the subject matter of training sessions. One method of reinforcing values is to hold a staff retreat focused on building and strengthening a customer service culture. At the retreat, participants may be asked to reflect on questions such as the following (Eubanks 1991):

- Who are our customers?
- What do our customers need, want, and expect?

- What values should we support to enable us to deliver these needs, wants, and expectations?
- What human resources practices may nurture our values?

Third-party facilitators (e.g., consultants, professional trainers) are often called in to help participants differentiate between personal values and institutional values, and reconcile the two if necessary.

Because every new hire brings some cultural assumptions based on his or her past experiences, leaders and managers must indoctrinate the employee into the culture and its values from day one. Quint Studer, former president of Baptist Health Care in Pensacola, Florida, required all new employees to go through a day-long orientation program. The orientation covered not only the obvious topics of organizational policies and procedures but also the cultural values of patient satisfaction and customer service. All employees were expected to remember the primary importance of customer service in their organizational decision making.

Studer ensured that Baptist's mission rested on the clearly defined values of service, quality, cost, people, and growth. Furthermore, he communicated these values early and reinforced them at appropriate times.

Aids Self-Management and Decision Making

The stronger the culture, the less necessary it is for employees to rely on the typical bureaucratic mechanisms—such as policies, procedures, and managerial directives—when making a simple decision about their work and themselves.

For example, a nurse faced by a complaining family member can be trusted to do the "right thing" to turn around the customer's negative attitude. The nurse does not need to find a manager to resolve the issue. In this sense, the employee is empowered. This is an important by-product of a customer-centered culture, given that so many aspects of healthcare happen during direct interactions (or moments of truth) between the patient and the caregivers (clinical and nonclinical personnel) that do not involve an immediate supervisor.

Unlike in the manufacturing business where the products are standardized and the production process is predictable, in healthcare every experience is unique. As a result, various types of complications come up for which the healthcare organization has not established a formal response, protocol, or policy. The more uncertain the task, the more employees must depend on corporate values to help them make decisions about what to do and how to do it because they cannot rely on previous training or formal instructions to guide their behavior (Davidow and Uttal 1989, 48).

Promotes Patient and Employee Satisfaction

Facilitative management, adequate resources, continuous training, excellent upward and downward communications, teamwork, aligned goals, and rewards are the hallmarks of a culture that involves its employees. Called a high-involvement work environment, this culture has been shown to improve service quality, patient satisfaction, and customer loyalty (Scotti et al. 2007). Furthermore, it results in greater employee satisfaction, which has been known to contribute to enhanced customer perceptions about the care they received. Various studies indicate that employee satisfaction is significantly linked to patient satisfaction (Atkins, Marshall, and Javalgi 1996; Corvino 2005; Leggitt, Potrepka, and Kukolja 2003), positive clinical outcomes (Leggitt, Potrepka, and Kukolja 2003), and greater market share (Zimmer, Zimmerman, and Lund 1997).

COMMUNICATING THE CULTURE

When customers lack the expertise to judge an organization's offerings, they turn into detectives, scrutinizing people, facilities, and processes for evidence of quality. When the service product is a healthcare experience, the patient becomes especially sensitive to every cue and clue about the healthcare provider. In other words, when no physical or tangible product can be seen and the clinical outcome cannot be experienced until after it occurs, the patient looks at everything and everyone in the environment to get an indication of how good the experience will be.

A healthcare organization should take every opportunity to leverage its cultural values through its laws and language; stories, legends, and heroes; symbols and rituals; and brand to communicate its customer orientation. This responsibility falls on leaders and managers. As Davidow and Uttal (1989) point out, "Leaders who take culture seriously are bears for internal marketing, selling their points of view to the organization much as they would sell a product or service to the public, with slogans, advertisements, promotions, and public relations campaigns. The largest single chunk of their time is spent communicating values."

Laws and Language

Every organization has laws—written rules, policies, and standards related to health and safety, human resources, clinical practices, and so on. These laws are based on larger governmental and industry regulations, and they detail the consequences of violations and deviations. An example of a healthcare organization law is the policy on safe disposal of hazardous medical waste.

Organizational language is the set of special terms or jargon used by insiders. This language is a type of shorthand that only members of the group can understand or follow, and as such it reaffirms that a person belongs (or does not belong) in the culture. For example, an emergency department doctor may say, "Palpate the axilla, and check for idiopathic pediculosis." Although this direction is in English, it may not be comprehensible to those not trained in medicine.

A common criticism from healthcare consumers is that healthcare personnel do not speak plain English, making them hard to understand. The same feedback is often given about brochures and other clinical literature. These customers have a valid point. A truly customer-focused culture ensures that organizational laws and language are as clear and simple as possible for the benefit of patients, families, and those without a clinical background.

Stories, Legends, and Heroes

In healthcare, stories, legends, and heroes abound. Leaders and managers can communicate the culture and its values through storytelling and highlighting the feats of people (employees and nonemployees alike) who have made remarkable contributions to the organization. These stories should be preserved and used at opportune times.

Most people love stories, and most people are more receptive to learning when the lesson is illustrated by examples, cases, and stories, not by dry concepts or theories. Lessons are more memorable this way, and employees are more inspired to apply the learning in various situations.

Here are two customer-related stories we obtained through our focus groups. We share them here not only to inspire and reinforce a customer service value but also to illustrate that such stories can be retold and embellished, if necessary, to urge improvement and guide behavior.

1. A nursing home resident, depressed and sullen, is refusing to eat. A nurse's aide is bothered by the situation and begins to look for a solution. The aide finds out that the resident is partial to peanut butter milkshakes. So the aide learns how to make the shake and prepares it for the resident. The resident is touched by this gesture and shows interest in eating again.
2. A nurse notices that a patient who just had a second leg amputation is extremely depressed. The nurse starts a conversation with the patient, and the

patient reveals that he is divorced and lives alone with his dog. Even though hospital rules prohibit animals (other than guide dogs) from entering the facility, the nurse arranges for the patient's dog to be brought in for a visit. The patient is overjoyed at the sight of his dog, and he is overwhelmed by the thoughtfulness and kindness of the nurse. The patient writes a letter to the hospital administrator, praising and thanking the nurse and other staff members. The patient has become an evangelist for the hospital, speaking enthusiastically about his experience at every opportunity.

The moral of these stories is simple: Telling an amazing story that employees can relate to can go a long way toward influencing good behavior, motivating better performance, and communicating the culture. For customers, such a story is an invitation to try the organization's services.

Symbols and Rituals

Symbols are physical objects or representations that convey an unspoken message. Examples of power symbols in the business setting include a large corner office with an administrative assistant at the door or a covered, personal parking space next to the entrance. In healthcare delivery, white coats and scrubs are the common symbols of a clean, germ-free environment. In healthcare management, office size and location are indicators of importance. For example, if a vice president who oversees customer service has a nicely appointed office, the message is the organization views service as a priority on par with other pressing demands (such as finances).

Rituals are symbolic acts performed to gain and maintain support of the culture and to remind group members of the culture's importance. In the service industry, including healthcare, a common ritual is to celebrate the achievement of milestones and goals. For example, if a nurse supervisor receives a letter from a patient about the wonderful job a nurse has done during her hospitalization, the supervisor may hold a quick unit-staff gathering to publicly acknowledge the nurse's performance. By doing this ritual, the supervisor is reminding all staff of the behaviors and values that should be practiced in daily interactions with patients.

Many healthcare organizations host elaborate rituals to acknowledge and celebrate service excellence. These rituals range from departmental pizza lunches to all-staff award galas. Such ceremonies communicate to members that the organization is paying attention to and is appreciative of accomplished goals. Ultimately, what the organization celebrates and rewards says a lot about what it values and believes. If it values customer service, it must celebrate and reward excellence frequently and enthusiastically.

Branding

The Mayo Clinic's powerful brand is based on its motto: "The needs of the patient come first." From the way it selects and trains employees to the way it designs its facilities to the way it uses care approaches, the Mayo Clinic delivers concrete evidence of its cultural strengths and values (Berry and Bendapudi 2003). Mayo built and hones its brand by systematically hiring people who share and/or support the corporate values. Incentives and rewards are in place to encourage collaborative, high-quality care. The design of the physical environment is intended to have a positive effect on the patient experience (Berry and Bendapudi 2003). All of these strategies communicate "patient first."

Be aware, however, that even a solid brand will not take much to tarnish. As mentioned before, just one dissatisfied customer can swiftly ruin a good image, especially in the days of the Internet and social media.

Guth and Deems (2008a; 2008b) suggest these practical approaches to taking a customer service brand to a higher level:

- Offer comfort items, such as blankets, pillows, and headsets.
- Ask patients their preferences on service delivery, such as whether they like conversation or quiet during treatment. If conversation is chosen, the focus should be on the patient, not the caregiver. Preferences on whether music (and what type) should be played should also be broached.
- Place cloth (not paper) towels and good-quality soap in clean restrooms/bathrooms.
- Make basic beverages available, such as bottled water, tea, and coffee, in waiting or reception areas.
- Smile and be courteous at all times.

TEACHING THE CULTURE

As mentioned throughout this chapter, teaching and reinforcing the culture are critical responsibilities of leaders and managers. Schein (1985, 9) posits that the only role of real importance to leaders should be "to create and maintain the organization's culture."

Following are strategies and examples from organizations with a thriving customer service culture. These methods may help a manager become more effective in teaching the service-focused culture.

- Scripting is a form of preparing employees to verbally respond to various scenarios common in their field of practice. Exhibits 5.2 and 5.3 offer timeless scripts that guide healthcare staff's interactions with patients and other customers. Scripts give staff a way to interact with and serve customers at a consistently high level.
- Bill Marriott Jr., is a constant teacher, preacher, and reinforcer of the Marriott Hotel's cultural values of guest service. He has logged millions of miles to visit Marriott operations worldwide and to spread the company's message (Albrecht 1988). His intense commitment to making personal contact with each and every Marriott employee is well known, and his mere presence on any Marriott property is a reminder to staff of the company's commitment to service quality. Bill Marriott demonstrates a focused eye for detail, even getting involved in the way his hotels are kept clean (Grugal 2002).
- In 1999, Greenwich Hospital in Connecticut initiated across-the-board changes that empower employees to do whatever is necessary to meet and

---

Exhibit 5.2 Housewide Scripts for Reinforcing the Culture of Customer Service*

- I'm sorry. Clearly we did not meet your expectations.
- You will receive a survey from us in the next few days. Please complete and return it, as your feedback is very important to us. If for any reason you cannot grade us "very good," please contact _____ .
- Is there anything else I can do for you? I have time.
- May I take you where you are going?
- I am closing the door (or pulling this curtain) because I am concerned with your privacy.
- I'm concerned about your comfort level. On every shift we will be asking you to measure your pain level.

*Only three or four housewide scripts were introduced originally. Others were introduced incrementally over time as associates became comfortable with the concept.

Source: Reprinted with permission from Baptist Leadership Institute, Pensacola, Florida. Originally included in a presentation, "Turning Customer Satisfaction into Bottom-Line Results," by Q. Studer and G. Boylan, July 2000.

Exhibit 5.3 Staff-Specific Scripts for Reinforcing a Culture of Customer Service

Position: Radiology technician

Script: We have purchased a blanket warmer, and I am putting a warm blanket around you. We are concerned about your comfort.

Position: Chaplain

Script: We are also aware that you may have spiritual concerns. We do have chaplains here around the clock.

Position: Parking attendant

Script: We will be asking you throughout your stay how we can do things better. Let me remind you that we do have valet parking for the convenience of you or your visitors.

Position: Department unit coordinator

Script: How may your nurse help you?

Position: Lab staff

Script: In the lab, we have done a study and looked at the best techniques and needles to draw blood. I understand that this procedure may not be pleasant, but I am using the best techniques and sharpest needles available, so hopefully, this will not bother you too much.

Position: Nursing staff

Script: Your physician cares about you very much, and he has asked that we get a blood sample very early so the results can be posted on the chart by the time he makes rounds in the morning.

Script: Hello, my name is _____ . I will be your nurse until _____ . Please let me know the moment we can do something better. My goal is to exceed your expectations and provide you with very good care. Any questions at any time, please let us know.

Position: Nurse leader

Script: Good morning, my name is _____ . I am the nurse leader on this unit. I want to assure you that we will do everything possible to exceed your expectations. I need your help. . . . This is my pager number and my phone number. Please call me the moment you find something we can do better, or let me know of an opportunity where we can exceed your expectations. Our goal is to provide you with very good care.

Source: Reprinted with permission from Baptist Leadership Institute, Pensacola, Florida. Originally included in a presentation, "Turning Customer Satisfaction into Bottom-Line Results," by Q. Studer and G. Boylan, July 2000.

exceed customer expectations. Various workshops, incentives, and tools were provided to push the initiative forward (Corvino 2005). The campaign hinged on seven standards of service excellence, including treating people as guests, respecting privacy and confidentiality, listening and acting promptly to address concerns, and maintaining a safe and clean environment. The results were phenomenal: Greenwich Hospital scored in the top 1 percent of hospitals nationally in inpatient satisfaction in 16 straight quarters, and employee satisfaction levels were at an all-time high at the 99th percentile (Corvino 2005).

- Herb Kelleher, former CEO of Southwest Airlines, set an example for the next generation of Southwest workers. Kelleher used to walk through airports, Southwest airplanes, and Southwest service areas to show employees that he cared about the quality of each customer's experience. Today, this tradition lives on. All Southwest managers are expected to observe and work in customer-contact areas for a given time.

- New York Presbyterian Hospital launched a Six Sigma initiative in 2003 to enhance patient, physician, and employee satisfaction. Employees were given training on the Six Sigma methodology, and a chief learning officer was appointed. Among the projects undertaken were inventory management, patient flow improvement, reduction of length of stay, and employee recruitment. This effort not only enhanced patient satisfaction but also garnered an American Hospital Association Quest for Quality prize in 2005 (Craven et al. 2006).

Mission and Vision Statements

The importance of customer service must be incorporated into the mission and vision statements. These written documents are visible representations of the organization's purpose and beliefs, and as such they are natural educational materials. Unfortunately, for some institutions, these statements are merely sayings. However, for a customer-centered organization, the mission and vision are carefully used to ensure that everything it says and does is aligned with the mission. Thus, as noted in Chapter 3, the institution's strategy, staffing, and systems should be made consistent with the mission.

Human Resources System

Human resource management should support a customer-focused culture. Job advertisements, descriptions, and interviews should reflect the customer service commitment of the organization (Crotts, Dickson, and Ford 2005). Beyond the recruitment and selection processes, orientation and training programs should also incorporate this cultural value. Senior leaders should be present at these sessions to add credibility to the effort and emphasize the importance of service excellence.

Once hired and acculturated, employees must be empowered to address and resolve patient complaints; afterward, they should be recognized and rewarded for doing so (Scotti et al. 2007). Research supports the argument that healthcare workers, by virtue of their frequent and close contact with patients, are reliable sources of insight into the needs, wants, and expectations of customers. Managers should acknowledge this reality and survey frontline staff to find out their perceptions about patient expectations and level of satisfaction (Fottler et al. 2006).

Customer Contact

Benchmark healthcare organizations fully understand and accept a basic truth: Patients are the sole reason healthcare institutions exist. For these organizations, investing time, money, staff, and other resources in patient care and satisfaction is the mode of operations, not just a corporate slogan. To this end, the leaders and managers build customer-contact time into their schedules, performing patient rounds and talking directly to patients and families to ask about their needs. All these hands-on activities serve as a model of behavior (and hence education) for the rest of the staff, and they communicate to the patients that everyone, even the senior executives, is committed to patient care and satisfaction.

CHANGING THE CULTURE

The culture must change with the times. For example, 30 years ago, the culture may have favored clinician needs over patient needs on account of the societal demands and industry standards at the time. That same culture cannot thrive in today's consumer-driven climate.

However, a fundamentally solid culture does not require a complete overhaul. The tools that allow a leader to create a culture in the first place are the same tools that allow a leader to change that culture. Communication tools (e.g., stories, legends, heroes) and human resources mechanisms that support customer service values may be used, while other cultural components, such as rituals, can be altered to fit changed circumstances.

A more arduous task is rebuilding a culture that has never been service oriented or has long ignored patient satisfaction (see sidebar for examples).

SIDEBAR: CULTURE CONVERSIONS

Baptist Health Care, Pensacola, Florida

In 1995, Quint Studer was appointed president of Baptist Hospital. When he arrived, the hospital was saddled with low patient satisfaction (close to the bottom in national surveys), high employee turnover, low employee morale, negative perception in the community, and a fiscal deficit. Studer knew that the hospital's survival depended on a massive cultural transformation (Studer and Boylan 2000).

Multiple large-scale initiatives were set in motion to boost employee morale, patient satisfaction, and occupancy rates; to minimize employee turnover; and to restore financial stability. Ambitious but measurable goals were set, and individuals were held responsible for attaining results. The transformation was successful, turning Baptist into a patient-centered organization. Studer (2007) notes that the key to sustaining service excellence is to embed values into the culture and key processes.

These nine principles were central to the transformation efforts at Baptist, but they can be applied to any attempt at culture building (Studer 2007):

1. Commit to excellence: Focus on measurable goals of excellence.
2. Measure the important things: What gets measured, gets focused on.
3. Build a culture around service: Use tools and techniques to drive performance.
4. Create and develop leaders: They are the flag bearers for any effort to achieve excellence.

5. Focus on employee satisfaction: The best barometers of problems are employees.
6. Build individual accountability: Create ownership with employees.
7. Align behaviors with goals and values: Leaders must be accountable for cultural change.
8. Communicate at all levels: Learn how to position others well.
9. Recognize and reward success: Behaviors that are acknowledged get repeated.

Tallahassee Memorial HealthCare (formerly Tallahassee Memorial Regional Medical Center), Tallahassee, Florida

In 1988, Duncan Moore began his new post as president and CEO of Tallahassee Memorial Regional Medical Center with a vision of the "ideal" hospital. At that time, each member of the executive team had a different expectation from and definition of the hospital's mission statement. With his team's participation, Moore developed a new mission statement and implemented an organization-wide change. Following are the strategies used in this process (Brinker and Phillips 1996):

1. Reach consensus on and ensure a clear recognition of a new mission focused on cost-effective customer service.

(continued)

---

2. Develop a vision statement that can be easily transmitted to staff and with which staff can identify.
3. Ask key staff members in each unit to visualize what their unit or service would look like if it disappeared overnight and if they had abundant resources to rebuild and reorganize it.
4. Assess the current conditions within the unit or service, including such factors as physician satisfaction levels, staffing mix, adequacy of supplies, and paperwork.
5. Superimpose the assessment of actual conditions on the ideal vision to identify gaps or areas in which change must occur for the unit or service to become the ideal.
6. Prioritize the changes cited in each area based on their relative importance, potential impact on patient satisfaction, and potential cost savings.

The hospital followed two basic implementation rules. First, all teams had to include members of stakeholder groups affected by the change. A manager, a supervisor, and direct reports rounded out the composition of the teams. Second, all plans had to state what means and resources would be used to accomplish the particular plan.

To maximize the impact of the interactive planning and management process and to promote an awareness of the mission and values among employees, the hospital provided education, communications, and rewards. For example, team members received intensive training in systems thinking, management styles, and systems model analysis (Brinker and Phillips 1996).

Moore (who retired from the hospital in 2003) has stated that a positive culture is personally enriching for employees and not too expensive to achieve and maintain.

CONCLUSION

Excellent leaders constantly and consistently display a personal commitment to the culture of customer service through their actions and words. They recognize the importance of serving as a role model for the rest of the organization. They realize that everything they do (or don't do), everything they praise (or don't praise), and everything they reward (or don't reward) is noted and emulated by staff across the organization. They give meaning to their organization's mission and values. They stress regular, two-way communication with all internal and external stakeholders, and they encourage and reward behaviors that reinforce the customer-focused culture.

A leader has many responsibilities, but perhaps the most important of these is defining and teaching the customer service culture.

Service Strategies

1. Integrate beliefs and values into every aspect of the employee/human resources management system, including recruitment, selection, performance appraisal, and rewards and compensation.
2. Develop customer-focused beliefs and values by actively involving employees in customer initiatives; coaching, training, and empowering employees; decentralizing decision making; and communicating with all staff.
3. Define and teach the culture by making a personal commitment to customer service. Regularly show this dedication with words and deeds.
4. Create reward systems, training programs, and measures of achievement that support and reinforce the customer-oriented culture.
5. Identify and adapt successful elements from other organizational cultures. Alter these elements to fit the realities of your own environment.
6. Interact with the outside world to promote an open culture that is receptive to new ideas and prepared for as many new challenges as possible.
7. Share stories of organizational legends and heroes to educate employees about the culture, reinforce the values, and inspire better performance and goal achievement.
8. Celebrate and reward excellent customer-oriented performance and behavior.

PART II

The Service Staff

There is a shortage of healthcare professionals across the country, as well as a shortage
of registered nurses, that is compromising patient care. This shortage will
reach crisis proportions in the twenty-first century.
—Kenneth Brownson and Raymond Harriman

CHAPTER 6

Staffing for Customer Service

Service Principle:
Find and hire clinically competent people who love to serve

A FATHER AND his small children rush to the emergency department (ED) to see
the children's mother. The mother has been critically injured in an automobile ac-
cident, and the prognosis is grave. Hospital rules, however, prohibit visitors under
age 12 to enter the ED. An ED nurse, seeing the family's grief and knowing the
dire condition their loved one is in, escorts them inside to the mother's room.

Clearly, the nurse is breaking the rules. What sets her defiant behavior apart
from blatant disregard of the rules is that it adds value to the family's experience.
The family will always remember and appreciate this nurse (and by extension the
hospital), regardless of their loved one's ultimate outcome.

Skilled, experienced, and thoughtful employees, such as this ED nurse, make a
tremendous contribution to enhancing the healthcare experience. Because so many
gray areas exist in healthcare delivery, leaders and managers should allow and encourage their staff to rely on their intelligence, training, and creativity, rather than
to strictly abide by the rules, to resolve service-related issues. In this way, employees
are empowered, which in turn motivates them to provide an outstanding service
experience. (However, clinical protocols must be followed every single time, given
that those standards are established to prevent adverse medical events.)

A healthcare organization that recognizes and applies the knowledge and capabilities of its human resources sends a significant message within and outside its
walls: We trust our employees to do the right things for our patients. This perception can be leveraged as part of a retention and recruitment strategy, especially for

people who entered the healthcare field with the primary intention of caring for patients. Feeling empowered to resolve service complaints without a manager's involvement is a reward by itself and can promote staff retention.

In this chapter, we address the following:

- All aspects of staffing a customer-focused culture
- The contributions of employees who are empowered to provide great service
- The challenges of building a pool of skilled and talented job applicants
- The concepts of job analysis and person–organization fit
- Approaches to retention and selection

CONTRIBUTIONS OF EMPLOYEES TO A CUSTOMER-FOCUSED ORGANIZATION

Much of the success of the service strategy hinges on the people who will implement the plans or do the actual work. To this end, new employees must be carefully recruited and selected for their service orientation, and existing staff who exhibit preference for and comfort with providing service must be retained.

Staff empowerment is critical. Employees who are given service training and are rewarded, encouraged, and appreciated for their service contributions should feel empowered to provide superior care. Such employees bring many advantages to the workplace, including the following:

1. They make the healthcare experience memorable for patients and their families. As a result, the organization is at the "top of the patient's mind" in a positive way and is likely to be recommended to others and to see the patient for a return visit if a healthcare need arises.
2. They represent the organization's competitive advantage. Plans and strategies may be duplicated, but empowered employees' personal commitment to high-quality service is unique and hence cannot be easily cloned.
3. They love what they do and thus tend to stay on the job. This high retention rate then attracts other service-minded workers.

When staff are insufficient in numbers, poorly trained, or poorly motivated, the gap widens between what customers expect and what customers receive. One Gallup study showed that 59 percent of employees are "not engaged" and 14 percent are "actively disengaged" (*Gallup Management Journal* 2006). Obviously, healthcare executives want more from their staff than simply being physically present;

they also want staff to be highly involved, motivated, and committed while on the job.

Health Professions Shortages

Recruitment and retention of healthcare professionals are important in the face of continuing shortages in key healthcare professions, including primary care physicians, nurses, and allied health professionals.

As noted elsewhere in the book, today's medical students choose to enter medical specialties rather than primary care because insurance reimbursement rates are higher and working conditions tend to be better in a specialty practice. As a consequence, retired/retiring primary care physicians are not being replaced by an equal or greater number of new primary care doctors. Compounding the shortage problem is the additional administrative burden on existing primary care physicians. As gatekeepers, these doctors have to coordinate patients, which is a challenging task in a time-stressed environment.

The American Hospital Association (2007) reported an average hospital nurse vacancy rate of 8.1 percent. This vacancy rate is related to an RN (registered nurse) shortage, which is estimated to be in the range of 340,000–1 million nurses by 2020 (Auerbach, Buerhaus, and Staiger 2007; HRSA 2006b).

Unruh and Fottler (2005) report data that suggest a more imminent and stronger decline in RN supply than initially projected by the U.S. Department of Health and Human Services. Their analysis documents recent gains and losses in the RN license pool; a decline in RNs working or looking for work in nursing; and a shift in RN supply from bedside nursing.

Nearly 17 percent of RNs were not employed in nursing in 2004, which was a 26.2 percent increase over the 1992 rate (HRSA 2006a). In one survey, 55 percent of nurses reported their intention to retire between 2011 and 2020 (AACN 2007), which would further contribute to the RN shortage.

Similarly, the American Hospital Association (2007) reported 6 percent to 11 percent vacancy rates among allied health professionals (e.g., occupational and physical therapists, laboratory technologists, imaging technicians). These shortages require current professionals to treat more patients and to work longer hours. Such conditions can contribute to emergency department diversions, increased patient wait times, decreased patient safety, and lower patient satisfaction.

These statistics raise a truth: If finding qualified clinical employees is difficult, finding qualified *and* patient-focused clinical employees is even more difficult.

Health professional shortages will force healthcare managers to work even harder at building a qualified and service-loving pool of candidates.

Service Lovers

Outstanding healthcare employees can easily be distinguished from the merely clinically competent. In his book *Positively Outrageous Service*, author Scott Gross (2004) calls such people "lovers" because they love to provide great service. In healthcare, these are the employees who connect with patients and build a relationship that make patients feel good about their healthcare experience. Although the relationship may be brief, it makes the patient believe that something is special and memorable about his total healthcare experience.

Gross estimates that people who love to serve others represent only one in ten of the available workforce: "Ten percent can't get enough of their customers. Five percent want to be left alone. When it comes to customers, the vast majority can take 'em or leave 'em" (Gross 2004). If Gross's percentages apply to the health professions, he raises two major challenges for healthcare managers:

1. Work hard to develop a process that will systematically find, recruit, and select those 10 percent of the clinically competent who are truly committed to providing excellent service.
2. Work even harder to develop an effective process for showing the rest how to provide the same quality of service that the "lovers" do naturally. Because naturally talented people are so rare in the labor pool, the organization must identify what service skills are lacking in the people hired and then train them in those skills.

Given the challenges of recruiting and hiring good employees in the healthcare industry, some organizations are tempted to place the "lovers" in the patient-contact jobs and hire the rest for support jobs that do not have direct contact with the patient. Because not all jobs in healthcare organizations require extensive patient contact, putting people who are not naturally good at service in these behind-the-scenes jobs may seem like a way out.

Excellent organizations, however, recognize the fallacy of this reasoning. They know that all employees are involved in serving customers (whether patients or co-workers). Knowing that service effectiveness depends on people in the organization taking their service responsibilities seriously drives great institutions to hire only candidates who are capable and have the willingness to provide outstanding service. Even the accountants must be sensitive to the needs and expectations of their customers—their colleagues. A hiding place does not exist anymore for those who may be outstanding technically or clinically but who have no service skills.

Jeffrey Pfeffer, a Stanford professor, conducted an extensive review of high-performance organizations in 1998. His examination yielded seven human resources management practices that are still relevant today. One of the seven practices is selective hiring. For healthcare organizations that wish to be customer focused, this practice means they need to identify staff traits that are related to customer service and then recruit and select the best. Although many healthcare organizations try to "select the best and train the rest," benchmark organizations have gained a competitive edge by developing recruitment, training, and placement programs that motivate all employees to provide outstanding service to both external and internal customers. If the organization is somehow able to attract and select the best potential employees, it will gain a significant advantage over its competitors that do not systematically seek out and find these service-focused people.

JOB ANALYSIS PROCESS

Job Analysis

Selecting the best person for the job should begin with a job evaluation. A careful, thorough job analysis allows the organization to identify the exact job specifications and required competencies for each job classification and type. A job analysis will reveal if you need physically strong people to assist patients in orthopedic rehabilitation, skilled nurses to monitor surgical patients, or multilingual people to speak to/translate for non-English-speaking patients.

The job analysis process generates two documents: (1) job description and (2) job specification. The job description outlines the duties and responsibilities of the position, while the job specification details the educational, experience, skills, knowledge, abilities, and personal requirements for the position. Sometimes, these two items are combined into one document.

Knowledge, Skills, and Abilities

Evaluating the job enables the organization to deduce the knowledge, skills, and abilities (KSAs) necessary to perform that job. Many organizations spend considerable sums of money identifying the KSAs associated with each major job or job category and then developing tests to measure the degree to which the applicants possess these KSAs. If this measurement process is done properly, and if the tests have been shown to be both valid and reliable, the organization has an effective and legally defensible means for putting the right candidates in the right jobs. Furthermore, by conducting a careful job analysis, the organization gets the added benefit of identifying training needs and building reward structures that are directly related to the critical KSAs for a job.

Measuring the technical competencies necessary to serve patients is easier than measuring friendliness, ability to stay calm when criticized by customers, professionalism, self-esteem, integrity, accountability, and willingness to help—all of which are necessary for excellent customer service. Even so, the organization must assess the attitudes and values of job candidates, not just their job skills. Because skills can be taught and learned more easily and readily than attitudes and values, new staffers must come in with a caring attitude. From the patient's perspective, the significance of staff attitude is expressed in the healthcare saying "Patients don't care how much you know until they know how much you care."

Staff Competence

According to The Joint Commission's (2007) publication *Assessing Hospital Staff Competence,*

> Ensuring the competence of individuals who work in all hospital areas is key to providing quality patient care and ensuring patient safety. Hospitals can achieve this goal through competence assessment, a process that involves using performance appraisal, credentials review, and privileging activities to evaluate and verify a person's capability of meeting job expectations.

The focus of The Joint Commission's competence framework is the employee's job skill and knowledge, not customer service ability or orientation. Thus, this framework does not assess staff's competency in providing excellent service.

A sound customer-focused model requires the management team of the hospital or department to define the customers, desired customer outcomes, and indicators of achievement for all outcomes. Generic core competencies in the area of behavior are defined for all employees, as are job-specific competencies in the area of customer service. Obviously, competencies cannot be determined without first defining superior performance. In the current market-driven healthcare economy, the outcome desires of both customers and healthcare professionals should be the standards of superior performance.

Competencies are characteristics that are causally related to effective or superior performance on a job. Pruitt and Epping-Jordan (2005) propose five areas of competencies:

1. Patient-centered care
2. Partnering
3. Quality improvement
4. Information and communication technology
5. Public health perspective

Obviously, the competency of patient-centered care is related to customer service. However, this area is too amorphous to serve as a guideline for finding candidates with a customer orientation. More specific customer-related skills, knowledge, and abilities should be sought.

Customer service problems and most management problems revolve around the hidden competencies, such as service orientation. This is not surprising given the historical emphasis on hiring staff for their KSAs and the fact that license and performance appraisal systems are based on task performance rather than customer outcomes. Competence cannot be determined without connecting customers' outcome expectations to worker characteristics such as motivation, interpersonal skills, and political skills.

Because motive, trait, and self-concept competencies are more difficult and expensive to assess and develop than knowledge and skills competencies, selecting a job candidate with these hidden competencies is more cost effective than cultivating these skills in the person after she has been hired.

Many possible clusters of obvious and hidden competencies can be developed, and Decker (1999) proposes the following:

- Customer service/communication
- Professionalism
- Decision making/problem solving
- Resilience
- Cost control
- Political/system awareness
- Support for the organization's values and goals

Decker (1999) identifies the following customer service/communication skills and competencies for benchmark healthcare organizations:

- Speaks courteously to customers
- Offers and accepts constructive criticism
- Practices active listening
- Writes legibly
- Provides and asks for feedback to confirm understanding
- Maintains eye contact when speaking to someone
- Provides timely and clear information and follow-up to requests from patients and other customers
- Identifies self to all customers at all times
- Answers phone in four rings and identifies service and self
- Offers assistance without being prompted
- Helps maintain a quiet environment
- Is not involved in private conversations in front of patients or other customers
- Asks permission to put caller on hold and returns in one minute or less
- Does not complain to customers
- Listens to and educates customers
- Treats everyone as an individual
- Does not talk down to others
- Addresses issues directly with the person involved in a calm tone of voice
- Greets people with a smile
- Focuses on customers' needs
- Shows dignity and respect for patients

RECRUITMENT PROCESS

Internal Candidates

Managers can fill jobs by recruiting from either inside or outside the organization. Most organizations prefer inside recruitment, if suitable internal candidates are available. The reason for this preference is that internal candidates have already demonstrated at least a moderate level of person–organization fit by staying and applying for the open position.

Simply, the internal candidate is a known quantity. Her everyday performance is displayed for observation and evaluation, and her strengths and weaknesses have been tested and are familiar to those with whom she works closely. These are true traits and talents that are difficult to assess in a job interview, as candidates may veil information to impress the interviewer. Even more important, the internal candidate has shown organizational loyalty by virtue of her ongoing employment and her desire to continue her tenure in the organization. In addition, assuming that the internal candidate is in good job standing, she has proven that she can interact well with the organization's customers, a valuable skill in healthcare, where building and maintaining relationships are critical.

If the job is managerial or supervisory, the internal candidate also has an advantage over the external applicant because she has performed the tasks and has worked with people on the unit, making her a natural contender for the position. Until a managerial candidate has experienced the hectic pace of healthcare work, felt the pressure of patient complaints, and resolved patient and staff problems on the spot, the candidate cannot understand what the job entails or be able to lead those who perform the work day in and day out. The internal candidate can definitely relate to these experiences. Although healthcare experiences acquired from employment at a different organization can be applied to the scenarios in another organization, they pale in comparison with the ones that occurred within the employing institution.

Cultural Compatibility

Internal candidates know the culture's beliefs and values and have proven themselves comfortable with them. The cultural learning curve for internal hires is substantially low. External hires, on the other hand, need a lot of cultural guidance in the beginning, as they get acclimated to what the organization expects and how things are done. As service expert Len Berry (1999, 45) puts it, excellent companies "hire entry-level people who share the company's values and, based on performance and leadership potential, promote them into positions of greater responsibility."

Church-based healthcare organizations promote people from within because these people often share the same religious values. For example, Baptist Health System in Birmingham, Alabama, gives preference to internal candidates who have demonstrated that they "live the mission." Another example is the Adventist System in Orlando, Florida, which also strives to select and promote job candidates who agree to live that system's Christian mission. Although internal candidates do not have to be members of a particular religious denomination, they must demonstrate by their behavior that they "buy into" the organization's value of Christian service.

Internal Search Strategies

A pool of internal candidates can be built in several ways. Many organizations use their intranet, staff newsletters, and other internal communication means to announce job opportunities throughout the organization. Most large hospital chains have an electronic version of a traditional job board that enables internal job seekers to scroll through a comprehensive and searchable job database and apply electronically. When a facility within the system has a vacancy, the hiring manager can post the vacancy on the system's intranet, and interested staff may respond by posting their qualifications, resumes, and other related material on the same site.

For example, a nurse manager is looking for a licensed practical nurse (LPN) who is geographically nearby, has five years of experience, and is a graduate of an accredited LPN program. The online job database generates a list of the top internal, eligible candidates, ranked according to the nurse manager's criteria. The manager then contacts the available candidates to explore the employment opportunity.

Online or electronic internal job boards have grown more sophisticated. Such systems not only provide real-time information, but they also can be set up to interface with college/university placement services, government job sites or programs, and industry hotlines. In this way, job seekers can identify opportunities with a "one-stop-shop" approach.

External Candidates

Not every job can be filled by an internal candidate, and organizations do not always opt to promote from within. External candidates are desirable when the particular competency needed for a vacant job is not possessed by existing employees or when the employer is seeking to inject fresh ideas and perspectives into an employee culture that has become too inbred.

Healthcare organizations must regularly recruit externally to maintain clinical skills and knowledge, most of which are taught in university programs. Among external job sources are the Internet, print advertising, professional associations, colleges and universities, employee referral programs, employment agencies, head hunters, career and job fairs, and social networking sites.

Creative Approaches

As noted, staff shortages will continue in the foreseeable future, which will make recruiting even more competitive. How can an organization find and pursue talented candidates when the competition is doing the same thing? The answer is simple: The organization must position itself as the employer of choice and wage a multifront effort that relies on all the available job sources in creative ways.

The typical job advertisement (in print or online) should be just one recruitment method, not the only one. After all, the typical job hunter does not look at ads only. Here are several creative approaches to recruitment (and by extension, retention):

- *Robust benefit package.* Offering only one perk or benefit, such as a sign-on bonus, is not enough of an incentive to keep the new hire on staff. Instead, present an attractive benefits package. The package should appeal to a wide range of workers and may include a competitive salary, medical and dental insurance, a flexible time-off and work schedule, and continuing education opportunities.
- *University collaboration.* Collaborate with universities and colleges to mine the supply of graduate students or to invite undergraduate students to become interns or fellows at the organization. The logic behind such a partnership is that after graduation, a student who has become familiar with and even made connections at the organization is more likely to stay on as a full-time employee than a student who has no previous association with the employer.
- *Finder's fee.* Staff, patients, and other company associates are a good resource for many things, including recruitment. Offer a finder's fee to a person who can recommend a candidate who successfully stays on for a specified period—six months, for example.
- *Focus group.* Invite current employees to give feedback on every aspect of employment at the organization, including the benefits package, culture, management, and growth opportunities. These responses may be used to design an attractive on-boarding program and a better recruitment and retention strategy.
- *Re-hires.* Seek out talented employees who left on good terms. Inviting them to come back to the organization presents low risk, as they already know the system and thus have no need for extensive orientation and training.

Following are major recruitment sources heavily used by healthcare organizations.

Professional Associations
Healthcare managers join professional associations to advance their professional interests, but professional associations can serve another purpose: They can connect their members with potential employees and/or sources of strong candidates. These membership organizations (e.g., American College of Healthcare Executives, American Organization of Nurse Executives, Healthcare Financial Management

Association, Medical Group Management Association) provide networking opportunities that may yield information, partnerships, referrals, and recommendations regarding a vast amount of issues, including finding good employees.

Students

An employer may attract young workers into the organization by developing internship and residency programs that target those who are either still in school or who have recently graduated. As mentioned, some organizations arrange for students to work for them through a partnership with a college or university. The arrangement may be in the form of field work for class or a student work program. For example, most health administration departments require graduate students to get real-world work experience while taking academic coursework. Some clinical programs count post-academic residencies or internships toward their licensing requirements.

The obvious advantages to the student are that she fulfills credit/licensing requirements and makes money in the process (that is, if the internship/residency is paid). For the healthcare organization, the benefit is gaining access to a pool of workers who are young, eager to learn, and academically trained but who do not expect a permanent employment commitment.

Smart organizations keep a close eye on student employees to identify the ones who have the potential to succeed in a particular position. They inform these impressive workers of their interest, and they even offer scholarships or give them special training in preparation for a full-time position after graduation. In turn, students seek out institutions known to have carefully designed work-experience programs that provide real-world learning opportunities and growth challenges.

Student recruitment programs can be a source of good employees who are willing to learn and contribute to the organization. In addition, these programs can function as a way for students to pay their dues in entry-level jobs until they learn enough to merit a promotion.

Employees

Long-standing, high-performing, and reliable employees understand the organization well and obviously like to work there. As such, they can recommend candidates who can fit the culture and do the job well. Employees who bring in their friends feel responsible for their friends' actions and performance. Thus, they exert positive peer pressure and encourage the new hires to do well, which works to the organization's benefit. As mentioned earlier, many employers give an employee referral reward if the new hire stays and does well through a probationary period. The reward varies, from money to weekend trips to a resort area.

Organizational Reputation

An organization's reputation can also aid in recruitment. As Schneider and Bowen (1995) note, employers who have a positive image in the community and a satisfied and motivated workforce have a deep applicant pool from which they can pick the best. These "employers of choice" are good neighbors to the community and have established their reputation for hiring and developing people for the long term. Their mentality, according to Len Berry (1995, 78–79), is to "recruit and hire well, offer a viable, expandable job, and expect most people to be productive, long-term employees. Invest in these people rather than save on those who leave." Lenaghan and Eisner (2006) argue, however, that further research is needed to determine the degree to which being an employer of choice is associated with having a greater number of qualified applicants.

Successful service companies that top the J.D. Power customer satisfaction surveys "recruit for values and personality, rather than technical skills alone; empower employees to act on their own; pay above market rate if necessary; attract career-minded individuals who care about the long-term satisfaction of their customers; promote from within; provide career ladders for everyone; and offer creative employee benefits such as telecommuting, flexible work schedule, and job sharing" (Denove and Power 2006).

In other words, if the company is known for offering high-quality services, it will attract high-quality applicants who prefer to work for it rather than for the competition.

The Competition

Watching employees at work at a different facility is a straightforward strategy that healthcare managers can easily pull off, given that much of healthcare work is visible. A visit to a competing clinic may yield possible contenders for an open position, as the manager is able to size up the clinic workers' ability to not only perform their tasks but also interact with peers and customers.

Most people like to be recognized for performing well. Approaching a potential candidate about a job opening on the basis of his demonstrated capability will flatter and compliment the person. If he pursues the opportunity and is selected for the position, the circumstance of his recruitment becomes a fond story that he and his manager can share. If he declines to apply for the position, the manager may ask him for a recommendation.

Callback

Candidates often enter the recruitment process but drop out before they can be interviewed or screened; some organizations call them back several months later to see if they are still interested. This callback is worthwhile because, often, people who opt out of the recruitment process do so because of another job offer. After several months on the new job, however, these people may already know whether or not they are a good fit for the job. For dissatisfied new hires, a callback serves as a "window of opportunity" to switch jobs.

Evaluating the Recruitment Process

This assessment depends on the availability of reliable and comprehensive data on applicants, a well-functioning human resources information system, the quality of applicants, the applicants' disposition, and recruitment costs.

Common measures of the success of a recruitment effort include the following:

- Quantity and quality of applicants
- Overall recruitment cost and cost per applicant
- Diversity of applicants
- Recruitment time or time to fill
- Percentage of interviewed applicants who are hired
- Percentage of those hired who are retained after one year
- Increase in customer satisfaction
- Decrease in customer complaints

SELECTION PROCESS

Customer-focused organizations cannot afford to have staff members who respond to customers in any of the following ways: "It's not my job," "It's against policy," "I'll have to check with my supervisor, but she's out to lunch," or "You'll just have to wait until the doctor gets here."

Selection of new staff should be done by the whole team, rather than a single individual, to allow for multiple inputs concerning customer service competencies. During the interview process, after candidates have demonstrated their clinical competence, the candidates should be evaluated on their hidden competencies such as self-esteem, personal accountability, communication style, and customer service. Applicants should be asked about how they have handled or will handle particular situations, such as a difficult patient or family member. The goal of this interview should be to uncover service competencies, which are usually possessed by 10 percent of the workforce.

Competency-Based Benchmarking

The intangibility of the healthcare experience and the uniqueness of each patient's expectations have frequently led organizations to use a secondary strategy for selecting good candidates: Identify the best performers, and determine the personal traits, tendencies, and talents that enable them to serve patients successfully. This approach reveals the necessary KSAs of great employees in jobs rather than the required KSAs of a particular job.

The logic of defining the person's, instead of the job's, KSAs is that doing so is easier, given that the customer service aspects of the healthcare experience defy precise measurement or definition. For example, putting together a meaningful and useful list of job-driven KSAs for a hospital chaplain is difficult. Thus, the alternative is to study or measure the KSAs that equip people (in all types and levels of jobs) for the roles they play in specific organizational settings.

The outstanding performers in a job category can then serve as the templates for the candidates hired for specific jobs. In essence, this process is benchmarking—comparing against the organization's best to hire the best. Simply, if you hire only those people who have KSAs that are similar to the KSAs possessed by strong job performers, then the new hires should be as successful. Many organizations have followed this strategy, which may be simplified as follows:

1. They assess the traits, tendencies, and talents of strong performers.
2. On the basis of this assessment, they create benchmark profiles for each major job or job category.
3. They use these benchmark profiles to screen new applicants.

The use of this benchmarking approach can be extended to ensure an appropriate mix of talents in the entire department. If an analysis of a particular department shows that the current composition of staff does not include a vital talent for departmental success, the selection process should be refocused to ensure that the next person hired into the unit possesses that missing capability.

Although a competency-based approach to selection offers advantages, it also presents disadvantages:

1. It is expensive and often has to be performed by a third-party firm. Consequently, this strategy is not cost effective if done for only one job or job category. The effort and the expense can be worthwhile, however, for an enterprise that desires to examine many jobs or job categories or is trying to find the best fit for a senior leadership position.

2. It is reliant on competency measures that constantly change with advancing technology and evolving job expectations. Selection measures must adjust to competency changes, thus creating the need for constant updating so that the measures do not become irrelevant.
3. It uses job-category competency measures that may not be aligned with measures and practices in other parts of the organization.
4. It could discourage diversity in KSAs. If only the KSAs of the best performers are used as an ideal for future hires, then diverse opinions, talents, and personalities are discouraged, making way for a homogenized structure consisting of just that particular type of "best."

General Abilities

In addition to assessing a prospective employee's KSAs, competencies, licenses, clinical training or experience, and customer service focus, healthcare managers should watch for certain general abilities. Doing so does not downplay the vital role of clinical competence, but it recognizes the equally vital role of personal investment—that is, caring about and effectively managing the customer's total healthcare experience.

General abilities include the following:

- *General mental abilities.* Patients require staff who are able to intellectually understand their concerns and figure out how their problems might be addressed and alleviated.
- *Enthusiasm.* Patients expect to be served by employees who are enthusiastic about the service, the organization, and the opportunity to provide service. Because enthusiasm is contagious, it positively influences patients' moods and satisfaction with the total healthcare experience.
- *Emotional commitment and conscientiousness.* Healthcare jobs require a heavy emotional commitment, a passion for service, and a readiness to be conscientious at all times. Employees must stay upbeat, cheerful, enthusiastic, and genuinely interested in serving the patient even when they do not feel like it, when they are having a bad day, or when a patient is not reciprocating the positive attitude. Not everyone, no matter how service oriented, can be expected to be continuously emotionally committed, especially employees whose jobs entail listening to complaints all day. For most employees, repeated negative experiences eventually exact a toll and result in burnout. For other employees, burnout is a consequence of having to do the same job in the

same way every day. At some point, many healthcare workers, including the receptionist, switch into an automatic-pilot mode, weary of the work and unable to make sincere emotional connections.

Staff who possess all three general abilities enhance the capability of the organization to satisfy and exceed the needs, wants, and expectations of patients. General abilities may be more or less important at various stages of an employee's career. For example, a study by Tracey, Sturman, and Tews (2007) found that general mental ability was a better predictor of performance for new employees, whereas conscientiousness was a better predictor of performance for experienced employees. These findings have direct implications for staffing decisions, employee training and development, and performance management.

Job Crafting

Although job analysis provides the basis for developing job descriptions and specifications, it does not outline job boundaries. *Job crafting* is the "physical and cognitive change employees make in the task or relational boundaries of their work" (Wrzesniewski and Dutton 2001). In other words, employees have the latitude to define or craft their job. They can use their knowledge of the organization's strategic goals to motivate their work and legitimize their membership in the group. Because job crafting is common among employees, the employer must hire people with a strong service orientation.

For example, the maintenance crew of one hospital crafted their cleaning duties under the "care of customers" rubric (Wrzesniewski and Dutton 2001; Wrzesniewski, Dutton, and Debebe 2003). They viewed their job as part of an integrated whole, rather than as a series of discrete tasks related to cleaning. Under this new framework, the maintenance crew functioned with an additional caring component, allowing them to relate differently with staff, patients, and families. Members of this group liked their jobs and felt the work required higher skill levels. They took on more tasks and timed their work to be maximally efficient to the workflow of their respective units. Also, they initiated or participated in warm, friendly interactions. As a result, the group helped the staff's jobs go more smoothly and the patients' day brighter (Wrzesniewski, Dutton, and Debebe 2003).

Nurses have also engaged in job crafting. By paying attention to the patient's world and conveying seemingly unimportant information to others on the care team, these nurses re-created their jobs to be about patient advocacy rather than simply about the delivery of high-quality technical care. They also expanded the job boundaries by including the patients' family in care giving (Wrzesniewski and Dutton 2001). The results were better clinical and service outcomes.

Job crafting will occur with or without encouragement from management. However, it will be undertaken more frequently if management rewards the practice and hires people who are willing to try it. Job crafting is beneficial for customer service because it empowers employees to mold their jobs in ways that meet and/or exceed customers' needs, wants, and expectations.

Person–Organization "Fit"

Person–organization fit is the extent to which an applicant's values match the values and culture of the employing organization. *Value congruence* is perhaps the overriding principle of fit (Kristof-Brown, Zimmerman, and Johnson 2005, 285). Furthermore, research suggests that serious applicants are likely to be as concerned as the employer about fit (Rynes and Cable 2003). However, selection methods for fit are far from perfect and are largely untested. Arthur and colleagues (2006) suggest that if fit is used as a selection criterion, then fit measures must be held to the same psychometric and legal standards as are more traditional selection tests.

While the idea of fit is appealing, researchers and managers do wonder if it contributes to job performance. Hoffman and Woehr (2006) found that fit is weakly to moderately related to job performance, organizational citizenship behavior, and turnover. In their meta-analysis of the studies in this area, Kristof-Brown, Zimmerman, and Johnson (2005) discovered that fit is strongly associated with job satisfaction and organizational commitment and is moderately correlated with intention to quit, satisfaction, and trust. However, the same study found a low correlation between fit and overall job performance.

This evidence should not discourage efforts to achieve fit, but institutions need to have realistic expectations regarding the link between great performance and fit. Certainly, hiring without concern for fit has led to poor long-term outcomes (Rosse and Levin 2003).

Targeted selection and behavior interviews are some of the human resources processes that have made hiring on the basis of person–organization fit possible. For example, Women & Infants Hospital of Rhode Island made an explicit effort not only to select employees on the basis of their fit with the culture, believing that a person must be qualified to do the job, but also to require the right personality to fit into its customer-focused culture (Greengard 2003). After starting a hiring program using behavior-based interviews and in-depth analysis of candidates, the hospital saw patient satisfaction rise from the 71st percentile to the 89th percentile, while turnover was reduced by 8.5 percent.

Labor disputes also decreased, while productivity increased (Greengard 2003). Similarly, UNC Hospitals use the Targeted Selection approach to assess employees' core values and attitudes in relation to those of the organization (DDI 2008).

SCREENING METHODS

Application Form

The application form, most of which can be completed online, is the first screen a candidate will go through. It serves as the hiring manager's preliminary check on whether or not the candidate possesses bona fide qualifications—an important detail to check to avoid charges of discriminatory hiring practices.

In developing an application form, managers should include enough work history and experience questions to enable a reasonable decision about which applicant should be called for an interview and which should be overlooked. Obviously, a major trade-off is involved here. The recruitment strategy should be designed to bring in as many legitimate candidates as possible. To attract a large number of qualified applicants, the job advertisement must be clear about minimum qualifications, work experience, service orientation, and education/training required.

Sometimes the application form is incorporated into a job hotline, an automated telephone line that lists job openings. With this method, the candidate responds to basic personal and work history questions. If the information given matches the employer's predetermined criteria, the candidate is asked to fax, e-mail, or mail a resume. Sophisticated optical character recognition or OCR systems can scan the resume, evaluate the candidate's suitability for the job, summarize the qualifications, and forward it to the manager.

Automated and online systems allow people to apply for a job 24 hours a day, 7 days a week and guarantee that each application is reviewed by the hiring organization. As such, they are equally useful for both applicant and employer.

Interview

If the applicant passes the initial screening, she will be contacted for an interview. The interview gives both parties a chance for face-to-face interaction, a powerful component of the selection process. More important, the interview is an opportunity to tell the candidate about the need to commit to the patient-focused philosophy of the organization and to ask questions about behaviors that are consistent with that philosophy.

During the interview, both parties can pose direct questions to each other and observe traits and body language that are impossible to discern over the phone or through the application form and resume. Discussions at this time focus on work experience and qualifications, job duties and expectations, the position's fit within the larger departmental and organizational contexts, and possibly benefits and compensation.

Obviously, the human resources department should verify the candidate's skill set and share the organization's standards of behavior (Studer 2008). For example, at Baptist Health Care, the questions at the first interview are focused on behaviors, and candidates are informed of the behavioral standards upheld at the organization. These standards were developed by employees and relate to such aspects as integrity, dependability, flexibility, and customer service.

Typically, if the first interview goes well, a second interview is scheduled. The unit or departmental leader (if not the same as the manager) makes the decision to let the applicant continue to the next round of interviews. At the second interview, the applicant should meet with at least two potential coworkers. Many times, the objective of the second interview is to determine if the candidate's personality, customer service orientation, and work style will blend with or complement those of the current staff members. Sometimes, however, the second interview is used to gain clarification on the items discussed during the first interview.

Determining an applicant's talent (inborn or natural capacity) has also been a focus of the second interview. The purpose of the talent discussion should be made clear (e.g., to address the applicant's customer orientation), and open-ended questions or scenarios should be posed (e.g., "What will you do if…?" "Give an example of…."). Hypothetical job situations should be broad enough to draw a range of responses. In addition, the candidate may be asked about specific responsibilities that he finds fulfilling.

Peer Interview

Peer interviews help reduce turnover. Because staff are intimately involved in the hiring process, they take a personal interest in and ownership of a new employee's success.

Before the peer interview, the structure of the interview (e.g., who asks a question first, is it formal or relaxed) should be decided and behavior-based questions related to the job's KSAs should be developed and selected. Questions may fall under such categories as integrity, communication, decision-making ability, dependability, and creativity. Peer interviewers should be prepared to answer questions from the candidates and to give feedback about the interview later on.

Structured Questions

A structured interview increases the likelihood that all candidates will be assessed according to the same criteria, regardless of who conducts the interview. Consistency is organizationally and legally important. Structured questions ensure that each interviewer collects the same personal and professional information from every applicant.

Probing questions—such as "Tell me about yourself," "Why are you interested in this job?" "What are your qualifications?"—may yield informative responses. But these questions are not universally interpreted; that is, one candidate may talk about his hobbies, while another may give a detailed history of his childhood hopes and dreams—neither explanation has anything to do with the job itself. Structured questions, on the other hand, are clear, job related, consistently scored, and posed to all candidates.

Three types of structured questions exist:

1. *Critical incidents skills.* These questions revolve around how the applicant works through a positive or negative event that occurs during a service encounter. For example, "What would you do if the patient constantly complains about your performance?" The response can be scored on the basis of the job description, which should be customer oriented.
2. *Clinical/task competency.* These questions address how the candidate performs technical tasks. For example, "What admission software are you familiar with?" "What admission procedures have you followed?" Scoring here can be objective (either correct or incorrect), depending on how specific the questions are.
3. *Willingness to work "healthcare hours."* These questions test the applicant's readiness for the irregularities inherent in healthcare work, such as overtime, long shifts, holidays, nights, and weekends. If the candidate is reluctant or uneasy about these hours, then he is not a good fit.

Psychological Tests

A variety of tests is available, including those that measure logical reasoning, intelligence, conceptual foresight, semantic relationships, spatial organization, and memory span. Tests of mechanical ability, physical ability, and personality may also be used.

Organizations have used these tests with mixed results. Physical and mechanical ability tests are more valid predictors of later job success than are mental or cognitive tests. Personality and other mental measures are much harder to validate against successful job performance. "What makes a successful manager?" or "What personality type makes a more effective leader in a particular situation?" are difficult questions to answer. Research has found that personality has five dimensions (Zhao and Seibert 2006):

1. *Extroversion*: the degree to which someone is talkative, sociable, active, aggressive, and excitable.
2. *Agreeableness*: the degree to which someone is trusting, amiable, generous, tolerant, honest, cooperative, and flexible.
3. *Conscientiousness*: the degree to which someone is dependable and organized, conforms to the needs of the job, and perseveres with tasks.
4. *Emotional stability*: the degree to which someone is secure, calm, independent, and autonomous.
5. *Openness to experience*: the degree to which someone is intellectual, philosophical, insightful, creative, artistic, and curious.

Of these five dimensions, conscientiousness is considered to be the most valid predictor of job performance. In studies that investigate the relationship between possessing these five traits and being a successful worker in the service industry, three dimensions are found to be critical: agreeableness, emotional stability, and conscientiousness (Dilchert, Viswesveran, and Judge 2007).

Results of personality tests may help managers gain an understanding of an applicant's service orientation. Certain personality characteristics, such as friendliness, are useful in a service-intensive field. However, more research is needed to support the contention that personality dimensions are strongly associated with a person's ability/inability to provide customer service.

Background and Reference Checks

No organization that sends out its employees to provide an unsupervised service can afford to send someone who has not been thoroughly checked out. Thus, most healthcare organizations routinely perform background checks to protect themselves and their patients. The healthcare industry is especially different from a manufacturing sector in this regard. A car does not care if a former car thief is part of the assembly team, but a hospital patient will not tolerate the fact that the housekeeper has gone to jail for assault and battery. Revelation of a staff member's criminal record not only can cause embarrassment but also can damage the organization's reputation. Worse, it can invite lawsuits from patients, who may find the organization liable for not exercising due diligence.

Reference checks may be more reliable and valid if a recent employer is contacted, the reference provider is the same gender and ethnicity as the applicant, and the old and new jobs are similar in content (Fried and Gates 2008). Some employers check professional networking sites, such as LinkedIn and Jobster, to get in touch with people who know the candidate personally and professionally (Athavaley 2007). Recruiters and hiring managers use social networking sites (e.g., Facebook, Myspace, Twitter) to find connections with whom they can talk about the candidate. Social networking sites have also added features that assist recruiters in finding more information about prospective employees (Athavaley 2007).

RETENTION

A weak retention system can compromise even the strongest recruitment and selection processes. Simply, hiring talented people is not enough; mechanisms have to be in place as well to ensure that new employees stay for a while. Experienced employees know how to get the job done, how to recognize and solve problems, and where to go for help if needed.

One factor shown to encourage retention and commitment is workers' belief that the organization treats them fairly, considers their interests, and shares financial success with them (National Institute of Business Management 2001). A healthcare organization that is driven to keep its best performers can easily turn this perception into a reality.

Relationship Among Staff Satisfaction, Customer Satisfaction, and Financial Performance

A strong relationship exists between employee retention and the organization's fiscal performance (Studer 2004). Specifically, the higher the retention rate, the greater the revenue (Glebbeck and Box 2004). Furthermore, worker happiness and satisfaction are found to be strongly correlated to patient satisfaction (*Marketing Health Services* 2004). The logic behind this is twofold.

First, turnover creates a staff shortage and/or the use of less experienced employees, which manifests itself in various types of inefficiencies, including longer wait times (Kacmar et al. 2006), underutilization of equipment (Shaw, Gupta, and Delery 2005), and higher costs (Marrow and McElroy 2007).

Second, inefficiencies lead to low staff morale, which ultimately leads to poor clinical outcomes and dissatisfied patients. This cycle can continue perpetually if turnover is not managed.

Again, satisfied employees stay, and they are well equipped to handle workplace relationships, stresses, and changes. There are no easy solutions to the staggering healthcare costs and reductions in reimbursements faced by healthcare managers and leaders. Inevitably, cuts in expenses have been and will be made, and these cuts have an impact on both staff workload and turnover. What is important for managers to consider is the long-term, multilayered effect of worker dissatisfaction. Operating in the red is difficult, but functioning without a clinically competent and service-oriented staff is impossible.

Role of Managers

According to Buckingham and Coffman (1999), "managers trump companies" when it comes to retaining employees. More recent data confirm this statement (*Gallup Management Journal* 2006). Simply, working for a great manager in a regular organization is better than working for a terrible manager in an organization that appears on a "best" list.

A great manager is defined as someone who informs employees of what is expected of them; provides the necessary tools, material, and equipment; allows employees to do what they do best; recognizes, praises, or celebrates good, not just exceptional, work; cares about each employee's personal life; and encourages the professional growth and development of every employee.

Studer (2008) argues that an employee's unfulfilling relationship with her supervisor can be the most important reason for her departure from the job. He identifies other factors as well, such as frustrating work processes, lack of tools necessary for the job, absence of career development and training, poor management of bad performers, and lack of appreciation. Studer recommends regular meetings between a supervisor and an employee, especially a new hire. A manager may ask the following questions during this meeting (Studer 2008, 179):

- How do we compare to what we said we would be like?
- Tell me what you like. What is going well?
- I notice you came from _____. Are there things you did there that might be helpful to us?
- Is there anything here that you are uncomfortable with?

- Do you know anyone who might be a valuable addition to our team?
- As a supervisor, how can I be helpful?

One study examined the strategies used by nurse managers who have succeeded in achieving low turnover rates and high satisfaction among patients, employees, and providers; good patient outcomes; and positive working relationships (Manion 2004). The study found that these nurse managers were able to develop a "culture of retention." Through their daily work, these managers created an environment where people want to stay because they enjoy the work and can contribute to sustaining this positive environment. These managers emphasized sincere caring for the welfare of their staff, forging authentic connections with each staff member and focusing on results and problem solving. Note that these strategies are not likely to succeed without a culture of retention.

Retention Strategies

Several general retention strategies have been shown to work:

1. Offer competitive compensation.
2. Structure jobs so that they are more appealing and satisfying. This can be done by carefully assigning and grouping tasks, providing employees with sufficient autonomy, allowing flexible work hours and scheduling, enhancing the collegiality of the work environment, and instituting work policies that are respectful of individual needs. In the nursing environment, job design encompasses elements such as the nurse–patient staffing ratios and mandatory overtime.
3. Put a superb management and supervisory team in place. Remember that people quit their supervisors, not their jobs.
4. Make opportunities for career growth available. Providing career ladders is increasingly difficult, as organizations become flatter and widen their spans of control. Alternatives to promotions need to be developed and implemented.

Becoming a Magnet healthcare organization seems to be another retention strategy. The American Nurses Credentialing Center established the Magnet Recognition Program to acknowledge and reward institutions that exhibit and provide excellent nursing care. Designated Magnet hospitals are characterized by fewer hierarchical structures, decentralized decision making, flexibility in scheduling, positive nurse–physician relationships, and nursing leadership that supports and invests in nurses' career development (Cameron et al. 2004). Magnet hospitals have been found to have better patient outcomes and higher levels of patient satisfaction (Scott, Sochalski, and Aiken 1999). Compared to other hospitals, Magnet institutions have lower turnover and higher job satisfaction among nurses (Huerta 2003; Upenieks 2002).

The Healthcare Advisory Board (HCAB 2002) conducted an extensive review of recruitment and retention strategies to determine each strategy's relative effectiveness. Findings are as follows:

- *Strategies that do not increase morale but improve retention:* Improving screening of applicants, monitoring turnover in key areas, and tracking turnover of key employees.
- *Strategies that increase morale and improve retention:* Establishing staffing ratios, providing career ladders, implementing buddy programs, and allowing flexible scheduling.

OTHER STAFFING CONSIDERATIONS

Diversity

A diverse staff composition is the moral and legal way to operate a modern, customer-focused enterprise, especially a healthcare organization. In the United States, much progress has occurred in race relations and many barriers to cultural, gender, and economic (to name a few) equality have been broken down. These advances, along with the rise of the global economy, have changed the demographic makeup of not only patients but also clinicians and other healthcare workers in many U.S. cities.

A diverse customer population expects a diversity-friendly service organization to provide culturally competent and sensitive care. Customers want talented healthcare providers and employees who represent their race or background and who speak their language, figuratively and literally.

An obvious staffing strategy for an organization located in a demographically diverse area is to recruit and retain employees who have the ability to communicate, interact, or empathize with patients from different cultures or ethnicities. For example, many healthcare facilities in Orlando, Florida, deliberately hire staff who are bilingual (i.e., English and Spanish) to facilitate communications with the large Latino population in the area.

The diverse workforce itself needs attention and consideration from healthcare managers. A typical healthcare employee no longer exists. Today's workplace is filled with dual-career couples, same-sex partners, single parents or grandparents, grown children with elder-care responsibilities, senior workers, female and minority senior leaders, and other modern-day realities. The manager must be sensitive to the needs and expectations of these employees and avoid designing one-size-fits-all selection, training, and reward systems.

Unfortunately, many organizations still do not fully appreciate, and hence underutilize, the diversity of skills and talents among their workers and within their diverse communities. A diverse workforce gives an organization a competitive edge, a reality that many institutions capitalize on by seeking out and recruiting people who not only are skilled but also have a customer service orientation. Such employees will deliver culturally and linguistically competent services and thrive on the challenge of taking care of a multicultural patient population.

CONCLUSION

Recruiting and selecting the right person is challenging for all organizations, but it is especially difficult in the healthcare industry. Job seekers in all fields must have skills that can be defined, measured, and tested. In the healthcare arena, however, job applicants must also possess interpersonal skills and creativity in handling patient problems. Often, the difference between a good and a great healthcare experience for a patient is the indefinable "extra" that an employee brings to the experience.

Retaining a high performer is the next challenge. The best healthcare organizations view staff recruitment and retention as the responsibility of each staff member and as an organizational priority. As such, these processes are included in the agenda at every board meeting and in the performance evaluation of each manager and supervisor.

Service Strategies

1. Empower employees to serve by giving them training, rewards, and encouragement.

2. Do not hire anyone who cannot or will not provide outstanding service. Customer service is everyone's responsibility, not just direct service providers.
3. Perform a thorough job analysis before undertaking the recruitment process.
4. Assess the attitudes and values of job candidates, not just their job skills.
5. Involve the entire team in the selection process, especially during the interviews.
6. Benchmark a high performer's knowledge, skills, and abilities, and then use this benchmark to screen an applicant and to create a model for a particular job.
7. Encourage and reward the practice of job crafting.
8. Weigh the pros and cons of promoting from within and recruiting externally.
9. Use all available recruitment strategies and sources, including creative approaches such as asking/recruiting past employees and studying competitors' employees.
10. Conduct a structured interview that relies on questions that are job related and can be scored.
11. Carefully consider the long-term, multilayered effect of worker dissatisfaction when making budgetary cuts that affect workload and retention.
12. Focus on retention of top performers by identifying and providing what they value most.

The dominant competitive weapon of the 21st century [is]
the education and skills of the workforce.
—Lester Thurow, former dean of Sloan School of Management,
Massachusetts Institute of Technology

CHAPTER 7

Customer Service Training

Service Principle:
Train employees, and then train them some more

THE CORE OF ALL customer service training is simple: Enable employees to view the experience through the customer's perspective and then act accordingly. With this perspective, employees are better equipped to create an outstanding service experience.

Service expert Len Berry (1995) identifies five key factors that customers use to judge the overall quality of service. Of these five, four are directly related to the ability of the service employee to deliver the service in the way the customer expects, and the fifth—the tangibles—includes the appearance of the service employee. These five factors are as follows:

1. Reliability: the organization's and employee's ability to deliver the service consistently, reliably, and accurately
2. Responsiveness: the employee's willingness to provide prompt service and help customers
3. Assurance: the employee's knowledge, courtesy, and ability to convey trust
4. Empathy: the employee's willingness to provide caring and individualized attention to each customer
5. Tangibles: service factors in the environment that are easily observed by customers

The nonhuman, inanimate aspects of healthcare, such as the physical product, setting, and equipment, are clearly important in forming the patient's impression of the total experience. But the individual service providers—from the nurse's aide to the specialized surgeon—are the ones who can either make or break the organization's relationship with the patient in each and every encounter or moment of truth. The patient-centric culture of the organization provides some strong cues on how to deal with patients, but customer–staff encounters cannot be left to cultural cues or the good intentions of employees.

For the medical staff to design an efficient clinical care system and the human resources department to select the right people are not enough. Healthcare organizations that consistently deliver high-quality healthcare experiences also extensively and continuously train their employees. Excellent healthcare organizations recognize the value of spending the necessary time and money on preventing service failures (and occasional disasters), and they know that an excellent way to do so is to invest in management and staff training and development. Emphasizing the significance of training by investing time and money into the process illustrates the organization's commitment not only to patient-focused care but also to its staff's development.

In this chapter, we address the following:

- Leader and staff development
- Customer service training
- Training methods

Although we provide principles and approaches related to general training, we focus the discussion on customer service training.

LEADER DEVELOPMENT

Most CEOs say that leadership development is a priority in their organizations. However, often, the hours of training that managers and leaders receive are inadequate considering the breadth of their responsibilities. Such development is vital to the organization's well-being, but it is typically forgone because of an alleged lack of time, money, and proof of its benefits. Instead, the development offered has vague objectives and applications and rarely yields sustainable results (Studer 2008). Studer (2008, 125) argues that leadership development must be treated as though it is the "premium tool that keeps the company's engine stoked and purring smoothly for the long-haul."

No organization can achieve excellence without great leaders. Great leaders do not appear out of thin air, as even natural-born leaders need coaching. Thus, organizations have to invest in leadership development that hones the skill sets necessary for accomplishing mission goals. Such training must be continuous, rather than episodic, so that lessons learned are reinforced.

Studer's Five Principles

According to Studer (2008, 129–32), leader development and training should be based on five principles:

1. *The CEO and other top executives must drive the training.* Senior leaders must be present from day one to kick off the training, observe it, participate in it, and wrap it up.
2. *All leaders must be trained.* Training only select members of the leadership group will not usher in significant changes.
3. *Leaders must be involved in designing the training.* Their input should reveal the inefficiencies, deficiencies, and difficulties encountered by management and staff on a regular basis. Organizational mission, goals, and challenges can be the starting point for identifying specific areas of development and training. For example, leaders may name the three top problems in customer service and then gear the training toward solving those identified issues.
4. *Training outcomes must be linked to organization-wide goals.* The new ideas and methods a leader takes away from the training must be relevant and applicable to her particular work and should improve her own performance, thereby enabling her to meet desired departmental and organizational objectives.
5. *Leaders must gain an acute understanding of the five phases of organizational change.* Phase one is the "honeymoon" period, where people are enthusiastic about learning. Phase two is the reality phase, where some employee expectations are not met and employees may view managers as "them." Phase three is the discovery stage, where performance gaps become apparent among employees, which may result in staff claiming unfair treatment and managers attempting to improve the performance of mediocre workers. Phase four is the intervention phase, where managers identify and address problems. Phase five is the action stage, where solutions and plans are developed and implemented.

Leadership development and training may focus on teaching leaders how to manage each phase. Phase one topics may include establishing behavior standards, communicating widely and regularly, and hardwiring key behavior expectations. Phase two topics may address recruiting former high-performing employees and preparing to have conversations with high/middle/low performers. Phase three topics may focus on responding to tough questions, completing conversations with all levels of staff, and ensuring the right people are in the right places. Phase four topics could revolve around innovation and standardization of key behaviors. Phase five topics could teach communication skills, including the art of high, middle, and low levels of interaction and the appropriate time and people to conduct them.

Example: Benefit of Leadership Training

Sacred Heart Hospital in Eau Claire, Wisconsin, is known for its commitment to patient satisfaction (Buckley 2007). One of the components of Sacred Heart's strategic plan was to start customer service excellence at the top: Provide leadership development.

With this focus, the hospital took its leaders offsite for training on the hospital's six pillars of success: quality, service, people, cost, growth, and congruency. Sacred Heart understood that beginning an organization-wide initiative with the leaders made sense because they serve as the role models of behavior for the rest of the institution. Next, the hospital created an accountability system to ensure that the newly trained leaders applied their learning. Service standards were established, using input from staff at all levels and benchmark information from other hospitals and the Ritz-Carlton.

After these initial efforts, Sacred Heart turned its attention to training its employees, which is discussed in the next section.

STAFF TRAINING

The average company spends approximately 2 to 2.5 percent of its payroll budget on training-related efforts, while the best organizations invest up to 3 percent (Killian 2009). Outstanding service providers make such a major investment in training and development because they receive a large return.

Customer service training programs for staff should include the following components (Business Research Lab 2007):

- Statement from the organization about the value of customer satisfaction
- Description of drivers of customer satisfaction
- Explanation of programs for measuring customer satisfaction and recognizing staff's contributions to its achievement
- Expectations of employees' role in keeping customers satisfied

Measurable increases in patient satisfaction and in competitive advantage are among the many benefits of providing training. Exhibit 7.1 discusses the lack of or inadequate employee training and development as a stressor.

Exhibit 7.1 Lack of Training and Development as Employee Stressors

Employees need adequate training. Training is a delicate subject for many employees because they are reticent to admit that they don't have adequate KSAs to complete their jobs. Training programs, even when they are based on some sort of clinical or practicum experience, are unable to address all the contextual nuances of a job. Thus, while many healthcare professionals may be technically sound, they still struggle on the job because of aspects of the work or tasks specific to the workplace. Lack of training in these areas sets them up for failure and is a significant stressor. Think about your own position. Did you know everything about the job when you started? How long was your learning curve before you felt up to speed? I have yet to talk with someone who was able to hit the ground running on the first day of his job; there are always things people could not know before starting.

Healthcare professionals crave true development, the kind that pushes them to think and broaden their horizons. In the same way that discussion with employees can pinpoint training opportunities, discussion with healthcare professionals can elicit development opportunities. Even more gratifying for employees is to have them create new development programs for others. Employees feel empowered when they are asked to develop the skills of other employees. This form of development is particularly enriching in that the ultimate learner in the process is the one doing the teaching.

Annual performance appraisals are a significant source of stress for all involved. Rather than scheduling that awkward annual meeting, document and give regular feedback that reinforces positive behaviors. Problematic behavior should be documented as well, but keep in mind that, according to learning theory and research, people react better to positive reinforcement. Punishment tends to prompt avoidant behaviors, not change for the better. When emphasis is placed on what employees do wrong, they don't know what they need to do to improve. Positive feedback guides people in the right direction.

Source: Adapted with permission from Halbesleben, J. R. B. 2009. *Managing Stress and Preventing Burnout in the Healthcare Workplace*, 88–91. Chicago: Health Administration Press.

Training Frontline Staff

Healthcare organizations have a dual challenge in training employees who have direct patient contact: They must teach staff not only how to perform their jobs efficiently but also how to interact positively with both external and internal customers. If the selection process went well, the employee hired can, presumably, do his job, so the training he receives should be focused on honing his clinical skills and performing his duties at a consistently high level and under the "supervision" of patients, family members, unit managers, and peers. On top of this, the employee must be trained on how to approach patient complaints in a creative and satisfactory manner.

A major undertaking, the training for patient-contact staff members goes far beyond teaching clinical protocols for drawing blood or administering medications.

Four Dos of Staff Training

- *Do empower staff.* No amount of training will matter if employees are not given the authority or encouragement to apply their learning in the workplace.
- *Do provide well-designed training.* Consistently poor training results in a domino effect: the employee's and the organization's performance drops, which causes high turnover, which leads to low company morale and job dissatisfaction, which negatively affects the customer (*ACHe-news* 2001).
- *Do make the training interactive.* No one wants to listen to a three-hour lecture; such a format discourages learning. Interactive training, on the other hand, allows participants to exchange ideas with the facilitator and the group. Active involvement in any kind of process is more memorable than passive attendance.
- *Do make training a regular occurrence.* Training an employee once (e.g., at the employee orientation) is not enough in a customer-driven healthcare environment. Managers should continually reinforce the organization's customer service orientation and the employees' role in this culture.

In addition, some healthcare facilities now provide training for patients. The purpose of such training is to give patients the information they need to enhance their overall experience with the facility and their level of patient satisfaction (see sidebar).

Impact on Retention and Turnover

Training is less costly than recruiting. When good employees leave, they take away knowledge, skills, and abilities, much of which they likely obtained during their tenure on the job. For the organization, this departure means two things: (1) recruiting and hiring a replacement and (2) investing money and time to train the new hire. A training strategy should be useful and well designed so that it helps minimize turnover and maximize retention.

More important, a robust training program conveys to employees that they are valued and not easily dispensable or replaceable. Such a perception then encourages staff to stay, to widen their expertise, and to perform their duties better. As a result, patients, their families, and other employees are served satisfactorily.

Managers of clinically excellent healthcare organizations may wonder if mounting a sustainable customer service training program is worth the time, effort, and

"We put patients first" was the theme of New York-Presbyterian Hospital's (NYP) 2007 strategic plan. To implement its patient-centered agenda, NYP partnered with a technology company to develop multimedia programs intended to enforce the message that patients are active participants in their own treatment (Liebowitz 2008). These programs are an innovative way to engage, educate, and empower patients, enabling patients to better understand the clinical procedures they are scheduled to undergo or to better manage their medical conditions.

NYP invested in these multimedia programs after learning of research that shows patients retain only 20 percent of the information they receive during physician consultations. Because the programs may be viewed multiple times, patients are likely to retain the information and share them with family members and caregivers. In addition, because the programs are Web-based, they can be accessed from any computer with Internet access. More important, patients can use the programs at their own pace and convenience.

This patient training tool is indeed beneficial to patients, easing their minds about an upcoming procedure and encouraging them to have more confidence in the care process and the care providers.

---

money. Exhibit 7.2 is an example of how Baptist Health Care confronted this concern when it underwent a customer service culture transformation.

Following are examples of how various organizations frame their training:

- Operating under the principle that happy workers lead to happy patients, Sacred Heart Hospital's employee training is based on customer perceptions—that is, patients' response to the question, "What do you need from staff to receive good care?" The answers are then incorporated into staff training (Buckley 2007).

- To improve their service and differentiate themselves from competitors, many healthcare organizations are seeking advice and assistance from customer-oriented hotels, such as the Four Seasons, Marriott, and Ritz-Carlton (Saranow 2006). Training topics range from maintaining service consistency across various locations to hiring staff with instincts for good service. Ritz-Carlton sensed this business opportunity several years ago and started to offer training classes at its center in Chevy Chase, Maryland, and at its hotels throughout the country.

   Ritz-Carlton's most popular class is "Legendary Service," a full-day program that teaches attendees about the Ritz-Carlton culture (with a motto of "We are ladies and gentlemen serving ladies and gentlemen"), the use of personality assessments in recruitment, and the role cash incentives play in motivating employees to go above the call of duty. Class participants also hear stories of employee empowerment, including the practice at the Ritz to allow staff to

Exhibit 7.2 Customer Service Training for Staff: Barriers and Benefits

Barriers	Benefits
1. We don't need to.	• Sets sustainable results
	• Lives values
2. We don't have enough time.	• It's the right thing to do
	• Helps improve employee and patient satisfaction
3. We cannot be gone from the department.	• Shares responsibility and creates ownership
	• Allows coordination and consistency within the leadership team
4. What more do I need to learn?	• Speeds the development of the skill set
	• Tailor-made for the organization
5. It's too costly.	• Not as costly as having poor leaders create lawsuits
	• Creates a team that can adjust to environmental changes
6. We already do it.	• Raises the bar
	• Networking builds relationships, trust, and support
	• Creates a "built-to-last" culture

Source: Reprinted with permission from Baptist Leadership Institute, Pensacola, Florida. Originally included in a presentation, "Turning Customer Satisfaction into Bottom-Line Results," by Q. Studer and G. Boylan, July 2000.

spend as much as $2,000 per day on problem resolution without supervisor approval (Saranow 2006).

• As described in Chapter 2, Walt Disney's guestology approach is an integral part of its customer strategy. Since the mid-1980s, Disney has been offering professional training through the Disney Institute (see www.disneyinstitute .com). Disney's customer service approach is summarized in its S.T.O.R.Y. method (Whittmore 2007):

  – **S**tudy the audience
  – **T**ailor the experience
  – **O**rchestrate the details
  – **R**elate
  – **Y**ield long-term relationships

ELEMENTS OF A GOOD TRAINING PROGRAM

First and foremost, employee training should cover the basics: the organization's service mission, culture, values, practices, strategies, products, and policies. Typically, this basic training is given at the employee orientation, but it should be provided repeatedly through various ways. Until all staff are clear on organization-specific information, they cannot fully understand the knowledge and behaviors expected of them. Furthermore, because the patient defines the quality and value of the healthcare experience, employees should learn about patient expectations, competitor services and strategies, industry trends and developments, and the general business environment (Berry 1995). Even an x-ray technician needs to know something more than how to operate the x-ray machine to meet the service expectations of the patient on the x-ray table.

Healthcare consultant Patrice Spath has helped many corporations improve their training. Spath offers five guidelines to developing a successful training program (Lau 2000):

1. *Set clear objectives.* If clear and specific objectives are not set, people will not know what to work toward. An example of a clear objective is to cut the errors that occur during the delivery of drugs to patients. According to Stencel (2006), the cost to hospitals of treating drug-related injuries is staggering, at approximately $3.5 billion a year (2006 figures). This estimate does not take into account the lost wages and productivity of those who suffered the adverse event.
2. *Show that training adds value to staff's lives.* Employees are more accepting (and thus less reluctant) of training if they recognize its contributions to their career and personal pursuits. Ultimately, these growth opportunities result in improved retention rates.
3. *Conduct role-playing sessions.* Role playing not only makes the training interesting (if not fun) but also enables a manager to assess the level of an employee's understanding of the material. One role-playing scenario is for staff to enact a problematic exchange between a patient/family and a nurse/clinical caregiver.
4. *Set safeguards.* Without safeguards, things can go wrong. Knowledge is a critical safeguard in healthcare. Physicians and nurses, for example, can spot errors or potential problems in medications or treatment plans if they are trained and expected to do so. Each person in the patient care process should be trained to spot and correct errors.

5. *Hold employees accountable.* Set measurements to see how well employees are performing and how much more training they need.

Len Berry (1995, 191) expands this list with five other strategies.

1. Focus on critical skills and knowledge
2. Start strong and teach the big picture
3. Formalize learning as a process
4. Use multiple learning approaches
5. Seek continuous improvement

Each of these methods is explored in this section. Berry's and Spath's recommendations can serve as the basis for creating effective training programs.

Critical Skills and Knowledge

Critical skills are the capabilities required of all service employees. An organization can identify these critical skills in two ways: (1) systematically analyzing the service product, delivery system, service environment, and staff and (2) asking patients, employees, and external experts.

Patients and their families can offer insights about the employee skills essential in satisfying customer needs, wants, and expectations, and employees can be trained to pose this type of questions to patients. Dedicated employees (whether clinical or support) are fully aware of the skills they possess, lack, and need for their positions, so they are a natural source for developing training activities. Just as in the case with leader development, employees must be invited or encouraged to participate in designing their own training as they are on the front lines or the receiving end of most customer service issues.

The Big Picture

The big picture includes the organization's overall mission, values, and culture as well as the employee's role in the organization's overall success. Typically, new employees are eager to learn how their jobs fit into the larger organizational context (the big picture), what is expected of them in fulfilling the mission, and how they can help contribute to achieving the goals. This employee attitude reinforces the need to incorporate the big picture into the training effort. Employees perform more effectively when reminded of the value they bring to the organization, including the impact they have on customers.

In many organizations, this big picture reinforcement occurs only periodically, mentioned at infrequent training sessions or at the annual company gathering. Understandably, the hectic pace of business makes losing sight of the big picture easy. But through available means of communication (e.g., staff meetings, customer/employee events, staff trainings, publications, intranet), leaders can regularly and proactively educate or remind staff of the specific ways they contribute to the organization.

For example, during the customer service turnaround efforts at Baptist Health Care, leaders discovered that patient satisfaction improved significantly if patients received a personalized phone call after discharge. Key staff members were trained in when to call, what to say, and how to record the responses. In addition, employees were shown data that linked the increases in patient satisfaction with the uptick in telephone follow-ups. Once staff realized the correlation between what they do and what the hospital wanted to achieve, staff made time to make follow-up calls regardless of their busy schedules.

After training, when an employee is confronted with a problem or situation that is not covered in the employee handbook or a procedure manual, she should be able to depend on the core values and service culture she learned and apply those to the issue at hand. Because so many situations in healthcare are unplanned and unforeseeable, teaching the big picture and the core cultural values is especially critical. People who are taught the organization's values and beliefs from the first day are far more likely to make the right decision for the patient and the organization when a situation calls for decisive action.

Formalized Learning

Formalized learning means

- building staff training and development into the job,
- making learning mandatory for everyone, and
- institutionalizing that expectation.

For example, on a regular basis, organizations should send employees to attend workshops, seminars, and other learning opportunities using company (not employee) time. By putting their money where their values are, organizations send a strong message that continuous learning is vital and all staff are expected to participate.

Multiple Learning Approaches

Using various training approaches is important because people learn or process information differently. No training opportunity should be left unexplored, and relying on traditional methods is not enough. Organizations should also promote learning through book clubs, site visits to exceptional service institutions, simulations, role playing, skits, case studies, and Internet-based training.

Continuous Improvement

The employee orientation is the official first training provided to employees. But training should not stop there. Superb organizations and dedicated employees both want continuing employee education and improvement, through on-the-job training, supervision, shadowing, external classes, and online seminars, to name a few methods. Cross-training also enables staff to expand their knowledge, skills, and abilities, which in turn makes employees more flexible and productive. Equally important is that cross-training affords a department or unit to function normally despite the absence of a staff member.

When an organization invests time and money into its employees' continuing education and improvement, it is conveying that it cares about the staff. The effectiveness (or ineffectiveness) of the actual training may become an afterthought, as employees recognize the organization's commitment to their personal and professional progress.

COMPONENTS OF A CUSTOMER SERVICE TRAINING PROGRAM

Developing a training program necessitates an understanding of its different components. These components are discussed in this section.

Needs Assessment

Needs assessment must always precede training so that perceived or observed problems and weaknesses may be identified first. These challenges then inform the focus of the training. Needs assessment also answers the question, "Will training solve this particular problem?" For example, some patients complain constantly about the slow and cold meal service at the hospital. At first glance, the problem may point toward the inability of the food service staff to prepare meals. A needs assessment, however, may reveal that the real culprits are the old elevators, which not only are slow but also do not have the capacity to carry a big batch of hot meals at once. If the root of the problem is mechanical or nonhuman, then no amount of staff training will correct the flaw.

Needs assessment takes place at three levels: organizational, task, and individual:

- *Organizational needs assessment* seeks to identify the skills and competencies the organization needs and to determine whether these skills already exist. For example, if the needs assessment finds that a unit can use more nursing supervisors but no current employees can fill those roles, then the organization can initiate a training program to prepare new or present staff to become nursing supervisors.
- *Task needs assessment* asks questions such as "What tasks have to be done?" and "Are duties being performed well, or is training needed?" Most task analyses in healthcare revolve around the clinical aspects of care, not the customer service components.
- *Individual needs assessment* reviews the job holder's work to determine if her performance is up to the established job standards. It also involves asking the employee to name the areas in which she thinks she needs training.

Once needs at these three levels (i.e., organizational, task, and individual) have been articulated, development of the training program can begin.

Heathfield (2008) recommends following this needs assessment process for staff who fill the same position (e.g., nurses, receptionists, billing personnel):

- Convene a meeting with the employees who hold the same job. This meeting should take place in a room equipped with a white board or flip chart.
- Instruct the employees to write down the ten training topics they need the most. These needs must be specific (e.g., how to manage an irate caller, how to handle multiple tasks). Capture these comments on the white board, making sure to avoid duplications.
- Ask the group to prioritize the items listed on the board, using a weighted voting process. In a weighted voting process, group members (using a magic marker or sticky dots) assign a vote to each item they perceive to be most important to their job. Members can vote as many times as they like.

- Tally the votes. The item that receives the most votes is considered first priority, the item that garners the second-highest number of votes is named second priority, and so on.
- Jot down the selected priorities, and keep a record or notes of the meeting. A laptop is handy for this exercise.
- Schedule another session with the group for brainstorming. The next session will focus on the desired outcomes and goals of the training, which will be developed on the basis of the priorities named.
- Also note one or two needs identified by each employee, especially if they are not selected as a group priority. These individual training needs may be incorporated into the employee's performance plan.

Training Objective

Needs assessment reveals an organizational, task, or individual deficiency. As such, the training objective should be to ensure that this deficiency is filled. For example, if patient comment cards show a general dissatisfaction with the effectiveness of the personnel who register patients, then the training objective should be to improve the staff's mastery of the registration procedures (assuming that the process itself is sound and does not need to be redesigned). The objective must be directly tied to the problem and must be measurable to enable improvement to be tracked.

Feedback from Physicians and Patients

Feedback from patients and/or the medical staff should serve as a trigger for training. These two groups serve as a check to employees' performance, so if they notice a deficiency in knowledge, skills, abilities, or processes, they are often vocal about their observations. Not all feedback is negative of course, but negative feedback can leave a lasting impression on employees.

Effective organizations constantly measure and monitor the performance of their staff (as well as their services, delivery systems, and setting), and feedback is one method of monitoring. The faster a manager hears this feedback, the faster a manager can institute corrective interventions, including training.

Presenting staff with current data on and future goals for patient satisfaction sets the stage for customer service training. However, this data presentation may be perceived as too impersonal, and the data may be too difficult to explain and comprehend. In this case, the raw data may be personalized in some way. For example, at a staff training in one facility, a videotape of a focus group attended by former patients and community members was shown. Instead of hearing the training facilitator read a transcript of the focus group or cite various customer ratings, training participants were given a chance to watch the customers' candid discussions about their experiences at the facility (Baird 2000, 89). This kind of presentation had a more powerful impact than a numbers-driven lecture would have had.

External Versus Internal Training

Training can be provided by persons inside or outside the organization. If the required training is in a general area or if only a few people are scheduled to attend, an internal program will probably not be worth the expenditure, so those who need training should be sent to an external trainer. Furthermore, many healthcare institutions do not have the resources (e.g., budget, staff, physical space) for an internal training department, so they turn to training experts and consultants. These external training companies range in size and scope, from small, highly specialized firms to large organizations that provide a wide assortment of topics in every imaginable field. Although many companies contract with training organizations that develop and deliver customized, onsite training, others send their employees to more generic and often less-expensive external programs.

Universities and colleges are another source of trainers. These programs employ faculty members who have academic training and/or management experience. Healthcare financial management techniques, information systems design and use, and marketing strategies are examples of special courses frequently offered by colleges and universities as well as professional associations. These programs are relatively inexpensive because they do not have specific application to a particular organization.

Many standard customer service training seminars and workshops are offered by professional associations such as the American College of Healthcare Executives, the Medical Group Management Association, and the American Medical Association. In-house training departments are widely found in large organizations, which usually have an internal unit that provides training to employees. Management consultants may be hired as well to establish a customer service training program.

Some organizations keep all training in-house to preserve organizational security and culture. However, the typical determinant of whether to outsource training is cost. Training cost depends on the number of employees who need training, the expense of transporting those employees from their current workplace (if the organization has different locations) to a central training site, and the level of training needed (the greater the expertise, the greater the cost). In addition, highly technical or specialized training costs even more. If only basic skills training is in order, presenting the course in-house is more cost effective. Also, the organization will likely hold the training internally if it involves many employees from many work sites.

Measurement

Measurement allows the training to be evaluated so that it can be improved if it is not accomplishing the goals. Ideally, the measurement will reveal whether or not the content of the training has been transferred from the trainer to the trainee. Following are the four basic measurement methods available, ranging in expense and degree of accuracy.

1. *Participant feedback.* This method is the cheapest and most commonly used for assessing training effectiveness. It involves asking the participants to fill out a questionnaire that asks them some general evaluation questions. Because responses to these questionnaires often tend to reflect the entertainment value of the training rather than its effectiveness, they have relatively little usefulness for accurate program evaluation. At least they tell you if the participants enjoyed the training.
2. *Content mastery.* If the training goal was to teach a specific skill, competency, or content area, then the participants' aptitude or understanding should be tested afterward. This testing can be as simple as administering a paper-and-pencil examination or as elaborate as requiring an on-the-job demonstration.
3. *Behavioral change.* Many people quickly forget what they learned in classroom settings, especially if they do not apply it; they "use it or lose it," as the saying goes. As many college students admit, they learn a subject well enough to get through the final exam and then they flush all the information out of their brains. To be effective in any meaningful way, training must be followed by real and lasting behavioral changes when the employee returns to the job. If the training is well designed and anchored to mastering specific service-related competencies or skills, and the behaviors are reinforced by positive results or what happens on the job, positive measurable behavioral change should result.
4. *Organizational performance.* Even if the training is well received, if the employees remember most of it on completion, and if they continue to use it on the job, the training is useless unless it eventually contributes to overall organizational effectiveness in some tangible way. To maintain the

organization's competitive position, the training objectives and the training program require constant monitoring to make sure that they continue to prepare employees to provide the level of service that ever-changing patients expect.

Using all four basic measurement methods is useful to determine whether the objectives of the training program were met. Each method is important because each one contributes unique information. As you move up the organization chain to higher job levels, the cost and difficulty of such evaluation increases. As a result, each organization needs to carefully consider which evaluation methods should be used for each program (Business Performance 2008).

TRAINING METHODS

The most common training methods are classroom presentation, video instruction (e.g., taped, live feed or streams), on-the-job supervision (e.g., residency, internship), independent/self-directed study (e.g., correspondence course), and computer-based learning (e.g., webinar). Many training programs use a combination of these methods, but emphasis has increased on computerized and multimedia methods, given that computers have become ubiquitous. A survey of 1,200 white-collar workers in 12 regions reports the following breakdown of training methods: An instructor-led class or workshop (i.e., formal training) was the format taken by 32 percent of respondents, while self-training via a trial-and-error process and peer training was the approach taken by 31 percent of survey participants; 33 percent completed a combination of both training methods (Danzinger and Dunkle 2005).

Classroom Presentation

Classroom training can follow a variety of formats, including lectures and interactive case studies.

Lecture
In a lecture, the assumption is that the speaker is an expert and thus can discuss all aspects of the subject and can provide insight or information pertinent to challenges faced by most, if not all, training attendees. Lectures are typically used when the goal is to impart the same information to a large number of people at one time.

Because they eliminate the need for individual training, lectures are cost effective (*Encyclopedia of Small Business* 2007).

Aside from being inexpensive, lectures are also time efficient and direct to the point. Lectures can supplement on-the-job training and mentoring to ensure that the employee also gets background information and/or theory about the work.

Lectures have a number of potential drawbacks. Personality or any other type of differences between the teacher and a student can disrupt the entire class and its learning goals; worse, this problem can rarely be anticipated or avoided. Additionally, if the facilitator does not mediate the pace of the training, more advanced trainees will get bored while beginning trainees may struggle to catch up (Stroisch and Creaturo 2002).

Interactive Case Study

The purpose of this classroom training is to have an open discussion about a particular case, which is usually selected by the trainer or facilitator. The material is relevant to an issue (e.g., deficient communication skills, barriers to workflow) that staff have to improve, or it may address broad topics such as better decision making or problem solving. In this format, trainees are active participants rather than passive listeners.

The main benefit of the case study is its use of real-life situations. Because the cases chosen for discussion are actual, the training becomes a practical learning experience rather than a collection of abstract knowledge and theories that may be difficult to apply to the real workplace (*Encyclopedia of Small Business* 2007).

The case-study classroom format works with team training as well. Here, the team (with or without a leader) explores a case that reflects the team's current dilemma, and each member may be required to give insight and submit a solution. Ultimately, this exercise can strengthen people's group orientation and ability to collaborate. In addition, team members discover and share a tremendous amount of knowledge and talent among them. Even in highly specialized training areas, teams can often teach each other specific skills more efficiently than a single instructor can, partly because the sum total of knowledge available in the group can fill in the gaps regarding how the skill is supposed to be performed. Smart managers take advantage of team knowledge.

Video Instruction

Videos are frequently used in conjunction with a classroom presentation as a way to bring in material for discussion or material that supports the trainer's teaching.

Video training enables learning to occur at any time, and it is cost effective. Video instructions can be created by a healthcare organization's training department. Alternatively, videos can be obtained through commercial training companies or professional associations. Either way, the videos are inexpensive, convenient, and relevant. For example, new employees can watch a video that describes the dos and don'ts of patient interaction.

One advantage of video instruction is that it presents standard, consistent material so that every trainee gets the same information regardless of when and how many times the video is played. The main disadvantage is that video instruction is typically not customized for a particular audience and offers no opportunities for discussion (*Encyclopedia of Small Business* 2007).

A well-designed and well-produced video can do an excellent job of holding the new healthcare employee's attention, portraying outstanding role models of expected service behavior, and stressing important points. With professional actors in a video showing the correct means of providing patient service, a new employee can see far more easily what the expected behavior is than if a trainer/lecturer talked for several hours. Truly, a picture is worth a thousand words when it comes to service training.

The making of training videos can function as an employee recognition and reward. That is, the organization can assign its best employees to produce a video of their job duties, highlighting ideal behaviors and interactions. Such an assignment shows these staff that the organization appreciates the quality of their work, respects their abilities, and views them as great role models for other employees. In addition, participation in making a training video is enjoyable and enhances the employees' status within the department and the organization.

Another type of video instruction is the live video that is broadcast to the trainees through a satellite feed or "streamed" on the Internet. Distance learning (e.g., webinars) frequently relies on live video technology, which allows interaction between the trainer and trainees even when they are in separate locations.

New technology, diagnostic procedures, and clinical techniques are all appropriate subjects for live video streaming. As such, video training can be considered "just-in-time" education that a rapidly changing environment such as healthcare needs.

On-the-Job Supervision

One-on-one supervised experiences are a typical on-the-job training method in healthcare. The trainee may complete an academic degree program and then be sent to a residency or internship program as part of the required preparation for a healthcare career. In such training, a supervising manager or clinician demonstrates, observes, corrects, and reviews the employee performing the required tasks.

This classic learning-by-doing approach is often essential in the healthcare industry; the skills required to render proper treatment are often so unique, complex, or dependent on the needs of particular patients that the only effective training method is to put new employees on the job and let them learn it by doing it under close supervision.

On-the-job training programs follow a formal sequence, and a process commonly used in training is the job instruction technique. The job instruction technique involves four steps for the trainer: (1) prepare to train, (2) present the material, (3) ask trainees to apply the concepts by role playing or by on-the-job demonstration, and (4) regularly follow up with trainees to ensure they are on track (*Encyclopedia of Small Business* 2007).

Some medical schools train interns to empathize with patients by having the students assume their patients' conditions. For example, in one class at the Mayo Clinic in Rochester, Minnesota, first-year medical students played the "Aging Game" to familiarize themselves with the physical circumstances faced by their elderly patients. Students were asked to wear "goggles to simulate cataracts, ear plugs to simulate loss of hearing, gloves to simulate arthritis, neck braces to simulate the nearly universal muscular stiffness of old age, and diapers to simulate adult incontinence" (Okrent 2000). Then, with these items on, students were asked to read the labels on prescription bottles and to count tiny pills with their fingers. By the end of the course's term, the students were divided into two groups: residents in a nursing home and workers at the nursing home. The "residents" were recipients of the "workers'" uncaring and poor service, including failing to bring food, shoving spoonfuls of applesauce into mouths already filled with marshmallows, and ignoring repeated calls for help (Okrent 2000).

These types of classes enable medical students to experience the care process from the perspective of those they will care for in the future.

Computer-Based Learning

"Computer-based training programs are designed to structure and present instructional materials and to facilitate the learning process for the student" (*Encyclopedia of Small Business* 2007). In other words, computer-based training can be both fun and educational, reach all types of trainees, and accommodate cultural and linguistic needs. Computers never get frustrated with a slow learner and will stay with the student until the educational goal is reached. That statement is still valid today. Computer-based learning provides a number of advantages, including reduced cost of training, instructional consistency, and wide access to trainees located in all parts of the world (*Encyclopedia of Small Business* 2007).

Some behaviors and skills can be taught through computer simulation of actual customer service scenarios. For example, the simulation could feature a patient who is irate about food service and is now berating the staff member. The software could offer several resolutions to this situation, and the trainee could pick the response she thinks is most appropriate. The software then could score or grade how well the trainee handled the scenario. Afterward, the software may present the ideal solution and explain the reasoning behind it. This interactive program can also offer rewards (in the form of points, perhaps) for good answers.

Computer simulation use shows the organization's commitment to patient service and investment in the employees. Simulations help employees develop their decision-making abilities, improve outcomes, and show the personal and organizational rewards gained from giving good service.

Even more exciting than simulations are the training opportunities available on the Internet, which a decade ago made Cisco Systems state: "One day, training for every job on earth will be available on the Internet." As mentioned, streaming training videos are now available on the Internet. With Internet technology and accessibility, updates to training content posted on websites can be quickly and easily made. In addition, the Internet has evolved to become a repository for all kinds of information, challenging and replacing the traditional repository of data—the library. Because Web technology enables any user to supply content, a lot of information on the Internet cannot be called educational or reliable. Despite this fact, however, it has become a training tool that rivals other nonvirtual educational tools, such as colleges and universities and training corporations.

Healthcare providers benefit from computer-based training. These institutions can avoid the expense of sending employees from different locations across the country to a centralized training program by merely telling the staff to go to their desks or a training room equipped with a computer with Internet access and/or training software. The amount of information and knowledge that can be obtained though this medium is enormous.

Other Training Methods

Training can be very specific or somewhat general. The specific is customarily used for entry-level employees who must quickly learn to perform a job skill well to justify their salary. General training can cover a wide variety of topics, ranging from literacy to operating complex electronic systems. Some healthcare providers even find it necessary to teach employees basic bathroom usage and hygiene, such as teaching food handlers how to wash their hands.

Following are other methods of training geared toward service excellence that can be either specific or general:

- *Customer service retreats.* Leaders and staff may go on a retreat that focuses on enhancing customer service excellence. For example, New York-Presbyterian (NYP) has developed a "commitment to care" philosophy that focuses on service expectations for staff. These expectations relate to all staff interactions (with patients, families, and colleagues) and are based on feedback from patients. NYP rolled out these expectations in a staff retreat, allowing an opportunity for staff to ask questions and even practice service behaviors (Liebowitz 2008). Customer service retreats should be full-day experiences to enable exploration of many customer service issues and to function as a reminder to staff of the reasons they entered the healthcare field (Liebowitz 2008).

- *Retraining.* This method is often made available to employees who have become burned out, have become unable to perform their current jobs because of technological developments, or whose jobs have been eliminated. The rapid pace of technological change in healthcare has made retraining an increasingly important issue. Retraining strategies range from sending employees back to school to providing on-the-job instruction in new procedures. Some organizations, like those selling laser eye surgery equipment, send medical doctors to the buyers to teach proper procedures.

- *Role playing.* This method helps staff learn how to best relate to customers. Different scenarios can be role-played for addressing a given customer service problem or issue, and then participants can select the most effective approach and role-play it. One example might be a patient who wants to go home today but needs to stay one more day. A question to consider in this scenario is: What are the options for communicating the "doctor's orders" and their rationale to the patient? The different approaches can then be role-played to determine the most effective one. Other examples might include what to do or say when the patient, a physician, or a family member is angry or when a patient's family makes a request that is contrary to policy. Role playing can be helpful in dealing with situations such as the following:

1. How to advise patients or physicians that their requests cannot be granted
2. How to deal with angry or difficult patients and other customers
3. How to praise patients and motivate them to continue desirable behavior
4. How to recognize unacceptable staff language and behaviors
5. Where and how to voice concerns and problems
6. What not to say in the presence of patients
7. How to address patients and other customers

- *Orientation.* This training is for new employees and can include a segment on customer service that covers the organization's mission and vision, the importance of customer satisfaction, measurement of customer satisfaction, the new employees' roles, customer service standards, and the link between customer service standards and performance reviews.
- *Cross-functional training.* This method enlarges the workforce's capabilities to become multiskilled healthcare practitioners. For example, a Florida hospital developed a patient-centered healthcare delivery system that relies extensively on multiskilled practitioners to perform a wide range of tasks to meet patient needs. As a result, patients receive just as much care but from fewer people. Employee–patient bonding has therefore increased, and patient satisfaction has risen to record levels. Cross-functional training provides task variety and higher interest levels for employees, which has significant benefits in improved employee motivation and morale. Cross-functional training is clearly a win–win situation for patients, healthcare organizations, and employees.
- *Special competencies training.* This method focuses on working as a team, creative problem solving, communications, relationships, and service orientation. Organizations using it realize that having clinical skills is only part of the service requirement for their employees. They know they must also show their employees how to handle the many types of relationships their patients will expect of them and how to solve the many problems that inevitably occur when different patients bring their different expectations to the healthcare experience.
- *Diversity training and attitudinal training.* These types of training focus on changing how employees view and interact with other employees and customers. With the changing cultural makeup of many communities, a heightened awareness of the issues, challenges, and opportunities faced by minorities is essential for those who provide healthcare services. As Rutledge (2001) reminds us, training is needed to ensure that caregivers recognize that "the 'one size fits all' approach does not work because all healthcare customers

have unique life experiences and histories that influence the nature and effectiveness of their participation in and interaction with healthcare delivery systems and providers." In today's competitive marketplace, healthcare organizations must educate their employees regarding such issues to expand services and programs to accommodate new markets.

Selecting a Training Method

Stroisch and Creaturo (2002) offer the following practical suggestions for selecting a training method:

- *Size of audience.* A larger audience often requires more formal training methods with less audience participation.
- *Maintaining attention through interaction.* Training methods that involve the trainees in the instruction have the advantage of maintaining attention and allowing all participants to be involved.
- *Variety.* Selecting and using various methods within a program often maintain the interest of the trainees.
- *Available resources/infrastructure.* When resources are limited, the opportunity to use resource-intensive techniques, such as field visits and demonstrations, may also be limited.
- *Duration of training session.* Training methods that involve discussions and casework take longer than more lecture-oriented methods.
- *Experience of the trainer.* The trainer must be comfortable using the chosen method.
- *Training aids.* Aids support the learning method and make the material more accessible.

Albrecht (2004) recommends that the following four ingredients be incorporated into the training method selected:

1. *Theory.* The essential data, information, and knowledge required to deal with a particular performance situation. It includes concepts, models, reference information, key facts and figures, and principles—all the elements that serve to inform a person's actions associated with a particular competency. Competency can range from simple facts to a complex set of concepts, principles, and/or protocols.

2. *Instruction.* The how-to part of the learning, specifying the actions, methods, procedures, rules, and decisions needed to deal with the performance challenge being learned.
3. *Modeling.* Providing observable examples of competent action. Examples include watching, hearing, or interacting with a person skilled in the desired performance, or observing an outcome or finished product.
4. *Experience.* The actual doing of the target behavior, under circumstances similar to those under which the performance challenge will typically arise, and with assessment and immediate feedback.

PROBLEMS AND PITFALLS OF TRAINING

Common problems with training include failure to establish training objectives, measure results, and analyze training costs and benefits (Business Performance 2008):

1. *Not knowing the training objectives.* Training programs can run into trouble if the precise nature and objective of the training are unknown or imperfectly defined, or if the outcome expected of the training is hard to define or measure. Such programs are hard to justify or defend when senior management reviews the training budgets. Typical examples of areas in which the effectiveness of training is difficult to measure are human relations, supervisory skills, and customer service. Because these terms are vague and situationally defined, knowing what and how much training to offer to improve effectiveness in these areas and how to measure results is difficult. Healthcare organizations quite naturally want their employees to have a service orientation, but the concept is hard to define, as is determining whether the training has resulted in such an outcome. What exactly that training should be and whether it is effective are much more difficult to determine.
2. *Not performing before-and-after measurement.* Although questions about effectiveness are difficult to answer, organizations should try to answer them. One measure of change in, say, patient-service orientation might be the number of patient complaints before and after training. Another approach is to use paid mystery shoppers to sample the level of service, both before and after the training. The point of any technique is to measure the value added by training. Without a "before" measurement,

the organization has little way to know if the measurement after the training represents any improvement. Here, larger organizations have an advantage, as they can use different parts of the organization to test different types of training and statistically determine whether or not one training type is more effective than another in terms of reducing patient complaints or increasing positive comments. Another strategy might be for the organization to measure the attitudes of its own employees toward patients, both before and after the training. Because we know that the correlation between the attitudes of healthcare patients and employees is positive, employee attitude may in general suggest how patients perceive the service level.

3. *Not analyzing costs and benefits of training.* Training programs have obvious direct costs, but they involve indirect or opportunity costs as well; the time that trainees spend away from their regular duties also costs money. Training is too expensive for the organization to train everybody in everything, so it must try to get the best value for its money by using those training programs that can be shown to give the greatest positive results in customer service and patient satisfaction for the training dollar expended. All too often, organizations are at the mercy of consultants selling programs of unproven usefulness and value. Organizations should make the effort to ascertain the value of each training program, whether internal or external, in terms of whether it results in greater patient satisfaction.

STAFF DEVELOPMENT

Training typically focuses on teaching staff how to do new jobs for/into which they have been hired/promoted or to overcome deficiencies they may have in performing their current jobs. Development, on the other hand, is typically focused on getting people ready for their future. Training looks backward to identify and correct employee deficiencies in performing the job today. Development, on the other hand, looks forward to identify the skills, competencies, and areas of knowledge the employee will need to be successful tomorrow.

The challenge with employee development is that knowing what the future will bring is difficult. Therefore, employee development programs tend to be more general, so measuring them and evaluating their effectiveness is even more difficult than for training programs.

Tuition Reimbursement

A good example is the traditional tuition-reimbursement policy many organizations use to encourage employee development. Is the organization doing the right thing for itself or its employees if it refunds tuition only for those courses that are directly related to the employee's existing job, or is it doing a better job if it pays for any legitimate course at any legitimate educational institution? In the first case, the policy looks quite practical as it underwrites courses that directly enhance the employee's ability to do a current job. On the other hand, paying for any course regardless of field expands the total pool of knowledge available to the organization.

Consider a group of people studying different topics in different majors who are brought together in a quality circle or problem-solving session to work on an organizational matter. This group's total knowledge will obviously be greater than if everyone had gone through the same educational program or had majored in the same subject. A variety of learning experiences expands the creative potential of both the employee and the organization and therefore increases the possibility of new and innovative ways to perform now and in the future.

General Education

Supporting any legitimate employee effort to improve, grow, and learn is in the employer's interest. Such support sends a message to employees that the organization values their potential as much as it values their current contributions; it is also a relatively inexpensive employee and organizational development strategy. More important, it supports a learning environment. An organization that actively promotes learning of all kinds sends a powerful message to its employees that it believes the only way it will stay competitive is to continuously learn. These learning organizations promote the active seeking of new knowledge that not only benefits the individual but benefits the entire organization by building its total pool of knowledge.

No matter how irrelevant the material may seem, the creative employee will use it to make organizational connections. The organization will eventually benefit from whatever creativity the educational experience spurred and from the increased loyalty and feeling of support that any employee gets from working for an organization that supports employee education. Forward-looking organizations understand that most of their revenues in ten years will be from products or services that they do not even know about today. Educational reimbursement programs that restrict people to those courses that the organization thinks are important today may be as silly as trying to predict which healthcare services will be important ten years from now.

Career Development

A good employee-development program should also include career development. Few people picture themselves doing the same thing in the future as they are doing today. An organization concerned about customer service should pay careful attention to its current employee-development efforts so that the people who are helping the organization meet customer needs today are prepared to continue doing so in the future.

Employees tend to believe that the longer a person is with an organization, the more that person is worth to it. Many organizations support that belief by celebrating anniversary dates with parties and pins to show that the organization recognizes and appreciates the employee's commitment.

Pins and parties, however, are not enough. The outstanding service organizations recognize that the individual's need for personal growth and development must also be satisfied by permitting the employee to travel along a well-designed career development path.

The entry-level healthcare manager should be able to see a path to the CEO's office that can be successfully traveled with hard work and dedication. The outstanding organizations provide career paths that give talented, ambitious people the opportunity to realize their dreams. The opportunity is symbolically important, even if not all employees choose to take advantage of it.

Mentoring

Mayo Clinic, MD Anderson Cancer Center, and the Veterans Health Administration are among the healthcare facilities that offer fellowship opportunities to recent graduates of master's in health administration programs. Fellowships allow senior-level executives to mentor young people who are just beginning their careers.

Typically, in a fellowship or mentorship program, inexperienced employees are paired with those with more tenure in an effort to encourage mutual learning and growth, both personally and professionally. In addition, mentors can serve as a sounding board for their protégés and can offer job coaching and career advice.

In this way, protégés gain a better understanding of their job roles, responsibilities, and expectations. Protégés are not the only ones who benefit from a mentor relationship; mentors gain valuable insights from their protégés and in the process become better managers (Levine 2008).

CONCLUSION

Employee growth can be facilitated by means of the many training and development techniques covered in this chapter. Organizations should give employees who have knowledge, skills, and abilities and who are willing to work hard the opportunity to grow personally and professionally. Career paths should be available and visible, and continuous learning should be encouraged. In fact, the philosophy that lifelong learning can lead to advancement should be an important part of the organization's culture.

Staff training and development begins with leadership development. Leaders must be the role models of career development. Ignoring the needs of employees to learn and develop may be a cost-effective strategy in the short run, but it is expensive in the long run. Simply, if employees are not growing, the organization is also not growing. The best employees leave this type of environment to offer their talents to an employer who can develop them.

Development is not just for staff. It is also a must for leaders, as leaders set the tone for the rest of the organization.

Service Strategies

1. Teach employees not only job-related skills but also interpersonal skills and creative problem-solving techniques related to customer service.
2. Use scripts related to customer service to teach staff how to respond to customers in a given situation.
3. Do not just train to be training; know what outcomes you expect from your training dollars, and measure your training results to ensure you get them.
4. Before training people, check the service delivery system; the problem may lie there.
5. Develop both leaders and staff for your organization's future.
6. Do not just believe in your people; champion their training and development.

7. Reward behaviors learned through training to keep them alive.
8. Relate training to employee job responsibilities, especially those related to customer service.
9. Make training and development in customer service an ongoing process.

Leaders think about empowerment, not control.
—Warren Bennis

CHAPTER 8

Motivation and Empowerment

Service Principle:
Motivate, empower, and reward employees
for achieving customer service goals

IN ALMOST ALL healthcare experiences, the patient-contact employees make the difference between a satisfied patient and a dissatisfied patient. Therefore, employees who provide the healthcare experience must not only be well trained clinically but also highly motivated and empowered to meet the patient's expectations and to do so consistently. A healthcare manager's leadership and managerial skills can influence employee attitudes greatly and are vital to employee empowerment and motivation.

In this chapter, we address the following:

- Motivating, satisfying, and rewarding staff
- Developing work teams
- Empowering employees to identify and solve problems

MOTIVATING EMPLOYEES

The challenge for healthcare managers is to discover what makes employees not only do their jobs efficiently and competently but also want to go the extra mile. Consider the following scenarios:

- For some time, a nursing home resident has been eating less and complaining more than usual. His exasperated family thinks his complaints are just another tactic to get attention, but an observant employee suspects the patient's reluctance to eat might have a physical cause and arranges for him to see a dentist. The dentist confirms the employee's suspicion: The resident's dentures are causing his discomfort, pain, and inability to eat. The situation is corrected, and the thankful resident begins eating regularly again.

- A chemotherapy patient is happily anticipating a trip to a dear friend's wedding, which was scheduled between chemotherapy treatments, when the patient could comfortably travel the long distance required. Then an attending nurse informs the patient that her high white blood cell count will require a change in the chemotherapy schedule, and the patient realizes she will not be able to go to the wedding. The attending nurse sees the look of dismay on the patient's face and asks the doctor to rearrange the treatment schedule. The change is made, and the patient attends the event and has a wonderful time.

In these examples, the nursing home employee and the chemotherapy nurse took a creative path to solving their patients' problem not because they had to but because they wanted to. Something or someone motivated these healthcare professionals to go above and beyond their clinical responsibilities and job descriptions to provide extra service to their patients. Benchmark healthcare organizations benefit from using the whole employee, from the neck up and from the neck down.

Every healthcare experience is unique, and any manager who believes it is possible to predefine policy and procedures for handling any and all healthcare experiences is mistaken. Employees should know they are encouraged, expected, and trusted to handle all the varied situations that come up in the patient-service areas for which they are responsible. Presuming they were properly selected and trained in the first place, management must make it possible for them to do their jobs with responsibility, skill, enthusiasm, and enjoyment. But how?

The answer is simple. It is based on the well-accepted psychological principle that behavior that is rewarded tends to be repeated, and behavior that is not rewarded tends not to be repeated. Implementing the answer, however, is the challenge facing every manager. The way to keep healthcare employees performing at high levels is to reward behavior associated with excellent healthcare experiences and to refrain from rewarding behavior that is not. In an intensely personal field such as healthcare, acknowledgment of employee contributions is extremely important (Studer 2008).

Finding the right reward is the hard part. Employees are as varied as patients. Just as patients differ in what they expect in terms of care, employees differ in what they expect in terms of rewards from their organizational relationships. In a sense, employees are the manager's customers. Employees define the value and quality of the employment relationship, just as the customer defines the value and quality of the healthcare experience. The managerial challenge is to determine the types of rewards each employee believes are equitable and appropriate, whether service awards, recognition for suggestions and improvements, or other incentives that recognize employees for serving customers well. Finding the right reward can be difficult because, over time, employees' expectations, moods, and valuations of the employment relationship change.

For the most part, healthcare employees look for four things in a job beyond the basics of competitive pay and benefits. It must be fun (in the sense of enjoyably fulfilling), fair, interesting, and important. Top organizations recognize that great employees are more likely to stay if they are allowed to have a little fun at work. For example, the unofficial mission of Paradigm Communication, a software developer, is "have fun or get fired." The company's owner also enforces a simple dress code and attendance policy: Show up for work, and wear something (McCann 2009).

Of course, many healthcare situations are no fun for anybody. Performing a clinical procedure that will be painful for the patient or telling a parent that a child is terminally ill is stressful and agonizing for a healthcare worker. Nevertheless, performing the overall job and accomplishing its goals should be fulfilling and enjoyable, if not exactly fun.

From an organizational perspective, the key to managing and retaining employees is to create job situations that employees perceive as fun, fair, interesting, and important. If the organization can successfully build these elements into the job situation, employees will be motivated to work hard and satisfy customers. The managerial challenge is that everyone's definition of these four traits is different.

Exhibit 8.1 indicates how healthcare managers can become transformational leaders to move their organization or unit toward outstanding customer service. They should start by first being effective transactional leaders. People's basic needs must be handled well in any successful organization, but there is more to a successful organization than a good pay plan, safe working environment, job security, competitive benefits, and working equipment. Truly successful organizations are also effective at finding ways to provide jobs that are fun, fair, interesting, and important (see Exhibit 8.1). This is how transactional administrators become transformational leaders.

Exhibit 8.1 Motivating Mission-Focused Employees

Job is ...	Because ...
1. Fun	Fun work environments communicate the organization's respect and appreciation for its employees; happiness is contagious.
2. Fair	Equity is important to workers as they compare what they are getting from the organization in terms of pay, benefits, development opportunities, and so on with what others are getting both inside and outside the organization.
3. Interesting	
Job content:	The job has autonomy, and workers are empowered and responsible for their own performance, work methods, and achievement of job goals.
Job context:	Work team and culture make the organization a friendly, supportive, and good place to work.
4. Important	The job has value in an organization with a worthwhile purpose that is valued by key stakeholders.

Fun

Fun is essential at work, because happiness is contagious. Employees who have fun tend to be less stressed and easygoing, qualities that spread to other people, including customers. Research has shown that customer calls made by employees who have a smile on their face are more likely to have a successful outcome than calls made by frowning or unhappy employees. A fun work setting improves employee retention, morale, and recruitment (Ford, McLaughlin, and Newstrom 2004).

Fair

The second contributor to a motivated workforce is fairness (Fulford 2005; Barsky and Kaplan 2007). People who are fairly treated are more motivated to perform on behalf of their organization than those who think they are not fairly treated. People compare the ratio of their outputs (what they get out of their effort) to their inputs (what effort they put in) with other people's ratio of outputs and inputs. If an employee thinks his output–input ratio is in line (he gets as much as he puts in) and is about equal with that of others, then he is satisfied. If the employee perceives he is getting less than deserved, he feels abused.

Employees who feel abused tend to steal, call in sick more often, and have low morale (Fulford 2005). Their unhappy attitude and demeanor are displayed to customers. On the other hand, employees who deem that they are paid more or given better benefits than their peers may feel guilty and opt to work harder (although not necessarily smarter), come to work earlier, or stay later to justify what they receive. However, such a reaction is temporary. Soon enough, these employees will come to believe they deserve everything that comes to them.

Employees want to be treated fairly by the organization, and successful managers seek ways to ensure this. The difficulty for a manager is not knowing the input/output measures that employees use to compare themselves with others. Managers must be alert to these comparison factors. Nothing undermines an employee's performance faster than a feeling of inequitable treatment.

Interesting

The third contributor to employee motivation is how interesting people find their jobs. Obviously, managers strive to hire skilled people who want to perform their functional responsibilities, and this desire can be motivated by intrinsic and extrinsic rewards most important to these people. After functionally qualified people are hired, however, the challenge becomes how to keep them interested in consistently and continually performing the specifics of their job.

No two employees are alike, but most employees share a common motivator. First, the job must provide an ongoing opportunity for learning and growth, both personally and professionally (Fiorito et al. 2007). People want to gain mastery in their area of interest, as it leads to increased personal ownership of their work and professional acknowledgment and respect for their knowledge, skill, and abilities. Second, the job must present an opportunity for group work (Fiorito et al. 2007), a concept discussed later in the chapter.

Important

Importance is the fourth motivating factor. This is an employee's perception that her job and performance play a key role in the organization's ability to fulfill its mission. If the community views the healthcare organization as a major contributor to the economic growth, health, and wellness of the community, the employees will feel proud of their association with the institution and their professional and personal input into this greater good. Simply, employees want to feel that what they do is valuable because it benefits other people.

Studer (2008) agrees that this perception of the job as important can lead to worker satisfaction. He expands this idea with three more employee desires (Studer 2008, 146):

1. Employees want to believe the organization has the right purpose.
2. Employees want to know their job is worthwhile.
3. Employees want to make a difference.

SATISFYING EMPLOYEES

Great leaders motivate staff, develop their talents, provide them with proper resources, and reward them when they succeed. If healthcare managers and supervisors offer appropriate incentives and fulfill employee needs, then employees will find their jobs to be fun, fair, interesting, and important; they will be satisfied in their work.

If employees are satisfied, they are much more likely to try to meet the needs of the customers they serve. Customer satisfaction obviously translates into a positive relationship with the healthcare organization, which translates not only into positive word of mouth but also community support and revenue enhancement. These interrelationships—the importance of leaders to employee satisfaction and the importance of employee satisfaction to customer satisfaction—make intuitive sense and are supported by research (Studer 2008).

Recent research by Zeithaml, Bitner, and Gremler (2008) supports the relationship between employee satisfaction and customer satisfaction and suggests that satisfied employees make for satisfied customers and satisfied customers may then reinforce employees' sense of job satisfaction. Unless service employees are happy in their jobs, customer satisfaction will be difficult to achieve.

Intervening When Necessary

Managerial intervention can turn a negative employee situation into a satisfying experience. Consider the case of a conscientious, hardworking nurse in a children's hospital. The nurse is a single mother with school-aged children, and she frequently misses work because of childcare issues. As a result of her absences, the nurse manager has informed her that she is being written up. She was already worried about losing her job, and this latest reprimand makes her feel insecure about her livelihood. Her personal problems and the threat of termination will likely have a negative effect on both the quality of service and the clinical care she provides.

This situation gives the nurse manager an opportunity to turn a negative situation around. What can the manager do to effect a change that will satisfy the nurse and the department? We offer the following step-by-step approach.

1. *Diagnose the problem.* The manager can determine the exact nature of the nurse's absences through facilitative listening. During this process, the manager should concentrate on actively listening, instead of giving advice, instruction, or solutions to the problem or, worse, interrupting.
2. *Clarify goals and expectations.* Specifically, the manager should discuss the organization's mission, vision, and goals and the department's expectations related to attendance, punctuality, patient care, customer service, and so on. Also, the manager may explain the rewards and penalties (including discipline and dismissal) for achieving or failing to meet these expectations. More important, the manager should relate all of these organizational and departmental goals and expectations to the nurse's specific job so that she can better understand how her role, behavior, and performance affect the functioning of the enterprise as a whole.
3. *Empower the employee to come up with the solution.* In this case, the nurse should be responsible for working out her childcare problem, and the manager should offer input and support as necessary. The goal here is to reach a resolution that is practical, achievable, and mutually satisfactory for both parties. If improvement occurs within the agreed-upon deadline, the manager may encourage continued progress by providing a personal note of congratulation or thanks for the nurse's efforts.

Coaching Versus Evaluating

A primary purpose of the traditional performance appraisal is to instill in employees the desire to improve their performance. Yet performance improvement often fails to occur for at least three reasons (Latham and Mann 2006). First, the appraisal is typically done on a fixed-interval basis—annually, biannually, or quarterly. Consequently, the feedback on performance that employees need to act on is often given too long after the fact. Second, because of myriad job duties, the typical manager cannot observe all her direct reports at all times. Consequently, many employees perceive their manager as an inadequate source of feedback about their performance. Third, and arguably worse, many employees think their manager's appraisals are biased. Consequently, staff are not inclined to change their behavior or performance on the basis of their supervisor's evaluation alone.

In the past decade, the prevalent view of a performance appraisal has been that it is conducted to fulfill an administrative requirement, not promote professional development. In fact, documented job evaluations can serve as a legal defense for promotions, demotions, terminations, transfers, layoffs, increase or decrease in salary, and other human resources activities that may be challenged.

Coaching has become the modern way of promoting career growth. It overcomes many of the problems faced in the traditional appraisal because it

- provides ongoing feedback,
- supports goal setting,
- clarifies the relationship between the job performance and the job expectations, and
- inspires the employee to take action to improve job performance.

As new generations of employees enter the workforce, the value of coaching will become even greater. Almost everyone wants feedback, but almost no one wants to hear negative feedback based entirely on a manager's subjective judgment. Coaching, in conjunction with the development of validated evaluation tools, allows managers to guide employees to help the organization achieve its mission.

As an unpublished study by one of the authors suggests, a mystery shopping approach can be used effectively for coaching. Mystery shoppers provide information that is objective, unbiased, and firmly anchored on key performance standards. Using such data allows the manager to coach, rather than judge, and thus to focus on desired behaviors rather than blame.

Asking Employees About the Factors That Motivate and Satisfy Them

Again, the most effective way of finding out what satisfies employees is to ask them. A well-designed employee survey can yield direct answers about staff's perception of the available motivators in the organization. Such a survey ought to assess employees' career interests and goals, identify changes that might improve working conditions and job satisfaction, determine the level of employee recognition and rewards, and name the key drivers of staff motivation (e.g., promotions, flexible work schedules, autonomy, increased responsibility, recognition, salary).

In their Baldrige applications, award winners Mercy Health System in Wisconsin and SSM Health Care in Missouri report conducting such surveys regularly and systematically. Yale-New Haven Hospital in Connecticut surveys employees every two or three years. Similarly, at Baptist Health Care in Florida, a systemwide employee task force conducts focus groups to gather information that can be useful in structuring employee incentive programs.

Baptist Health Care surveys all of its employees every two years and conducts mini surveys every 90 days on the job aspects they know lead to job satisfaction or dissatisfaction, such as employees' relationships with their supervisors and employees' feelings about pay and working conditions.

The organization understands the direct relationship between employee satisfaction and morale, turnover, and quality of the healthcare experience. Managers whose employees have low satisfaction scores are reminded of the low scores in their performance evaluations and compensation. The satisfaction scores are also posted for all employees to see. Employee satisfaction has led to increased patient satisfaction and productivity at Baptist Health Care.

Exhibit 8.2 lists 12 questions that measure key factors associated with attracting, focusing, and keeping employees satisfied with the job and the organization. The questions are based on extensive work by the Gallup organization confirmed

---

Exhibit 8.2 Questions Assessing Core Work Elements

1. Do I know what is expected of me at work?

2. Do I have the tools, materials, and equipment I need to do my job right?

3. At work, do I have the opportunity to do what I do best all day?

4. In the past seven days, have I received praise or recognition for doing good work?

5. Does my supervisor, or someone at work, seem to care about me as a person?

6. Is there someone at work who encourages my development?

7. At work, does my opinion count?

8. Does the mission or purpose of my company (organization) make me feel my job is important?

9. Are my coworkers committed to quality work?

10. Do I have a best friend at work?

11. In the past six months, has someone at work talked to me about my progress?

12. This past year, have I had the opportunity at work to learn and grow?

---

by a meta-analysis on more than 100,000 managers in 24 companies (Buckingham and Coffman 1999). Still valid and valuable in today's workplace, the list suggests that employees do not quit organizations, but they do quit their managers. As mentioned in Chapter 5, transformational managers know this simple fact and strive to get the answers to such questions so that the right people who can help the organization fulfill its mission are retained.

REWARDING THE DESIRED BEHAVIOR

Most managers focus on their problem employees and tend to ignore those who perform competently. Their employees quickly learn that "the squeaky wheel gets the grease." Rewarding the wrong behavior is as big a mistake as not rewarding the right behavior. The organization's reward system needs to be constantly and carefully reviewed to ensure that the behaviors being rewarded are aligned with the behaviors that the organization supports.

For example, many hospitals say employees should make every effort to satisfy the patients, but many of these same hospitals evaluate and reward employee performance only according to the budget numbers and clinical results. This practice has been called "rewarding A while hoping for B." Most employees will naturally focus on the numbers and not on the patient-satisfaction ratings. Similarly, if healthcare managers tell employees that team performance is important but only reward employees as individuals, employees will realize that team effort does not really matter that much.

For example, say a hospital hires Roberta Hunter to serve as a receptionist at the hospital's information desk. The manager tells Roberta explicitly that her primary responsibility is to greet and welcome patients and their families and to provide them with any information they need. As time goes on, however, to keep Roberta busy when patients are not entering the hospital, the manager adds responsibilities to the position: doing routine but important paperwork.

Roberta quickly realizes that the manager never compliments her for cheerfully greeting patients or giving helpful information, nor does the manager say anything when she does not speak with a customer promptly because she is too busy with other duties. But if Roberta fails to get the paperwork done, she is strongly reprimanded. By action or lack of action, the manager has redefined Roberta's job description. By his actions, the manager has made the real priorities clear, and Roberta adjusts her actions accordingly.

Identifying the Rewards

Managers must learn techniques that accurately identify the rewards employees want. Quint Studer (2008, 163–68) calls this process "knowing your employees' 'what'—the factors that workers perceive to be rewards, which promote motivation and commitment. He suggests finding out these needs by the following means:

- Conducting an employee satisfaction survey
- Paying attention to issues during daily or weekly rounds
- Sending out a "what's your what" e-mail to all employees
- Asking each employee directly

Well-designed employee questionnaires, such as Exhibit 8.2, can make managers aware of the rewards most likely to motivate or satisfy a given category of employees. Effective performance is a result of employees being rewarded in ways that recognize both what they personally value and what their work contributes to the organization. These rewards keep them energized to perform their jobs efficiently and enthusiastically.

As mentioned in previous chapters, one form of reward that has been successful in enhancing employee retention is flexible scheduling. AARP's 2008 "Best Employers for Workers Over 50" included two healthcare organizations that offer flexible scheduling: Inova Health System in Falls Church, Virginia, and SSM Health Care in St. Louis, Missouri (AARP 2008).

NECESSARY MANAGERIAL SKILLS

Managers must have certain skills to support and motivate employees, including both the administrative transactional and the leadership transformational skills. Administrative or transactional skill is the ability to take care of routine tasks, including paperwork, administrative procedures, and policies that directly influence each employee's ability to perform the job. A manager who forgets to submit the proper payroll, who fails to provide the necessary information for employee decision making, or who schedules too few people to work in the emergency department on a Saturday evening creates situations in which even the most enthusiastic, energetic employee cannot succeed. Managers must effectively administer the basic job-related requirements of employees.

Transformational leadership skill is the ability to identify and provide the rewards individual employees want to move the organization to a higher level of performance along some dimension. It often means transforming some aspect of the organization to better align it with the changing external environment (i.e., changing some aspect of the culture). Although fear and the threat of punishment may be powerful short-term motivators, the ability of the organization and its managers to fulfill employee needs is what yields energetic employee commitment to organizational goals in the long run. What managers offer in return for employee contributions are inducements that make the job fun, fair, interesting, and important; are fairly distributed; and affirm the job's value to the organization and society. These inducements can be referred to as eager factors.

Eager Factors

What makes employees eager to join the organization in the first place? People join organizations to fulfill their needs. Although individual needs are infinitely varied, they usually include the need for financial security, the need to belong to an organization that matches and enhances one's self-image, the need to associate with people who think and feel the same way, and the need to grow and develop as a person and as an employee. Although every organization will have poor performers, most people work hard when they are doing what they love in a job that satisfies their needs.

Salary
Financial compensation policies should be carefully designed. Competitive salary and benefits are important to any worker, but pay is not the only driver of good performance or willingness to stay. Sometimes, pay could present a negative snowball effect. Consider a group of employees who receive a bonus for successfully completing a project. The group will probably be highly motivated to perform on the next project, perhaps even doing a better job. If their performance on the next job is of higher quality and they receive a lower bonus or no bonus, their motivation for future projects may decrease.

Sense of Belonging
Many years ago, studies at the Hawthorne Plant of the Western Electric Company showed that a sense of belonging or not belonging greatly influences what people will or will not do in the workplace. Well-formed work groups can help managers give direction to employees and guide behaviors in the workplace. To this end, managers

should work in harmony with the group and support its efforts, because the accomplishment of the group's goals facilitates the achievement of the organization's goals.

If a group offers its members an opportunity to achieve something greater than individual members could alone, then the group's value to its members becomes greater than merely satisfying people's belonging needs. Membership in a group with a strong corporate culture and a widely respected mission is beneficial for both the individual and the group. This esteemed and admired mission becomes itself a powerful tool for motivating and retaining the members. The concept of team is discussed further in the next section.

WORK TEAMS

By nature, healthcare work can profoundly change people's lives. Healthcare workers who understand this fact and are committed to their work are the ideal members of a team charged to identify service quality problems or patient care improvements.

In the last section, we discussed the need of people to feel a sense of belonging. A work team satisfies this need without any organizational intervention. Most organizations, however, are unaware of the interrelationships between individual goals, team goals, and organizational goals. That is, individual efforts help the team reach its goals, which in turn enables the organization to achieve its mission.

If the organization enables the team to satisfy its higher-level need (e.g., sense of belonging), then the organization and its efforts will gain support from the team and its members. Although this sounds easy to do, it is not. Most organizations do not know how to tap into their connection with work teams and their many benefits, as discussed in the next section.

Building strong work teams is worth the effort. Exhibit 8.3 sums up the characteristics of a well-functioning work team. A manager can use these guidelines to strengthen a weak work team and improve its performance.

Benefits of Teams

An organization can reap many benefits from supportive and productive work teams:

1. *Access to the team's innovative ideas.* Few healthcare managers know everything or are capable of identifying the ideal answers to every customer problem. Using team problem-solving processes generates a wealth of new ideas and frequently a better perspective than the manager alone might have. After all, those who deal with customers and the problems serving customers may create know the details of those problems better than do the managers, who typically have multiple responsibilities.

2. *Improved employee behavior and productivity.* If the team has a performance objective, the group is better equipped to monitor and oversee each member's contribution than managers are. The team's approval of the member's work will likely have greater weight for the individual than the supervisor's because the individual works more closely with the team.

Exhibit 8.3 Successful Work Team Characteristics

The successful work team…

1. Has a meaningful team purpose that inspires and focuses the members' efforts

2. Has goals and objectives that are measurable, specific, realistic, easy to understand and with defined areas of authority

3. Is small enough to act as a true team (5–15 members)

4. Has members with the necessary skills to operate as a team (functional/technical skills appropriate for the decision area, problem-solving/decision-making skills, and interpersonal/ team skills)

5. Has clear, well-organized work procedures and rules of behavior that are enforced by the team

6. Has a cultural value of mutual accountability, where only the team, not any one team member, can fail or be a hero

7. Is supported by the organization's leadership and led by a team-building coach who builds a performance culture

8. Has enough group time to allow members to interact and learn how to care about one another

9. Understands the extent of its authority

10. Is provided with the resources necessary to succeed

---

3. *Shared learning and decision making.* When teams are brought in to help with organizational efforts, shared learning occurs. Team members learn more about the organization and its strategies. In turn, leadership gains a better understanding of what it wants to do and how to do it. Also, members learn more about the task or goal at hand, the reason it must be done a certain way, the contributions of others toward its accomplishment, and its relationship with the overall organizational goal. Involving teams provides management a clearer picture of the problem; after all, a manager who lacks insight about an issue cannot explain it to anyone else nor determine the best resolution. Lastly, team involvement enables employees to be more accountable for their own work.

4. *Ownership and responsibility.* When a team is charged with a project, its members take ownership and responsibility for every aspect of the project, including analyzing the issue, communicating with stakeholders, identifying solutions and implementing the best one, and monitoring the outcomes.

   For example, a work team is formed to resolve the problem of too many dishes breaking during meal deliveries. The team discovers that the plates break because the food trays are stacked without spacers in between. When the service carts roll over tile floors, the trays rattle and then slide off, spilling the plates to the ground. The team's solution is to place rubber spacers between the trays.

   Because the team came up with this idea without managerial input, the members work harder to ensure it is viable. They push the service carts loaded with trays with rubber spacers, wriggle the trays to ensure no slipping occurs, talk with the kitchen staff to get their input and cooperation, and assess the effectiveness of the intervention several weeks later. In the end, this solution is noted a success.

   Often, such problems are given to industrial engineers or outside consultants, who come up with elegant but impractical solutions. This move does not usually solve the problem and only frustrates employees.

By using a work team, managers enable those who do the actual work to participate in making improvements. Also, it sends the message that employees are trusted and their capabilities are valued. Possible results of this approach include a boost in morale, a reduction in absenteeism, and enhanced recruitment and retention. (See Sidebar A for another example of a work team in action.)

Self-directed work teams drive the services at Kansas Neurological Institute (KNI), a residential facility for people with developmental disabilities. KNI has 24 self-directed teams, each of which is composed of 8–14 support staff and is led by a coach. Teams offer 24/7 support to residents and may call on KNI's clinical staff, including therapists, at any time.

Teams provide a lot of services, including assistance with personal care, meal preparation and shopping, and entertainment. In addition, team members are sensitive to residents' lifestyle preferences and consider those needs when extending any kind of support. KNI's self-directed teams advance KNI's mission. (See www.srskansas.org/kni for more information.)

Nursing Teams

Nursing care teams have emerged as a common approach to organization design and acute care in U.S. hospitals (Dreachslin, Hunt, and Sprainer 1999). A typical nursing care team includes one registered nurse, who serves as the team leader, and one or two nonlicensed caregivers, who help the nurse deliver care. Like other team approaches, complementary skills and commitment to a common purpose characterize a nursing care team. The difference between a nursing care team and a traditional nursing team is that the boundaries of the latter are rigid whereas the boundaries of a nursing care team are permeable. Nursing care team members are able to perform duties as needed to serve the patient, unhampered (within legal boundaries) by rigid role definitions. This design allows team members to experience more empowerment in terms of decision making in patient care.

Possible Problems with Teams

Potential problems with the team approach include the following:

- Teams do not always work as fast as individuals do.
- Teams require managers to take on a new mind-set and change behaviors related to employee leadership.
- Teams require investments of money and time.
- Teams are limited to tackling one problem, situation, or task, all of which must present opportunities for member participation.

Many of these disadvantages are discussed in the following section.

Team resolutions take more time than those reached by an experienced manager. Most team members do not intuitively know how to make decisions systematically or how to collaborate with others to build a consensus. Teaching members these skills adds to the limited time afforded for problem solving. Also, explaining the who, what, why, when, where, and how of an issue to a group of people with varying degrees of team skills and organizational experience takes time.

Team decisions cause confusion and fear among current managers and supervisors. Most managers and supervisors were promoted because they were the best at doing whatever job they now supervise—the best nurse becomes the head nurse, the best x-ray technician becomes the department head, and so forth. If the organization assigns a promoted manager to coach a decision-making team, the manager will become confused and wonder why she was promoted at all if the organization did not intend for her to make decisions. Simply, the message here is mixed, and many managers have a difficult time shifting gears to be coaches instead of doers or decision makers. The other consequence for managers is fear. Managers may feel insecure about their future role and responsibilities when their direct reports are now able to do their job. If a manager's job is to oversee all aspects of his department and employees, what value does the manager offer if those employees are empowered to manage themselves and make departmental decisions? Because of this threatened feeling, many managers have found ways to discourage (or even sabotage) empowerment programs and team efforts.

Team decision making is neither cheap nor always effective. Taking employees out of their normal routine to work on a special task or project has a cost. Furthermore, teams are incapable of making decisions (or making them well) on matters that are beyond the authority, concerns, interests, or expertise of their members. For example, a team of pharmacists is not equipped to establish a sound corporate policy for nurses. Even if the pharmacists receive extensive training on nursing issues, they will still be unable to grasp the details and implications of their decisions.

Following are some additional problems with teams:

- Decisions that require technical expertise beyond that typically available to the involved team members will not likely be successful.
- Employees who are not on a team may feel left out and become resentful when teams are rewarded for good ideas and/or successful implementation.
- Some team members may become freeloaders and not contribute their fair share to the team.
- Not everyone can work successfully in a team format.

When to Use Work Teams

An organization needs to determine the answers to four critical questions before it uses team-based decision making:

1. *Is management comfortable letting work teams make decisions about their job responsibilities?* Although this sounds easy to answer, it is not. Many managers are uncomfortable letting go of their managerial prerogatives. Even so, they often have to in healthcare because so many healthcare activities, such as strategic planning, can only be accomplished by teams. No one person has the time or skills to perform every task and make every decision.

2. *Is management ready to let teams be accountable for their efforts and decisions?* Because most managers are evaluated on the basis of their unit's performance, this is a hard question also. If the manager is accountable for the decision, how can the manager be comfortable allowing the group to make a decision that might come back to haunt the manager if it turns out poorly? If they have to be accountable for the results, most people believe they might as well make the decisions themselves, and they have a hard time trusting another person or group to make the decisions for them.

3. *Is management ready to share the benefits of the decisions?* This question leads to others: If the group makes good decisions and saves the organization money, will management share the rewards with the group? In a related way, will management share the glory and other benefits that result from high levels of performance in an organization? If the team makes the decision that wins the boss the big bonus and the trip to Hawaii, will they ever work that hard on behalf of the organization (or that manager) again unless they too benefit in a meaningful way?

4. *Is management ready to let team decision makers grow and develop?* If the group and its members do not get the opportunity to grow and develop, but see management getting these opportunities as a result of the group's efforts, they will lose their interest in and enthusiasm for the team decision-making process. Management who wants team decision making to succeed must be ready to let the team and its members participate in growth and development opportunities and organizational rewards and must be willing to trust them with the authority and responsibility for decision making.

Although work teams offer an important benefit to employees by providing a sense of belonging, effective work teams do more for their members. They provide a sense of self-worth, the opportunity to grow and develop, and a means to recognize and share achievements and failures and to reinforce each other's values and beliefs. In brief, they help satisfy each group member's need to grow and develop as a person and as an employee.

For an organization to garner the benefits of teams, success in achieving customer service goals needs to be celebrated in public. Not only do data need to be shared but team success also needs to be recognized publicly because it reinforces the culture of excellence. Public praise played a major part in the successful turnaround of Baptist Health Care (see Sidebar B).

EMPOWERING EMPLOYEES

Teams need to grow and develop, but so do individuals. One great asset a team provides to its members is the opportunity to grow within the group setting. But the organization should provide additional opportunities for its members to satisfy this important need. The most widely discussed strategy for doing so is empowerment. Becoming empowered may add to the fun and value of the job for employees. It may also add a sense of fairness because well-trained employees may think it is only fair that they be given some responsibility for making decisions related to their own work.

The main benefit of empowerment is that a job that offers opportunity for growth and development through empowerment is more interesting. The organization also benefits from interested, empowered employees. An empowered

---

SIDEBAR B:
TURNAROUND AT BAPTIST HEALTH CARE
Baptist Health Care, a 456-bed, not-for-profit pediatric teaching hospital, formed a patient satisfaction committee to evaluate and monitor its service performance (Stavins 2004). The committee conducted telephone surveys for inpatient, outpatient, emergency, and day-surgery departments. These surveys enabled the team to identify problems, reward outstanding service, and initiate innovative and improvement practices.

For example, when waits and delays were determined to be a concern to patients, the staff were asked to inform patients and families whenever there was a delay and how long the wait would be. Later, the committee's work branched out to departments with little or no patient contact. The purpose for this expansion was to improve service between departments and among all staff.

Formation of the committee created a unified, organization-wide approach to customer satisfaction. It emphasized the importance of customer service, even among those who usually did not provide direct customer care. It also brought out and involved employees who have extensive yet hidden/underused skills, such as knowledge of survey tools and statistical processes and a passion for customer service.

---

healthcare provider can personalize the healthcare experience to meet or exceed each patient's expectations and can take whatever steps are necessary to prevent or recover from service failures. Organizational success or failure can hinge on the quality of a healthcare experience.

Empowerment is the assignment of decision-making responsibility to an individual. It requires sharing information and organizational knowledge that will enable the empowered employees to understand and contribute to organizational performance, rewarding them based on the organization's performance, and giving them the authority to make decisions that influence organizational outcomes. Empowerment is broader than the traditional concepts of delegation, decentralization, and participatory management. Empowerment can stretch decision responsibility beyond a specific decision area to include decision responsibility for the entire job and for knowing how the performance of that job fits within the organizational purpose and mission.

Managers of some organizations talk the talk of employee decision input but do not give employees any real power or authority to implement decisions. The purpose of employee empowerment is not only to ensure that effective decisions are made by the right employees but also to provide a mechanism by which responsibility for job-related decisions is vested in individuals or in work teams. Empowerment also means management is willing to share relevant information about and control over factors that impinge on effective job performance.

Empowerment is not an absolute; it has degrees. Managers may find that more empowerment is not necessarily better. For example, a manager can choose to provide higher degrees of empowerment for some individuals and teams doing certain tasks than for others. Indeed, even within a given person's job or a given group's task responsibilities, different decision areas can be empowered to different degrees. A clinic, for example, may empower its nurses with complete authority to regulate who may visit patients and when, within a certain range of variation, to meet the level of patient satisfaction offered by competing clinics. However, the clinic might not be willing to let the same nurses make minor modifications in clinical protocols or hours of clinic operation.

The Job Content/Context Grid

Healthcare managers may need help in seeing how to use the empowerment concept in their own organizations. They may also need help with managing the delicate balance between giving employees control over their own work processes while retaining some supervisory control over what employees do. What would happen, for example, if management empowered a work group by assigning the group authority and responsibility over a job and the group decided to do nothing at all related to the organization's goals? Obviously, empowerment must occur within some limits, and where to place them becomes a major challenge in implementing any empowerment strategy.

An organization wanting to empower its employees must first analyze its jobs. All jobs have two dimensions: content and context. Job content represents the tasks and procedures necessary for doing a job. Job context refers to why the organization needs a job done; how one job interacts with related jobs; and how a job fits into the overall organizational mission, goals, objectives, and job setting. Managers trying to use empowerment will find it helpful to view decision making not simply as an act of making a choice among alternatives but as a five-stage process:

1. Identify the problem,
2. Discover alternative solutions,
3. Evaluate the pros and cons of those alternatives,
4. Make the choice, and
5. Implement and follow up on the effects of that choice.

Employees can be empowered to participate in one, some, or all of these stages.

Exhibit 8.4 shows a grid with the job context on the vertical axis and the job content on the horizontal. The horizontal axis shows the way in which the employee's or team's decision-making responsibility over job content progressively increases in relationship to the decision-making process. For example, at the far left of Exhibit 8.4, in the first step of the decision-making process, employees have little responsibility; but the level of responsibility and the decision involvement increase as one moves to the right. Similarly, as one moves up the vertical axis, responsibility and involvement over decisions related to job context increase. A manager seeking to empower employees may wish to increase decision responsibility over job content, job context, or both. The five points (points A through E) identified on the grid allow a better understanding of varying strategies for empowerment available to managers.

Point B (Task Setting) is the essence of many empowerment programs used today. Here, the worker is given a great deal of decision responsibility for the job content and little for the context. The worker is empowered to make decisions about the best way to get an assigned task accomplished. In these cases, management defines the mission and goals, and the worker is empowered to find the best way to reach them. Management hopes the empowered workers will apply their job knowledge and intellect to discover ways to improve what they do in their jobs.

Exhibit 8.4 The Employee Empowerment Grid

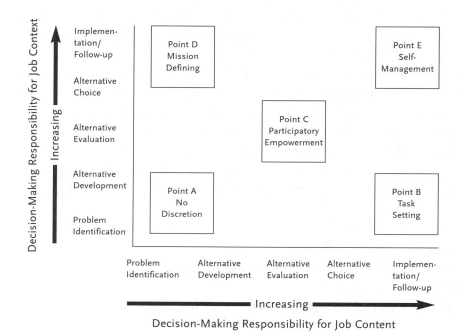

Source: Reprinted with permission from *Academy of Management Executive* 9 (3): 24, 1995. "Empowerment: A Matter of Degree," by R. C. Ford and M. D. Fottler.

Many healthcare jobs are in this category. Patient-service employees, for example, must do the job as defined by the clinical protocol but have flexibility to do it in a variety of ways to meet the needs and expectations of varied patients. An admissions representative may be given the decision responsibility to prioritize patient treatments based on some triage protocol, for example. Hospital nurses also follow strict clinical protocols but have a certain degree of flexibility in how they deliver care.

For example, a nurse on the maternity ward may give an educated, married mother of four a copy of the postoperative instructions as clinically ordered but may choose to spend more time explaining instructions to an unmarried teenager having her first child. Nurses must make care decisions based on their judgments about the needs of each individual. A 90-year-old man with a broken leg requires different care from an 18-year-old football player with the same condition.

Point B represents a significant departure from Point A (No Discretion) because employees are totally involved in making decisions about job content. Jobs at Point

B can be redesigned by employees or even teams of employees. They may redesign their tasks to add more content or develop a variety of new employee skills. Many Point B employees find such enriched jobs more motivating and satisfying, leading them to do higher-quality work. Even when management confines empowerment to job-content decisions, employee motivation may be enhanced for those who strongly value feelings of accomplishment and growth. The success of the Point B strategy, however, will partly depend on factors beyond employee control, such as the design of the service delivery system, organizational structure, patient expectations, clinical protocols, reward systems, and support of top management.

Point B and the Healthcare Industry

Point B empowerment perfectly suits many healthcare organizations and many healthcare employees. The clinical requirements define the job, and employees are expected to meet those requirements to achieve the desired clinical outcome. Some organizations expect employees to do the job strictly by the numbers, but benchmark organizations empower employees to provide service in a variety of ways. For example, even if a nurse in a burn ward has 25 patients who need their dressings changed every six hours in the same way, the manner in which that care is given and the interaction patterns that take place with each patient make each occasion somewhat different and potentially interesting for the nurse. Each occasion also presents an opportunity to perform a routine task with personalized care and attention.

Benchmark healthcare organizations know patient satisfaction increases when employees are empowered to decide if they need to spend more time with patients and are able to go the extra mile to make them feel comfortable. Allowing staff to exceed patient expectations is particularly important when patients have complaints. Benchmark organizations empower all employees to provide token restitution (up to a certain dollar amount) when a patient believes some type of service failure has occurred.

For example, at Baptist Health Care, each employee can go to the hospital gift shop and spend up to $300 to replace a patient's lost belonging or buy flowers to appease a complaining patient. Studer (2008, 155–56) gives an example of a hospital cashier in a cafeteria who notices that some patients who are admitted have no family to help them. She realizes they will probably have to leave an inpatient stay with the same clothes they arrived in. For such patients, the cashier will offer to take their clothes home to launder and will return with clean clothes the next day. Studer describes this person as an "owner" because she attends to her customers, thinks innovatively, makes personal sacrifices, and goes beyond her job description to keep customers happy. Studer suggests that all managers should identify such employees, hold them up as an example to others, and do everything possible to empower them to serve customers.

All in all, a Point B empowerment level is the most suitable for many patient-contact jobs in the healthcare industry. This level gives healthcare providers the flexibility to meet and exceed the patient's expectations and to prevent and recover from any service failures while maintaining the proper clinical protocols.

Implementation

Successful implementation of an empowerment program requires knowledge of the available strategies and the determinants of their successful application and an awareness of the situations and people who can benefit from empowerment. Implementation of empowerment should begin by focusing on decisions related to job content and then moving gradually through the various decision-making stages from problem identification through implementation to follow-up. Later, after employees and managers become comfortable with empowerment in job content, increasing levels of empowerment in job context can be added by raising the level of decision-making authority from problem identification up through implementation and follow-up.

At each step, management can determine what difficulties were created; how they should be addressed; and whether or not the individuals or teams were ready, willing, able, and trained to move on to the next stage of decision involvement and responsibility. Alternatively, a company might empower employees to identify problems and develop alternatives simultaneously for job content and job context.

For either of these approaches or any other mid-range strategies, management needs to determine first where it would like to be on the grid in Exhibit 8.4 and then develop a plan to move its employees gradually toward that point. The grid simply illustrates the stages of employee empowerment, which allow managers to decide what level of empowerment their organization is ready for and what can be done to implement that desired degree of involvement in making job-related decisions.

Following are five key ingredients to any successful empowerment program:

1. Training in knowledge areas, patient service, and decision making; if empowering a group (see the work team discussion), training in group interaction

2. Measurable goals or standards, so empowered employees and their managers have a means to test whether their decisions are good or bad
3. Methods of measuring progress toward goals, so empowered employees and their managers can tell if what they are doing is heading toward the job goal or away from it
4. An incentive system to reward the employees for making good decisions and to make it worth their while, both financially and in terms of other eager factors, to take on decision responsibility
5. Willingness of employees to make decisions and willingness of managers to take those decisions seriously

Limitations and Potentials

Of course, employee empowerment has some organizational limitations. Employee empowerment may be less appropriate under the following conditions (Bowen and Lawler 1992):

1. The basic business strategy emphasizes low-cost, high-volume operations.
2. The relationship with customers tends to be short term.
3. The technology is simple and routine.
4. The business environment is highly predictable.
5. Employees have low growth needs, low social needs, and weak interpersonal skills.

Alternatively, employee empowerment can be highly rewarding under the following circumstances (Bowen and Lawler 1992):

1. Service is customized or personalized.
2. Customer relationships are long term (this is sometimes but not always true in healthcare).
3. The technology is complex.
4. The environment is unpredictable.
5. Employees have high growth needs, high social needs, and strong interpersonal skills.

Regarding item 5, employee empowerment alleviates the uneasiness and awkwardness staff feel during many patient-contact situations, especially when those situations are negative. Within all organizations, including healthcare organizations, some departments, employees, or jobs may be better suited for employee empowerment than others. Managers hoping to gain the benefits of empowerment can initially implement a limited form of empowerment in areas where the match appears potentially fruitful. From here, problems can be worked out and the empowerment process gradually expanded. Indeed, those healthcare organizations engaged in total quality management efforts, organizational reengineering, or attempts to reenergize their corporate culture's commitment to service through the introduction of more participatory management styles may find the incremental strategy useful.

Because the workforce is so diverse, some employees will be better suited for empowerment than others. Part-time employees or contract (temporary) employees may not be interested enough in the goals of the organization or their long-term relationship with the organization to be good candidates for empowerment programs. For example, doctors sometimes build strong relationships with patients. These relationships motivate patients to come back again and again; seeing familiar physicians adds value to their healthcare experience. A major problem with health maintenance organizations (HMOs) is that their managers seem unable to use appropriate motivation and empowerment techniques to keep physicians on their panel. This physician turnover is one reason for widespread customer dissatisfaction with HMOs. HMOs need to empower physicians to practice in the patients' best interest rather than question and penalize their clinical decisions.

The art of good management is in determining which employees should be empowered to do which task or to make which decision. Admittedly, this is a daunting challenge, especially if the wrong call on the manager's part leads to a decision that presents a disadvantage to a large number of people. For example, if an empowered employee allows patients to check out two hours late, the housekeeping staff may have difficulty preparing the room for the next patient, especially if another empowered employee allows the next patient to check in early. Empowering one employee must not be allowed to negatively affect how other employees perform their jobs.

Ultimately, a successful healthcare manager knows the vital importance of motivation and empowerment if the organization is going to retain the employees it worked so hard to recruit and train.

CONCLUSION

All employees seek certain types and amounts of inducements from their organizations; that is why they joined. A manager who is able to provide those inducements can elicit effort, productivity, enthusiasm, and other contributions the healthcare organization seeks from all employees. Determining the mix of rewards or motivators most important to employees or a group of employees is a critical managerial responsibility. These factors enable employees to view their jobs as fun, fair, interesting, and important.

Service Strategies

1. Set clear, measurable standards that define expectations for job performance in all areas, including customer service. Constantly reinforce these standards by setting examples. Let employees know the standards are important, and reward employees when they meet them.
2. Walk the talk. Set the example. Employees respond more to what is done than to what is said.
3. Make all tasks and goals measurable; people like to know how well they are doing.
4. Pay attention to communication; people cannot do what they do not know about or do not understand.
5. Be fair, ethical, and equitable. People need to believe they are being treated fairly. If you do not show people why distinctions are made between employees, they will assume the worst.
6. Focus on frequent, ongoing feedback geared toward improved job performance (i.e., coaching).
7. Reward desired behaviors. Among the most important rewards are public celebrations of individual and team success in serving customers.
8. Identify and provide the types of rewards most desired by various subgroups of employees.
9. Praise, praise, praise. Give public reinforcement to employees who are doing the right things. Re-educate and coach, in private, those who are doing the wrong things.
10. Show employees the relationships among their personal goals, group goals, and organizational goals. Find win–win–win situations.
11. Support and trust frontline employees.
12. Give people a chance to grow and get better, and then reward them for it.
13. Make employees' jobs fun, fair, interesting, and important to the extent possible.

God helps those who help themselves.
—C. Simmons

CHAPTER 9

Involving the Patient and Family in Coproduction

Service Principle:
Empower patients and their families to help meet their own
healthcare needs

PATIENTS AND THEIR friends and families may participate in coproducing almost any healthcare experience. This involvement can take many forms, no matter how seemingly minor. For example, patients are encouraged to walk after surgery to facilitate their recovery, are required to bring their own test results to a follow-up visit, and are put in charge of regulating their own medications. In addition, friends and family members are increasingly called upon to assist the patient at home or at the hospital.

Assigning specific tasks to patients and their informal caregivers (e.g., family, friends) is part of a broader trend to actively engage consumers in their own healthcare. To this end, healthcare providers and their staff must spend time and effort investigating where and how patients can participate. Successful coproduction of a healthcare experience relies on the effective coordination of care processes, a responsibility of management and staff.

Prahalad and Ramaswamy (2004a) advise consumers and organizations to think of themselves as joint creators of value. They can do this by creating personalized healthcare experiences that take into account the uniqueness of individual patients. Organizations that allow everyone to participate in this process will encourage communication-rich transactions and open dialogues.

Prahalad and Ramaswamy (2004b) note that the role of consumers has changed. They are now connected, rather than isolated; informed, rather than unaware; and active, rather than passive. These changes are manifest in patients' readiness to access information, participate in networking activities, and experiment with care modalities.

In this chapter, we address the following:

- The reason healthcare organizations should promote the involvement of patients and their families in coproducing service experiences
- Ways to facilitate consumer involvement
- The advantages and disadvantages of coproduction from all perspectives

PATIENTS AS QUASI-EMPLOYEES

Traditionally, employees think of their job as the producers of a consistently flawless healthcare experience while coping with the anxieties of patients and their loved ones. In this view, employees do things *to* patients.

Managers, in turn, help employees handle patient confusion and uncertainty by providing training in customer relations techniques. A more effective strategy is to treat patients and their families as quasi-employees (Ford and Heaton 2001). In this view, employees do things *with* customers.

To enable a successful quasi-employee approach, the organization must design the service product, environment, and delivery systems in a way that takes advantage of the knowledge, skills, and abilities (KSAs) of patients and their friends and family. The organization must figure out how to enable quasi-employees to participate in their care. (Although the quasi-employee role may be played by the patient, a family member, a friend, or all three, for the sake of simplicity, the role will refer to the patient in this chapter.)

Managing quasi-employees follows a four-step strategy:

1. *Carefully and completely define the role.* In effect, do a job analysis: Define the KSAs required to perform the jobs identified as desirable and appropriate for the patient. Make sure the patient is physically able, mentally prepared, and sufficiently skilled for the tasks.
2. *Communicate and clarify the role.* The quasi-employee should be clear on the role's expectations. Set goals, and show the patient the benefits of the role. This will give him a reason to do the tasks well.
3. *Evaluate the quasi-employee's ability and performance.* In effect, conduct a performance appraisal on the patient to ensure that the experience being coproduced is meeting expectations. If it is not, identify what needs fixing

and fix it. Does the patient need further training? Is the environment or delivery system impeding the patient's ability to successfully perform the assigned tasks?

4. *Provide resources and support for coproduction and follow-up care in the form of care coordinators.*

Of course, no one should be allowed to coproduce the experience if learning the necessary skills is too dangerous, time consuming, or difficult. By carefully assessing the care processes of a healthcare experience, the manager or provider can identify those aspects where patient participation should be discouraged, encouraged, optional, or required. For example, a physician may require a patient to take her blood pressure at home or to walk to the cafeteria for meals, instead of waiting for the food to be delivered to her hospital room. These aspects of the healthcare experience are within the patients' capabilities and can aid their healing.

Ordering patients to resume physical activity during hospitalization or after surgical procedures has become common. In the past, patients were expected to stay in bed after an appendectomy, for instance, but today they are encouraged to get up and walk, a move that promotes healing. Today, the linkage between physical activity and postsurgical healing is so well accepted that patients have to participate to get better.

Again, not all aspects of the healthcare experience call for patient involvement. Sometimes it may even be harmful. The challenge for managers and providers is in distinguishing between when participation makes sense and when it does not.

Beverly Johnson, president of the Institute for Family-Centered Care (see www.familycenteredcare.org), provides a succinct call to action: "If we could make only one change in healthcare it should be to change the notion that families are visitors. Families are allies and partners for safety and quality" (Beck 2008).

STRATEGIES FOR INVOLVING PATIENTS

Patients can get involved in their care in several ways: as consultants or sources of expert information, as part of the environment for other patients, as coproducers of the experience, or as managers of the service providers and systems. Some of these coproduction roles may sound unlikely, but they are all common.

As Consultants

One of the best ways for healthcare organizations to enhance their performance in customer service and customer satisfaction is to bring customers into the decision-making loop by allowing their input on devising new services and improving existing services. Today, fierce competition has forced most organizations to become more flexible and creative in their dealings with customers to give them exactly what they want (Berry and Seltman 2008).

For example, in 2008, GE won the prestigious NorthFace ScoreBoard Award for the seventh year in a row. This award recognizes GE's excellence in customer satisfaction and loyalty. In receiving the award, Mike Battuello, general manager for GE Healthcare's Life Systems Services, said,

> Our organization is devoted to understanding and improving the customer experience at every interaction. You will never see us rest on our laurels. For example, after receiving last year's NorthFace Award, we launched an initiative called the Raving Fans program, in which our field personnel had business review meetings with many of our customers beyond the time of service. It is a great opportunity to have a dialogue, listen to customer input and learn about the initiatives at their hospitals to make us an even better partner. Winning this award is a reflection on the team's ability to turn customer input into customer delighters. (Cram 2008)

When an organization asks its patients what they liked or disliked about their healthcare experience, the patients become unpaid consultants (Kotler 2004). Because patients have gone through the experience, they are experts and good sources of information related to the service, environment, and delivery system. Using customers as consultants is not unique to healthcare businesses; in other industries, past and present consumers are invited to provide systematic feedback and review about their product and service. Customers are also asked to participate in focus groups.

Today, benchmark companies give customers the tools to design/redesign products and to serve as collaborators (Heckscher and Adler 2006). Pitt County Memorial Hospital in North Carolina gives family and patient advisory groups a voice in designing new facilities and in interviewing physicians who apply to practice at its hospitals. Initially, some staffers worried that this process would take up valuable time, but it saves time in the long run because doctors and nurses have more information to work with (Beck 2008).

One way the patient-as-a-consultant idea can apply to healthcare is to invite patients and families to speak with a team of administrators, physicians, nurses, and other staff after a service encounter. Also, customer input may be collected through a 24-hour hotline, comment cards, telephone interviews, and the organization's website.

In many healthcare organizations, no real collaboration exists between patients and providers. Collaboration requires mutual contribution, but in healthcare the patient does not feel like an equal partner because she relies on other people and probably lacks clinical knowledge. Caregivers are more dominant in the traditional system of care. To change that system, providers have to see it from the patient's point of view and redefine it on the basis of patient concerns.

Focus Group

A focus group is one method for learning the patients' point of view and concerns. For example, the orthopedic unit of a major hospital in Florida conducted focus group sessions to identify areas of improvement. The unit learned that patients were troubled that they could not file a complaint about the same people on whom their care depended. Patients wanted to complain about the night nurses who disregarded their requests for help or left them unattended for lengthy periods. Patients were afraid that their complaints would lead to retaliation. As a response to this finding, the unit's management created a new channel of communication that gives patients direct access to someone who can intervene on their behalf (Fottler et al. 2006).

Another finding from the focus groups was that patients did not appreciate being uninformed while awaiting treatment; this uncertainty only created more anxiety. This and other findings led to improvements in various areas such as patient involvement, provider punctuality, complaint process, patient access to information, and patient–provider communication. A focus group serves as an excellent way to create a successful partnership between patients and healthcare providers.

As Part of the Environment

Each patient invariably influences the healthcare environment, whether positively or negatively. Research has shown that, when in a group, patients endure pain better and display a more positive attitude. The same observation may be true for negative experiences, illustrating the saying "misery loves company."

There is an appropriate and inappropriate time for making the patient part of the environment. Because of the intimate nature of many healthcare experiences, privacy is a must. For example, when one patient is undergoing a physical exam, no one else beside the physician and the patient should be present in the room, regardless of how much support and encouragement another patient could offer the patient.

As Coproducers of the Experience

As discussed, a patient's coproduction of a healthcare experience can take many forms, including something as simple as pouring his own water to something as complex as monitoring his own glucose level or heart rate and reporting the results to the physicians using Web-based software. For about a decade now, many providers have been enabling their patients to participate in their care by giving them information that can be used to make decisions on treatment options, medications, providers, diets, and so on (Friedewald 2000). Such information may be accessed through organizational websites, audiotapes and videotapes, guidebooks, and 24-hour hotlines. Even more information is available on the Internet. A Google search or a visit to WebMD will yield an amazing number of links.

How can hospitals ensure that patients continue to coproduce care beyond the institution's doors? Let's consider the issue of readmissions. According to Landro (2007b), U.S. hospitals see about 5 million readmissions a year, and approximately one-third of these occur within 90 days of discharge. Instituting transitional programs can prevent as many as 46 percent of these readmissions (Landro 2007b). Identifying patients at risk for return, scheduling follow-up doctor's appointments, and sending nurses to patients' homes are also good strategies for reducing readmission rates. Educating patients and their families on self-care should be added to these reduction strategies. Patients can be given practical tips on how to adhere to medication schedules and how to monitor their symptoms at home.

Another area in which coproduction is beneficial is palliative care. The fast-growing field of palliative medicine is gaining respect from doctors and appreciation from patients. The number of medical centers offering palliative care has doubled since 2000, growing to 1,240 programs in about 30 percent of hospitals (Szabo 2007).

Because palliative medicine relies on a team approach, involving doctors, nurses, psychologists, social workers, dietitians, and physical therapists, it is only natural that it involves the patients and their friends and family, who play the role of informal caregivers. In many cases, family members of cancer patients without a care coordinator end up serving as the patients' administrative assistants, chasing down lab results, keeping track of prescriptions, facilitating communication among providers, and managing other care-related tasks. People in this role should be taught the proper way to assist and care for the patients.

As Managers

Patients can take on the role of a quasi-manager, acting as the unofficial supervisors and motivators of employees. They may also educate other patients by discussing treatment options that have worked or not worked for them personally or any other service-related problems and resolutions.

Patients who have had a long or repeated history with a unit or a clinic are ideal as managers because they are familiar with the operations, staff, providers, and procedures. They have had a chance to observe employee behaviors through direct contact or conversation, perhaps more than the supervisor has. As a result, such patients can provide good ideas and motivation to employees. The more familiar patients are with the organization, the more they know about the current level of service and the more qualified they are to provide improvement recommendations.

Seasoned patients are not the only ones who can act as managers, however. When an unhappy new patient tells an employee that he is not providing the service properly, the patient is in effect performing a supervisory function—giving immediate feedback. The typical patient "feedback" to a caregiver consists of grimaces, smiles, screams, or some other nonverbal response. These responses are far more effective guides about the quality of the experience than any instructions a supervisor can give to the employee. Supervisors monitor staff's behavior as they perform their clinical duties. They should also observe the patients' reactions to gauge satisfaction or dissatisfaction with the service. Facial contortions, verbal directions, and direct complaints are definitive cues from patients to staff and managers.

Patients can also be motivators. Most healthcare employees find great satisfaction in meeting and exceeding the expectations of their patients. Employees usually enjoy the opportunity to be challenged by a patient who shares an interest or expertise in the subject of the experience, just as college professors often find the students who ask the most difficult questions are the most fun to have in the classroom. Most employees are constantly tested by the variety of patient expectations and the variety of responsibilities in the service delivery process.

Patients can also supervise each other. For example, caregivers try to help patients cope with a terminal illness, but it is an enormous challenge that patients may think the staff, whose lives are not at risk, are not equipped for. After all, those who have not faced such an illness cannot possibly understand the degree of emotional and physical pain that these patients must endure. As managers, patients who have or have survived similar diagnoses and treatment options can get together with other patients to talk about their experiences.

Most patients, like most employees, are anxious to fulfill their responsibilities and do whatever is needed to relieve their suffering. These patients often watch others to learn how to help themselves. For example, many pregnant women go to birthing classes to learn breathing techniques that can minimize pain during childbirth. Similarly, many amputees and breast cancer patients and survivors attend group gatherings to gain insight from each other. Also, videos of experienced/former patients can be shown to inform or "train" current patients on various subjects.

Savings in cost and time of patient participation can be substantial. Often, no one is better able to help patients than the patients themselves.

ADVANTAGES AND DISADVANTAGES OF COPRODUCTION

Coproduction of the healthcare experience presents advantages and disadvantages, each of which is explored in this section.

Advantages for the Organization

First, coproduction can reduce employee costs. Every time patients serve themselves, they are replacing personnel the organization would otherwise have to pay to do the same thing. The more the patients can do for themselves, the fewer employees that need to be hired.

Second, coproduction enables the organization to better use the talents of its employees. For example, at some hospitals, families are allowed to lead exercise routines for their hospitalized relative. If patients (or loved ones) are allowed, encouraged, or forced to take care of some of their own basic needs, employees are freed up to attend to more complicated services or deal with life-threatening situations.

In 2007, Emory University Hospital began inviting family members to move into the ward to assist in caregiving for their respective relative (Landro 2007c). Emory is among the first U.S. hospitals to meld an intensive care unit (ICU) with family living quarters, testing the healthcare grounds for coproduction. A wave of recent studies shows that critically ill patients may benefit from having family present. A case may also be made for having loved ones present for resuscitation, brain catheter insertions, and other life and death procedures.

In early 2009, the Society of Critical Care Medicine, the largest international society representing intensive care professionals, recommended that ICUs open visiting hours and increase family involvement. This recommendation comes as hospitals nationwide are set to spend $200 billion over the next decade to upgrade aging facilities. This massive investment should include physical structures that provide better accommodations to families and friends who coproduce the care. Providing space for these quasi-employees may increase their participation, which may reduce length of stay, costs, and caregiver liability from errors. (See Sidebar A for an illustration of this point.)

Advantages for the Patient

First, coproduction can lessen patient disappointment in the healthcare experience while increasing the perception, and perhaps the reality, of service quality. Because patients define an experience's value and quality, their involvement could mean that they are more satisfied with the outcomes they helped produce. For example, if a patient adjusts his medication schedule according to his body's reaction to the drug, he is likely to comply with his own changes and to think that the drug works better at a given time.

Second, coproduction can reduce the time required for service. A simple example is using home-testing kits instead of visiting a doctor. A patient's participation in her own care often means she is using the most convenient and easiest method. As a result, she will not likely travel any distance if she could complete her share of the healthcare tasks in the safety of her home and with assistance from a family member or friend. In this way, the doctor's and staff's time is saved for patients who need immediate attention.

SIDEBAR A:
FAMILY SPACES

In 2003, MCG Health System in Augusta, Georgia, transformed the shared patient rooms in its neuroscience ICUs into private rooms with family living areas. As a result, the average length of time a patient spent in the unit fell by 50 percent. One year after the unit opened, medication errors dropped to six, from an annual average of 13 in the two previous years. In addition, patient satisfaction rose and nursing turnover dropped (Landro 2007c).

The mounting evidence was enough to sway the Institute for Healthcare Improvement (IHI). In a 2004 editorial published by the American Medical Association, IHI head Donald Berwick and Meera Kotagal (2004) called on hospitals to open ICUs to unrestricted family visitation.

Third, coproduction minimizes unpleasant surprises for patients. If nursing home residents are allowed to eat in the cafeteria instead of being expected to eat whatever is delivered on the tray, they are given a choice. This choice reduces the likelihood that the residents will complain about the food or the delivery time.

In ICUs, family members who witnessed resuscitations or emergency invasive procedures on their loved ones reported it helpful to be in the room, instead of waiting outside and not knowing anything. The experience allowed them to see what doctors had to do to save the patient's life (Landro 2007c).

Disadvantages for the Organization

First, coproduction exposes the organization to legal risk, especially in this litigious society. A patient walking, instead of being wheeled, into the x-ray room can lead to a lawsuit if the patient falls and sustains an injury.

Second, coproduction requires more training (and hence more expenditure) for employees, who will need to know how to give directions to patients or family members so they can participate in the care process. These careful instructions must be given so that patients do not cause harm or damage to themselves.

The organization has to understand that every patient has different needs, wants, and expectations and varying degrees of KSAs. Employees must be alert to these patient differences so that they can properly coach each patient, not use blanket instructions. When hiring laboratory workers, for example, an organization could look for qualities that may, down the road, help the worker teach a patient how to read his own test results.

Third, coproduction requires the organization to ensure that the delivery system is user-friendly, which costs money. If the organization wants the patient to follow a predetermined sequence of steps to create the desired experience, it must assign employees to guide patients and ensure that excellent directions are in place or the sequence is intuitively obvious to people from varied cultures and backgrounds. Only then can the organization be reasonably sure that all types of patients will do what they are supposed to do when/where they are supposed to do it.

For example, signs and directions must clearly point out where the entrance or exit is, how to reach a particular unit or room, what times the unit/room operates, what payment methods are accepted, and so on. These details may be well known to staff and current patients, but they would be unfamiliar to a newcomer. Staff must be alert for confused-looking or wandering patients if the signs and directions are unclear or not helpful. Today, more patients are directed to organizational websites to conduct self-service transactions, such as scheduling an appointment.

Organizations must keep websites user-friendly as well to lessen patient frustration and promote the use of the self-service technology.

Fourth, coproduction may require the organization to make back-of-the-house areas look as presentable as front-of-the-house areas. Making the back of the house a part of the healthcare experience has an obvious impact on how the equipment is laid out; how shiny it is kept; and how the staff dress, behave, and interact during service production.

In lab testing, for example, coproduction may mean that lab technicians, who typically do not interact directly with patients, will need to hone their communication and interpersonal skills and take note of their general appearance and the orderliness of the laboratory. The costs of the uniforms, the extra training in interpersonal skills for back-area employees, and the rearrangement and upkeep of the back area can all add up.

Fifth, coproduction may cause conflicts from patients who are unwilling to disengage from their role. Some patients enjoy coproduction so much that they refuse to move on when necessary. An organization that accommodates this refusal ends up needing to add extra capacity.

Clearly, when patients become coproducers, the traditional role of the provider is redefined. The provider needs extra training in assessing the coproducer's KSAs and coaching this quasi-employee so that she is capable of performing her tasks. If the patient insists on playing a role for which she lacks the capability, she will invariably introduce a conflict and may force the organization to spend more money, which is not ideal in tough economic times.

Sixth, coproduction can be risky. For example, if a patient or family member is injured during coproduction, the person may sue. Good organizations make every effort to ensure that patients succeed as coproducers, but the risk of failure is always present. If the costs of failure are too high, the organization must tactfully intervene to stop the coproduction. The organization must be astute enough to recognize when coproduction will not be successful, such as when the patient does not possess the right KSAs to monitor his own vital signs or to comply with physician orders. In this case, the organization or provider must take over before a negative event occurs, and must do so with grace so as to not embarrass the patient or anyone else involved.

Disadvantages for the Patient

First, paying patients may resent having to produce any part of the service for which they are being charged. Some task-oriented patients do not particularly want much service provider interaction; they just want a health service. A production-line approach suits them just fine. Other patients, on the other hand, insist on and require close personal attention. If shifting part of the healthcare experience to patients themselves results in less TLC (tender loving care), those patients will be dissatisfied.

Second, patients may fail to coproduce the service or any associated product properly. If patients find the physical therapy routine they engage in boring, they will quit and view the experience as unsatisfactory; worse, they will not have a provider or staff member to blame for this failure. Healthcare organizations try to protect patients against self-service failures, so they let patients try again or they offer help. Nonetheless, the risk of a negative outcome is ever present.

Patients should participate when they have the necessary KSAs, and are motivated to do so if they know that the outcome is beneficial or the service itself cannot happen without their involvement, such as in the case of losing weight, stopping smoking, lowering cholesterol, or even saying "Ah" during a throat examination or pushing during childbirth. In addition, many medical conditions are first diagnosed when the patient clearly describes the symptoms.

Many patients are motivated to participate because of their personalities, their familiarity with the experience being offered, boredom, or a desire to get well. By contrast, those who are not motivated to get well or even to survive will not want to participate in their own healthcare. Some patients simply want to be a part of whatever they are involved in at the moment, no matter what, and constantly look for such opportunities. Some people always park their own cars, carry their own luggage, or walk up the stairs because they like to demonstrate for themselves (and anyone else who cares to watch) that they are physically fit enough to do these things. Others do things, such as complex medical research using the Internet, to showcase their mental fitness or technical adeptness.

A Perspective on Coproduction

A cynical view of coproduction (or self-service) in our society is reflected in this quote from nationally syndicated columnist Ellen Goodman (2008):

> The outsourcing of work to other countries had produced endless ire. But what about the outsourcing of work to me and thee? For every task shipped abroad by a corporation, isn't there another one sloughed off to that domestic loser, the consumer. For every job that's going to a low-wage economy, isn't there another going into our very own low-wage economy?... In this self-service economy, we also serve (ourselves)

by having intimate and endless conversations with voice recognition machines, simply to refill a prescription drug or check our bank balance. We are expected to interact with "labor-saving technology" without realizing that it's "labor transferring" technology. The job has not been "saved," it's been taken out of the paid sector...

She goes on to give specific examples:

- Patients now buy do-it-yourself kits to test and track everything from human immunodeficiency virus (HIV) to blood pressure.
- Every operation short of brain surgery is done on an outpatient basis.
- Nursing care has been outsourced to family members whose entire medical training consists of TiVo-ing "Grey's Anatomy."
- We've become our own computer geeks as help lines become self-help lines.
- We are expected to be healthcare analysts, determining which drug prescription plan covers our ever-changing prescription drugs.
- Outside of healthcare, customers now make their own airline reservations and print their own boarding passes.

Goodman's points are overstated to emphasize that the self-service movement is not a positive development for time-stressed consumers. However, healthcare is not just another product that consumers can passively receive without any personal investment of time, money, and energy. In addition, much research evidence shows the benefits of patient involvement. The lesson here for healthcare leaders and providers is to be cautious in deciding which healthcare services and experiences are appropriate for the patients and families to coproduce. See Exhibit 9.1 for a summary of these advantages and disadvantages.

DETERMINING WHEN PARTICIPATION MAKES SENSE

Sometimes coproduction benefits both the organization and the patient; sometimes it benefits no one. Determining the who, what, when, where, why, and how of patient participation depends on a variety of factors. Generally speaking, participating in the service is in the interest of patients when they can gain value, improve quality, or reduce risk. Participation is in the organization's interest when it can increase patient satisfaction, save money, enhance operational efficiency, gain a competitive advantage, or build patient commitment and loyalty. Each opportunity for patient participation should be assessed on these criteria.

Exhibit 9.1 Advantages and Disadvantages of Patient Coproduction

For Patient		*For Organization*	
Advantage	**Disadvantage**	**Advantage**	**Disadvantage**
Reduces service costs	Could be frustrating	Reduces labor costs	Increases liability risk
Increases interest	Could diminish service quality	Improves patient satisfaction about outcome	Increases patients' training costs
Saves service time	Patient knowledge, skills, and abilities are inadequate	Reduces service failures	Increases employee costs
Improves service quality	Learning curve too steep	Opens new market niche	Increases design costs
Reduces risk of disappointment		Enriches employee jobs	Interferes with work of other units
Could enhance satisfaction		Increases patient loyalty	Too much variability in patient KSAs and motivation

Value, Quality, and Risk

Almost every patient is happy to coproduce if it adds value to the experience. By definition, value can be added by reducing patient costs (for the same quality), increasing healthcare quality (for the same costs), or both. Costs include not only the price but also the other costs incurred by being involved in the healthcare experience. For example, if a potential patient sees that the parking lot or the waiting room of her walk-in clinic is full, she may go to a different clinic if the cost of waiting is too great. With this choice, the patient risks experiencing a decrease in quality but expects a decrease in time cost to compensate for it.

Similarly, patients who want to be sure of service quality may want to participate in providing the service. Those patients want to know they are getting the service tailored to their specific needs, wants, and expectations. Patients can participate in providing the service without actually handling instruments or reading charts, such as in discussing with their physicians what clinical procedures and treatments might lead to the desired clinical outcome. In the past, patients followed doctors' orders without question; today, patients are more involved in this type of decision making. If the doctor says, "Take two aspirin and go to bed," the patient may ask, "Why?"

Many consumers, including healthcare consumers, have become activists regarding the goods and services they buy. Patients believe they can improve the quality of the healthcare experience when they can choose among available options offered or described by the provider. Computer-savvy patients often derive their own second opinions from medical advice on the Internet. They may also visit medical websites or chatrooms and news groups to interact with people with the same medical conditions. Such information empowers many patients' decision making.

Customer and Organizational Reasons

Some research suggests that two factors are of primary importance to patients: time and control. When patients can save time and/or gain control, they are more likely to want to participate in their own care.

With time, the perception of how long a procedure takes is as important as the actual length of time of the procedure. The same is true for control. The perception of control over the quality, value, risk, or efficiency of the experience is as important in determining the value of participation as the actual control. For example, patients are sometimes given real control over their pain medication. They are allowed to administer more pain medicine when they decide the pain is too great; having this control adds to patient satisfaction.

From the organization's point of view, the most obvious reason to encourage or require coproduction is to achieve higher levels of patient satisfaction; another reason is to save money. As noted earlier, whenever a patient produces or coproduces a service, the patient is providing labor the organization would otherwise have to pay for. A third reason is to enhance operational efficiency or increase capacity utilization.

If patients are allowed or encouraged to do more for themselves, the staff can attend to other patients with more immediate needs. In this way, the organization can maintain a constant staffing level while still being able to accommodate the variability in patient demand. Simply, letting patients coproduce part of the healthcare experience increases the number of patients who can be served.

An organization can also use patient or family participation to boost its competitive advantage. For example, a hospital may distinguish itself from others by using nurse midwives, instead of the typical obstetrics team. Another example is a real-time, secure website from which patients and family members can get information about their test results or interact with their providers.

A final reason for coproduction is to build patient commitment and repeat business. If a patient believes the organization trusts him enough to let him participate in his care, then the patient feels a bond and a commitment. He feels ownership in that experience, which leads to feelings of loyalty to the organization that offered this opportunity (Berry and Seltman 2008).

Many service organizations try hard to build such relationships because they recognize the lifetime value of a loyal repeat customer. Frequent flyer and "frequent patient" programs are both designed to build this attachment so that customers come back time after time to the organization that knows them. Frequent patient programs provide various rewards to repeat customers, such as preferred rooms or locations and facilitated intake and discharge. Benchmark healthcare organizations understand that their customers have many choices concerning where they will receive health services. Consequently, these organizations offer more incentives to keep the loyalty of their customers.

Costs Versus Benefits

The key to deciding when to offer the patient the opportunity to participate is to do a simple cost–benefit analysis. The organization needs to be sure that the benefits of participation outweigh the costs. The costs and benefits of patient and family involvement need to be reviewed to find the point beyond which the incremental benefits are outweighed by incremental costs (Prahalad and Ramaswamy 2004b).

The organization should ask itself the following questions (Elwyn et al. 2000):

- What are the KSAs necessary to perform successfully as a quasi-employee?
- Are all, some, or none of these KSAs likely to be found in the quasi-employee?
- What is the motivation for a patient to participate, and how does the organization appeal to that motivation?
- What are the training requirements for successful performance in the quasi-employee role, and does the organization have the time and staff to train the quasi-employee in that role?
- Will the quasi-employee come back and use the training the organization provided? If so, the investment of time, money, and staff may be worthwhile.
- Is it cheaper, faster, or more efficient for the organization to provide the service or to allow the quasi-employee to do it?

- Are role models (especially other patients) available to help with training the quasi-employee, and how can the service environment be physically structured to take advantage of these role models?
- Will letting patients produce their own experience interfere with service to other patients or with other parts of the organization?

For patients to be effectively used in the healthcare experience, they must have the motivation and ability to participate, training, and KSAs. Also, their specific functions need to be clearly defined. Organizations that see mutual benefits to coproduction and hence encourage it must always have a backup plan to accommodate the fact that some patients will not want to participate in the experience. Those organizations that find ways of using patients and their families as much as possible will, however, decrease their costs and increase the value and quality of the service for the participants.

Letting Patients Decide

Many situations lend themselves to using some self-service or patient participation. An organization can follow two strategies when leaving the participation decision to patients:

1. *Communicate to the service population that every patient is expected to participate in some of the interventions.* Clarify the degree of involvement—for example, patients who seek counseling must agree to share information and cooperate with the therapist. By clarifying the level of involvement, patients are aware that they will not be expected to do manual tasks, such as clean their own bathrooms.

2. *Offer segments of the patient population a choice to participate.* For example, group therapy patients might be told that verbal participation, although it is to their advantage, is not required. Physical therapy patients might participate or not, depending on their energy levels and the extent of their injury; if patients are unable, therapists can continue to exercise the muscles for them. As an additional example, some patients may prefer to visit the organization's website, or they may opt to receive information from a human being. If the patient chooses the latter, the organization should provide contact names and phone numbers.

Firing the Patient

In a sense, all patients coproduce, or have the potential to coproduce, the health-care experience for other patients simply by being in the vicinity. A well-mannered, well-dressed patient sitting quietly in a waiting room is an enhancement to the setting, even a role model for other patients. On the other hand, a boisterous and obnoxious patient in the same waiting room will scare off other patients.

Extreme behaviors from staff or patients—being verbally and physically abusive, refusing to comply with reasonable organizational rules and policies, making outrageous demands, or endangering themselves and others—are unacceptable in any healthcare setting. Not all employees work out, just as not all patients work out. The organization can do something about both groups.

If the patient's performance as a quasi-employee is unsatisfactory, the organization must, as a last resort and employing clearly defined procedures, "fire" the patient. A quasi-employee may also be fired for deliberately damaging or stealing equipment and for disrespecting and abusing the staff. The organization should, of course, give the patient the benefit of the doubt, and the dismissal should be accomplished with minimal harm to the patient's physical or mental well-being and dignity. A patient who feels unfairly treated and who is angry about being terminated may become a source of long-term negative publicity and even lawsuits. (See Sidebar B for example.)

SIDEBAR B:
FIRING THE PATIENT

Firing the patient may be inconsistent with the organization's mission, as this real-life example illustrates.

Doctors and nurses at Highland Hospital in Oakland, California, complain about the irresponsibility, rudeness, and bad smell of a patient who has serious heart and blood pressure problems. She begs lunch from hospital staff and bums cigarettes from strangers. She has been jailed for belligerence in the emergency department (ED), and a restraining order has been placed against her, banning her from the hospital unless she is receiving medical care. She refuses to coproduce her healthcare experience and throws her prescriptions in the trash to ensure further trips to the ED. The patient seems ready for a pink slip.

But Highland is a public county hospital with a mission to serve all who come in with a medical problem, whether they can pay or not. As a result, the hospital cannot "fire" the patient, who has presented in the ED more than 1,200 times, costing taxpayers close to $1 million (Foster 2001). While the patient has reduced her use of the ED, the hospital still continues to serve her. Highland also cannot police difficult patients or prevent them from using the ED because of its mission to serve everyone who shows up at its door.

In some instances, patients are "fired" not because of inappropriate behavior, but because of financial reasons (i.e., limits on reimbursement for specific services) or because of the organization's inability to provide needed care for the patient's changed condition. Assisted-living facilities "fire" their patients when they need nursing care services. Nursing homes "fire" their patients when their health benefits run out. Hospitals "fire" patients when their doctors think they are ready for discharge, whether the patients agree or not, or when their HMOs refuse to make further payments. HMOs fire their Medicare patients due to excessive regulation and inadequate reimbursement by the federal government.

Although firing a patient may be a response to a patient failure of some kind, the organization must sometimes realize that it has also failed in some way. The rude, troublesome patient had expectations, whether reasonable and realistic or not, and the organization failed to meet them.

CONCLUSION

Coproducing the healthcare experience offers many advantages for both the organization and the patient. However, these advantages will not be realized if the organization does not provide training and support for the staff and the quasi-employees or informal caregivers. In addition, the organization must gauge patients' KSAs and willingness to participate in their care. To achieve this kind of motivation, the organization needs to make clear how coproduction benefits the patient.

Providers should be encouraged to attend to the interpersonal aspects of their interactions with informal caregivers to promote coordination that will ultimately benefit the patient's health. This can be done through building shared goals, sharing knowledge, and developing mutual respect among employees, patients, and other informal caregivers, but dedicated resources and support are needed to facilitate this process.

Service Strategies

1. Hire and train your service personnel to coach, monitor, and supervise customers' (e.g., patients, family, friends, clergy) coproduction.
2. Train patients to participate, and be sure they have the required knowledge, skills, and abilities for coproduction.

3. Restructure patient rooms to encourage family and friends to visit, coproduce, and share an adjoining room.

4. Motivate patients who derive value and quality from participation to coproduce.

5. Determine which patients, family members, and friends are motivated to become informal caregivers and to coproduce a healthcare experience.

6. Encourage patients to help monitor the service behavior of employees.

7. Encourage all patients and families to become informal caregivers. Always provide an option for staff service if that is preferred by patients and their families.

8. Structure healthcare experiences in ways that encourage patients to train other patients; provide pretreatment videos or prepare patients to engage in the experience.

9. Preserve the patient's dignity if you need to "fire" him.

PART III

The Service System

Communicate everything you can to your associates.
The more they know, the more they care.
—Sam Walton

CHAPTER 10

Communicating Information Internally and Externally

Service Principle:
Keep the patient, family, and employees informed

WHEN CONFRONTED WITH uncertainty about a medical condition or any phase of the healthcare experience, most patients seek information to reduce their anxiety. Although they can readily obtain information from various sources, including the Internet, patients often look to their healthcare providers for answers. Thus, providers have to be prepared to meet the information needs of not only patients and their families but also employees, payers, and other stakeholders.

Sharing information is a big challenge in healthcare, as the field is not known for its pioneering use of information technology and is restricted by many privacy protections for patients. Ideally, providers and delivery systems must find the right balance between facilitating a health information exchange and safeguarding patient privacy.

In this chapter, we address the following:

- How health information systems are integral to the three components of the total healthcare experience: product, setting, and delivery system
- The use of Internet technology in information access, healthcare decision making, medical practice, and cost reduction
- How information systems can meet all the needs of the organization's stakeholders, not just the business needs of the organization or the clinical information needs of providers
- Advantages and disadvantages of health information systems

THE VALUE OF HEALTH INFORMATION SYSTEMS

A well-designed information system gets the right information to the right person in the right format at the right time. In this way, the system is viewed as adding value to a person's decision. A system is useless if it does not deliver the right information to the right person in the right format at the right time. For example, an x-ray image that arrives after a doctor has already prescribed a course of treatment is a useless piece of information.

Patients, staff, clinicians, other caregivers, payers, and other stakeholders all have information needs that the organization must meet.

Informing Consumers

The information the organization provides to patients helps make the intangible service tangible. This is an underdeveloped but critical concern of a health information system. What information should the organization provide, in what format, and in what quantity to help create the experience the patient and other stakeholders in the healthcare experience expect? For example, if the experience is a surgical procedure, the operating team should organize all the information it provides to enforce the perception that the procedure is proper and will result in an excellent outcome.

The surgical theater should be a sterile, well-equipped, well-laid-out room, and clinical team should be wearing clean surgical gowns, gloves, and head caps. Such environmental cues send this message: "Relax. You are in the hands of a skilled surgical team in a high-tech hospital." One of the authors of this book remembers being wheeled into surgery and noticing the clinical team standing around the room chatting and drinking Cokes. They did not seem to care that the message their casualness was communicating was not of reassurance or professionalism. Because most patients cannot differentiate a surgical team with a good record from a surgical team with a bad record, the onus falls on the organization to carefully manage the preoperative procedures, facilities, patient-contact employees, and any other aspect of the care to ensure all these elements of the care communicate clinical competence. Whatever the patient tastes, touches, hears, sees, and smells makes up the information the patient receives, which in turn influences her perception of the total healthcare experience.

All of the informational cues in the service setting should be carefully thought out to communicate what the organization wants to communicate to the customer about the quality and value of the experience. The less tangible the service, the more important these cues will be. Information can glue together the product, the environment, and the delivery system that make up the total healthcare experience. By managing this information with the use of an appropriate, reliable health information system, the organization can ensure that the service is seamless and the customers' needs, wants, and expectations are met or exceeded.

Similarly, an organization should also pay attention to the information needs, wants, and expectations of its internal customers—physicians, other clinicians, managers, and other employees—in designing and implementing a health information system. Clearly, organizations can use information to add quality and value to the total healthcare experience.

THE GROWING ROLE OF WEB-BASED TECHNOLOGY

The Internet has greatly expanded the ability of healthcare organizations to communicate with their many customers. Exchange and dissemination of information and services are easier, cheaper, and faster on the Internet, which is rapidly changing the dynamics of healthcare delivery.

In 2000, futurist Russ Coile Jr. summarized the Web-based strategies and activities in which healthcare providers and healthcare-related business would engage. Clearly, many of Coile's predictions have come to pass and are still relevant today:

1. *Advertising*: Healthcare providers will communicate to consumers directly and inexpensively through the Internet.
2. *Providers*: Healthcare consumers will use the Internet to identify the best local, regional, and national providers.
3. *Customer information and referral*: Health insurers will use the Internet to communicate with their enrollees about benefits, referrals, physicians on their networks, and medical information.
4. *Shopping*: Health-related products and services will be sold online more quickly and at lower prices. Examples include prescription and over-the-counter drugs, medical supplies and equipment, vitamins, and home fitness equipment.
5. *Internet pharmacy*: Discounts and home delivery will encourage many consumers to get their prescription refills through online pharmacies.
6. *Health insurance*: Health insurers will provide online functions for consumer registration, eligibility verification, and transaction processing.
7. *Electronic medical records*: Hospitals will become virtually paperless. All stakeholders will be able to get medical information online, which they can

use to diagnose, treat, or make a decision about their care. Patients will be able to access their own health records electronically, which will help them monitor their own health status.

8. *Health advice and telemedicine*: Health advice will be available through a variety of websites, although not all such advice will be valid or evidence-based. Telemedicine will allow institutions to provide diagnostic, consultative, and clinical services.

9. *Customer service*: Most health insurers and delivery systems will offer transactional capabilities for consumers on their websites. Examples include verification of health plan eligibility, explanation of benefits, search for plan-approved providers, after-hours inquiries, online enrollment, and appointment scheduling.

Just one year later, an article in the *Wall Street Journal* (2001) also forecasted the practice of medicine in the twenty-first century, in particular the growing role of technology:

> Within a couple of years, patients all over the U.S. could have secure electronic medical records and go online to schedule appointments, shop for the best hospital, look up lab results, track the status of a claim, order a new drug or consult with a specialist. With existing technology, doctors can interview and examine patients hundreds of miles away or teach colleagues computer-aided surgery via the Web. There are pilot electronic monitoring systems to keep track of chronically ill people at home, and portable medical-alert devices that can monitor them on vacation. Computerized ordering systems in hospitals can help eliminate medication errors. Powerful data systems, if specially designed to link hospitals around the country, can analyze huge amounts of medical information and share it over a network to help identify and treat public health threats before they spread. Unfortunately, the chances that any of these innovations will actually show up at your local hospital anytime soon are remote. Unique among American industries, healthcare lags so far behind in adopting the latest in information and communications technology that some experts say it may never catch up.

The number of advances in information technology since the Russ Coile and *Wall Street Journal* articles published, along with the call to action for the health-care industry to embrace more innovation, has turned most of these predictions into a reality. The growth in information technology use is important for three major reasons: It reduces costs, improves patient safety and healthcare quality, and increases patient access to healthcare knowledge.

Many Web-based patient services save time and money for both the provider and the patient. Cleveland Clinic, for example, gives its patients secure access to its website to view their test results and medical records and update their personal data. This is just the beginning of patient-controlled Web-based healthcare databases. Several websites, including Google Health, Dossia, MEDecision, Microsoft Health Vault, and Revolution Health, allow patients to post their own medical data and designate who can access it; they also provide links to relevant sources of health information (Kornblum 2008; Green 2007). Kaiser Permanente offers e-visits (virtual doctor office visits) to make 24/7 healthcare access possible. Relay Health is another resource for virtual doctor visits (Wessel 2008). In developing countries and rural/remote areas where healthcare is not easily accessible, telemedicine offers a low-cost option (Scott 2006; Wallauer et al. 2008).

Information technology also improves patient access to healthcare knowledge (Laing, Hogg, and Winkleman 2004). Websites on just about every healthcare aspect are available for consumers, including those that help with the following:

- Diagnosing symptoms (e.g., WebMD.com, Familydoctor.org)
- Keeping medical records (e.g., www.mychartlink.com)
- Determining what questions to ask a doctor (e.g., www.ohri.ca/decisionaid)
- Finding experts on medical conditions (e.g., MyConsult on www.eclevelandclinic.org)
- Evaluating medical practitioners and healthcare providers (e.g., www.ratemds.com, www.HospitalCompare.hhs.gov, www.QualityCheck.org)
- Giving family and friends updates on a patient's condition (e.g., www.caringbridge.org)

Social networking sites—such as Facebook, Plaxo, and Twitter—may also be used to put a patient in constant communication with family, friends, and other associates about personal and health issues. In addition, specific websites exist for the following:

- General health topics (e.g., www.healthfinder.gov, www.webmd.com, www.mayoclinic.com)
- Prescription drugs (e.g., www.pharmainfo.net, www.ditonline.com)
- Heart conditions (e.g., www.americanheart.org)

- Cancer (e.g., www.oncolink.com, www.cancer.org)
- Health plans (e.g., www.ahcpr.gov/consumer)
- Personal health profiles (e.g., WebMD.com; see Sidebar A for more on personal health records)
- Health screenings and comprehensive health awareness initiatives (e.g., www.impacthealth.com)

Consumers must exercise caution when visiting these and other websites because not all such sites provide valid, accurate, and up-to-date information. Some of these websites may violate patient privacy rules, and their databases may be tampered with or hacked, providing access to names, credit card numbers, health records, or other personal data.

In spite of these efforts to better use information technology to improve the effectiveness and efficiency of healthcare, these improvements cannot come fast enough. According to Noor (2007), healthcare is the largest industry in the United States, representing about 16.5 percent of the gross domestic product, and it is estimated to grow to 20 percent by 2015. This is a large resource commitment, and any improvements will translate into very big numbers. "An estimated 30 to 40 percent of healthcare expenditures go to inefficiency involving duplication, systems failures, unnecessary repetition, and poor communication" (Noor 2007). Creating a system that manages information effectively is one of the most important and challenging issues facing any healthcare organization.

The Internet as a Powerful Tool

Online bookstores, newspapers, travel agencies, schools, and other services have transformed their respective industries in numerous ways. The same is true for healthcare, as the examples earlier illustrate.

SIDEBAR A: PERSONAL HEALTH RECORD

A personal health record (PHR) not only improves patient–physician communications but also enables the patient to take control of her medical files and thereby become an active participant in her care (Tang and Lansky 2005; Ball, Smith, and Bakalar 2007). Ongoing research at the Cleveland Clinic confirms that patients like the flexibility of reporting blood pressure measurements at their convenience and as they are needed (Moore 2009). This entails moving the patient's information from the doctor's office to the patient's home. Adoption and ongoing use of PHR can facilitate this clinic-to-home link. The PHR represents a fundamental change in our traditional system (Tang and Lansky 2005).

The data contained on the Internet are immeasurable, and no one really knows how many health-related websites exist. The search engine Google has become a primary tool for many healthcare consumers and providers who seek information and resources about medical conditions. In 2007, 56 percent of American adults— more than 122 million people—sought information about a personal health concern, up from 38 percent in 2001, according to a national study by the Center for Studying Health System Change. From 2001 to 2007, use of the Internet for information purposes doubled to 32 percent (Tu and Cohen 2008).

Tu and Cohen (2008) report that significant increases in Internet usage were observed across all consumer categories of age, education, income, and race/ethnicity, and health status. Although elderly Americans—65 years and older—sharply increased their information seeking online, they still trail younger Americans by a substantial margin. Consumers who actively researched health concerns widely reported positive impacts: More than half said the information changed their overall approach to maintaining their health, and four in five said the information helped them to better understand their illness (Tu and Cohen 2008).

Medline, the National Library of Medicine's online search service, was visited by nearly 50 million visitors in the second quarter of 2008 (Kronstadt, Moiduddin, and Sellheim 2009). Medline is a gold mine of healthcare information, providing access to more than 10 million articles published in medical and healthcare journals. MedlinePlus also offers extensive information on more than 750 diseases and conditions from the National Institutes of Health and other trusted sources. The website includes a listing of hospitals and physicians, a medical encyclopedia and a medical dictionary, information on prescription and nonprescription drugs, health alerts from the media, and links to thousands of clinical trials. (See also the National Library of Medicine, National Institutes of Health's website at www.nlm.nih.gov or the Medical Library Association's website at www.mlanet.org.)

Decision-Making Aid

The Internet is also breaking barriers to competition in healthcare because it enables patients to seek alternative treatment options, discover medical developments, and question the quality and cost of healthcare services. Such information is empowering, making patients less inclined to have blind faith in their doctors' ability, knowledge, and recommendations. In fact, many patients seem to trust Google more than they do their doctors. Physicians are being confronted by patients who are fully informed about cutting-edge treatments and the various implications of their medical conditions or symptoms. Some patients may even know more than their physicians about drugs and interventions that are little known, under investigation, or in clinical trials.

Further, consumer-initiated/hosted websites allow patients who share a disease or an ailment to directly communicate with each other to ask questions, explore treatment options, and evaluate the treatment they currently receive. Nearly every disease has a dedicated website, and their impact on the practice of medicine has been growing (Landro 2007d).

In some states, including Ohio and New Jersey, patients can even go to a website to find out if their doctors have been disciplined (e.g., www.state.oh.us/med). Similarly, those interested in the quality of specific nursing homes can now make that assessment by visiting www.medicare.gov/nhcompare.

Information on physicians and their practice, health insurance companies, and medications are also available online:

- Physicians and practices: www.ama-assn.org; www.bestdoctors.com
- Health insurance companies: www.ncqa.org; www.ehealthinsurance.com
- Prescriptions: www.nabp.net; www.rxaminer.com

Some healthcare providers may view the availability of this much information with alarm, but the Internet has a huge potential to improve health as it presents information that may prevent illness, complications, and even death. The Internet helps providers find more resources (e.g., medical research and data, disease experts, community partners) and extend their connections with patients well beyond the physical setting—all in a cost-effective way.

Telemedicine

Telemedicine is the practice of providing medical care and advice or performing a medical procedure from a distant location. It relies on electronic connection, such as the telephone, the Internet, or some other communication device. For example, patients with severe chronic wounds, such as those associated with diabetes and circulatory diseases, may consult with their doctors via the Internet. A patient may take a picture of the wound and transmit the image electronically; on the basis of this picture and a conversation with the patient, the physician may make a decision to ask the patient to come into the office for further consultation or to instruct the patient to monitor the wound at home. The benefits of such an approach include a reduction in visits, prevention of hospitalizations, access to remote medical services, and lower costs.

Sentara Healthcare has an electronic ICU (intensive care unit), a system that takes advantage of Internet technology to ensure that all of the system's ICUs (spread across a wide area) are appropriately staffed with specialists at all hours. Using video feeds and real-time connection, the electronic ICU ensures no lag in services—that is, an ICU patient in a different location receives timely, high-quality care from a physician many miles away (Mullaney 2006).

Medem is an example of a growing number of companies that run websites to facilitate physician–patient communication. The company established the Health Care Notification Network to deliver urgent patient-safety alerts—such as medication and device recalls, warnings, and label changes—to their physician clients. Medem's system also helps doctors manage their increasing use of e-mail to communicate with patients. Physicians can check on patients and give diagnoses through e-mail instead of office visits to manage time more efficiently. (See www.hcnn.net for more information.)

Electronic Recordkeeping

The use of Internet-based information technology to eliminate paper errors in hospitals and clinics is advancing rapidly as well. For example, SingHealth in Singapore created the Digital Hospital, a cutting-edge innovation in healthcare informatics. The Digital Hospital is supported by three main pillars: (1) digital ward; (2) digital clinic; and (3) telecare, telemedicine, and home care. The Digital Hospital works in the following way (Stockholm Challenge Event 2008):

1. *Information sharing.* Inpatient discharge summaries, allergy information, and medical alerts are exchanged between clusters. Such a system facilitates clinical decision making, which improves patient safety and care management.
2. *Empowerment.* Clinicians and patients have anytime, anywhere access to knowledge and information.
3. *Improved patient–doctor relationships and care provision.* Secure messaging between clinicians and patients allows patients to manage their diseases or check in for a medical review. Clinicians can institute early treatment to reduce or prevent hospitalization and/or refine medication dosages.
4. *Access to medical records.* Clinicians have convenient access to patients' health information.
5. *Time savings and convenience for patients and staff.* Up-to-date patient information is accessible online on a 24/7, 365-day basis, freeing up patients' time spent calling laboratories for test results. Nursing staff are spared from retrieving and collating patient information to be reviewed by physicians. SingHealth estimates a cost savings of $750,000 per ward.
6. *Improved quality of care.* System alerts for abnormal results, duplicate medication orders, and drug interactions and allergy contribute greatly to patient safety and appropriate interventions.
7. *Cost savings.* Patients can save as much as $100 each by avoiding repeated laboratory tests and radiology procedures if they transfer to another institution connected to the Digital Hospital.

Provider–Consumer Connectivity

The Internet can link the many players in healthcare delivery, including patients, families, doctors and other clinicians, pharmacists, hospitals, clinics, laboratories, consultants, equipment and drug suppliers, and insurance companies.

For example, WebMD.com posts health news, alerts, and other information; hosts message boards and blogs; promotes wellness and healthy eating; advertises health and medical products, including prescription drugs; and offers practice-management software to doctors. Similarly, Aetna debuted a website in 2008 called SmartSource, a search engine designed specifically for health and medical information, including disease risks, costs, and local providers (see www.aetna.com/showcase/smartsource).

Web-enabled provider–consumer connections can enhance clinical quality and outcomes, prevent medical complications and errors, and improve patient satisfaction. They can also reduce costs, as they arm health consumers with information and alternatives.

Personalized Service

Information can enable organizations to personalize the service to make each customer, client, or patient feel special. For example, the use of direct linkages can allow a nurse who is monitoring many patients at many locations to contact a person whose vital signs are deviating from normal. Patients may be unaware that their vital signs are being monitored until they receive a phone call from an off-location nurse, who greets them by name and gives them personalized attention and instructions.

Information and information technology can improve the service itself. A bar code on a prescription drug label includes a wealth of information. For example, the bar code contains a real-time record of the medications disbursed, enabling the pharmacy to automatically reorder more so that the drugs are available when requested. Bar codes on patient records and wrist bands with radio frequency identification chips allow the hospital or local pharmacy to monitor the types of drugs one physician is prescribing so that other physicians can be alerted to potential interaction problems. Such technology can also help providers identify patient needs. For example, if a doctor prescribes the blood-thinning drug Coumadin, the system can suggest that the patient purchase a blood-monitoring device. (See Sidebar B for another example of a personalized technological intervention.)

A 60-year-old male is rushed to the emergency department. He is unconscious and thus cannot provide any information to the emergency medical technicians (EMTs). Luckily, the EMTs find a smart card in his wallet.

A smart card is a credit card–sized device that stores a person's health information, including his condition, medications, and treatments received. When inserted into an optical reader, the smart card enables a physician or any other clinical caregiver to access the person's information. Like the PHR, smart cards are most effective when loaded with updated information. Such information is electronically transmitted to the card by authorized people, such as a primary physician during routine checkups and emergency department staff in the event of an emergency.

Because the smart card is portable and holds critical medical data, it helps providers give appropriate and timely interventions.

INFORMATION AND THE COMPONENTS OF THE TOTAL HEALTHCARE EXPERIENCE

The challenge of information systems is to figure out exactly how to gather the right data, organize that data into the right information, and distribute that information to the right people when and in whatever way needed. Effective healthcare organizations recognize that quality information is often as important as quality clinical service. Therefore, managers must identify the information needs of all internal and external customers who receive or produce the three components of the total healthcare experience—the product, the environment, and the delivery system. In this section, we explore the role of information in each component.

Information and the Service Product

Sometimes, information itself is the service product (see Sidebar C for an illustration of this concept). At all times, however, information provides cues that guide customers' favorable or unfavorable perception about the quality and value of the product.

For employees and clinicians, generally, information is the product. It is the thing they need to deliver a service or to make a decision about next steps. For example, consider a rehabilitation therapy manager who must decide whether to revitalize or replace a rehabilitation room full of outdated, obsolete, or underused equipment. The manager will need data related to the service, such as rehabilitation patient counts, room utilization rates, and wait times; she will also need patient survey results and forecasts of future rehabilitation demand. Each set of such information is a product produced and delivered by another employee or unit.

Providing information is the service activity of many employees, and benchmark healthcare organizations aim to be effective and efficient at this activity because they understand its significance to the total healthcare experience. Indeed, the entire movement toward patient-centered care depends on clinicians and employees having easy access to all patient-related information. Prompt, appropriate, and high-quality patient care is impossible without a systematic way for staff to obtain or exchange patient information.

Information as *the* product enables careful decision making, outcomes measurement, and patient-centered approaches.

Information and the Service Environment

An information-rich service environment is useful to patients and other customers. For example, in an outpatient imaging center, patients need instructions on how to find the x-ray room, how to prepare for the x-ray procedure, and what to do after the x-ray image is taken. Directional signs should be placed and should be visible throughout the center to facilitate the patient's travel to the x-ray department. Instructions should be given at the reception desk to tell the patient what to do before and after the procedure.

On the organization's website, pictures of the setting help potential patients see the intangible product as a tangible service. Such graphic representations inform patients of the quality to be expected from the facility. Many organizations post images of patient rooms, the lobby, waiting rooms, staff and clinicians at work, the equipment, and views from room windows. In a larger sense, the environment itself can be thought of as an information system by the way it is designed and laid out. That is, the presence or absence of navigational tools can enhance or detract from the service experience. This information ranges from a simple orientation map to interactive, computerized kiosks.

Information and the Service Delivery System

Information is required to make the service delivery system work. That system includes the people and the processes by which the service and any accompanying tangible product are delivered to the patient. The nature of the service product, setting, and delivery system will determine the ideal information system.

For example, in a routine checkup at a physician practice, the patient is seen by a nurse or nurse assistant first. The nurse takes the patient's vital signs, asks the reason for the visit, and makes notations in the patient's chart. Then, the nurse communicates the information to the physician, who goes into the examination room where the patient is waiting. After the checkup, the physician leads or instructs the patient to go to the reception area, where the patient may receive prescription orders from the doctor or set up a follow-up appointment. This example illustrates the information system generally in place in a doctor's office.

Many doctor's offices use color-coded flags to indicate the stage to which the patient has moved along the delivery system. At each stage, the patient receives information that will guide him through the next steps.

Information on Service Quality

One important use of a health information system is in the systematic gathering of information on service quality. Acquiring this information, organizing it into a usable form, and disseminating it to managers and providers aid in identifying and resolving problems. Entering complaints into the information system about patients' annoyance with the constant paging of doctors over the intercom, for example, is a first step. But this step is worthless unless the manager and all others involved are alerted promptly of the complaint as soon as it is entered. An effective information system is designed to issue notifications and reminders so that someone can follow up on any concerns or problems.

The information system should be designed to ensure that all the people involved in delivering a service have the information they need to do their jobs in the best possible way. Here is where the most powerful applications of modern information technology have been developed. Providing the healthcare employee with the information necessary to satisfy and even impress the customer is an effective way to add value to the healthcare experience.

Customers today are used to fast service. They can pump gas at a self-serve station 18 seconds after paying. As patients, these same customers get frustrated when they have to wait 10 minutes for their prescriptions to be refilled or for a nurse assistant to fetch an extra blanket. The difference between a gas station service and a clinical service may not be readily apparent to many patients.

Consider the task of checking a patient's insurance coverage in a doctor's office. To the patient that task should be as simple as presenting his insurance card, which generally contains all the necessary information. The office, however, needs more information than the insurance carrier's name, the plan number, and the copay amount. Unless the patient is receiving the same services as in previous visits and unless the office has a current master list of all services covered by all insurers and all their plans, the process of checking will take time and may cause delay. Patients are naturally unhappy about such waits.

The situation, however, is changing rapidly for insurance verification tasks. Information systems, especially Web-based systems, make it possible for the healthcare staff to provide service to customers quickly and efficiently in many situations. Indeed, this is the area in which the healthcare industry has worked the hardest to capture the benefits and economies of technology without losing the human contact that is so vital to the healthcare experience.

It is a high-tech world, but because technology has taken over so many functions that used to be performed by people, patients value a high-touch experience even more than before. Healthcare organizations try to use as much technology as they can both behind the scenes and in direct patient contacts; this gives employees enough time to offer the personal attention patients value so much while still offering efficient patient care.

Electronic Expertise

In a number of innovative ways, information technology allows organizations to provide expert skills without paying experts to provide them. Rural hospitals, for instance, can have online access to major teaching hospitals where expertise is available around the clock. Rural hospitals do not use specialists enough to make it cost effective to have them on-site all the time.

The evolving availability of evidence-based medicine databases, such as the Cochrane Collaboration's Cochrane Library (see www.cochrane.org/reviews/libintro.htm), is also making greater expertise available through an online connection. This powerful tool allows clinical providers from the local general practitioner in a remote town to the specialist at the university hospital to log in from a bedside and access the best available knowledge and expertise on a medical condition and its treatment (Carey 2006). If this knowledge can be provided through an Internet connection in the patient's room, through a touch-screen device, or even through an employee who can easily access a computerized database, the cost to the patient and the organization of providing that expertise is reduced and the quality of the information and the ease of access are increased. This is an exciting illustration of how information and information technology can be used to enhance the organization's ability to provide a valuable service for the patient.

Customer-Contact and Healthcare Support Groups

Another major part of the healthcare service delivery information system ties together the customer-contact group (those people and functions serving healthcare customers) with the healthcare support group (those people and functions serving the people who serve the customers). Coordination between these two geographically separate groups in the service delivery system is critical to providing a seamless experience for patients. Patients do not care if the communications system between the pharmacist (who belongs to the healthcare support group) and the nurse (who belongs to the customer-contact group) is faulty. Patients care only about the quality of the total healthcare experience, and the organization is responsible for providing the quality by ensuring that things happen the way they should, such as the right prescriptions getting to the right patient at the right time.

To illustrate, say a patient undergoes a physical exam in a primary care physician's office. If the physician does not have a laboratory to do medical tests on-site, the patient might be asked to visit a medical laboratory, have certain tests done under certain conditions (e.g., after eating no food for eight hours), and have the lab fax/e-mail back the results to the physician's office. The probability of seamless service in such a situation is low even when directions for both the patient and the lab are extremely clear.

Information Flow Across and Between Organizational Levels

The last major requirement of the information system in service delivery is to move information between organizational levels. This level-to-level flow of information can take the shape of a simple employee newsletter or a document with a routing slip, or it can be embodied in a sophisticated online, real-time, wireless data retrieval and decision system. Information can also be provided through a centralized database or intranet that is accessible to all employees, allowing them to retrieve specific information on corporate policy, dates and places of training opportunities, or availability of job openings within the organization.

All of these methods of communication, whether on a piece of paper or through increasingly sophisticated electronic devices, are additional ways healthcare managers can reinforce cultural traditions, motivate employees, and educate them to enhance the healthcare experience. Of course, many other communication channels flow up and down between management and employees. Employee-of-the-month programs, for example, allow the organization to communicate to all employees the types of behavior desired and rewarded. Employee suggestion programs are another way for management to pick up new ideas and other types of information from their employees that enable quick identification of problem areas in the service delivery system.

Perhaps the most problematic example of information flow between levels is the chronic miscommunication problem between nurses and physicians. For example, illegible physician handwriting can result in a nurse misreading the orders, which can then result in tragedy. John Kerry and Newt Gingrich, in a 2007 joint editorial arguing for e-prescriptions, noted that medication errors kill at least 7,000 Americans annually. Furthermore, of the more than 3 billion prescriptions written annually, more than 1 billion, or one third, require follow-up between the provider and the pharmacies for clarification (Kerry and Gingrich 2007). Noor (2007) reports that 98,000 patients die each year because of medication errors, many of which result because the nurses could not decipher the physician's handwritten prescription.

Technology can provide an avenue for improving such problems by providing a common database that records and tracks everything the physicians order for a patient's care and everything all the clinical employees do in executing or implementing those orders. Indeed, in more sophisticated systems, orders can be automatically forwarded to other units and logged into schedule books so human error is eliminated in information transmission. Handheld devices and computers can link doctors' various databases to ensure that patients get the right medication. Such devices can also alert doctors if one of a patient's drugs conflicts with another.

The Leapfrog Group encourages healthcare organizations to practice transparency and to make healthcare information more easily accessible. Leapfrog also recommends giving rewards to hospitals that have a proven record of high-quality care. (See www.leapfroggroup.org.)

Information technology also allows organizations to effectively outsource functions that are beyond the core competence of an organization. McKesson, for example, can operate a pharmacy for a hospital and ensure compliance with all rules and regulations and provide service at a level of quality that is consistent with the healthcare organization's mission.

A study reported by Kim (2005) found that outsourcing the supply-chain management system for drugs enabled hospitals to improve the procurement processes and inventory control of pharmaceutical products and decreased total inventory by more than 30 percent. Because the drug wholesaler can share information with hospitals, it can gather more timely and exact data about inventory status and drug usage volumes of hospitals. This allows the company to forecast the demand more accurately and supply needed products more cost effectively and quickly.

ADVANCED INFORMATION SYSTEMS

Two types of advanced information systems that do more than simply provide information are decision systems and expert systems, which help users analyze information and choose between alternatives. Decision systems are particularly useful to organizations that want to establish lasting relationships with patients. Expert systems are sometimes called artificial intelligence. Both systems constitute the informatics infrastructure of benchmark healthcare organizations.

Decision Systems

Decision systems help clinicians make decisions, and sometimes, they replace the decision maker altogether. An example of a decision system is a monitor at the nurses' station that sounds an alarm when a critical care patient's blood pressure is too low. A decision system can replace a decision maker when real-life situations can be accurately modeled. In these cases, the decision system is programmed with information. The system will automatically respond according to the information it received.

For example, an intravenous drip programmed to increase the glucose percentage if the monitor registers a certain drop in the glucose level will respond without the prodding of a clinician.

Other models of decision systems include inventory reorders of medical supplies, pre-preparations of surgical trays on the basis of statistical projections, and home monitors that automatically dial 911 when certain vital signs register in the danger zone. All of these activities can occur without any human intervention and based solely on the data gathered and organized by the information system.

Decision Modeling

Decisions may be modeled when the relationships among the measured factors are generally predictable. However, typically it is not worth an organization's time and trouble to do the necessary research and data gathering to develop a mathematical model describing the situation and to discover the appropriate decision rule unless the decision is one that occurs frequently or comes up in a large number of patients.

For example, an inventory system might have a built-in, preprogrammed reordering capability that ensures the continuous availability of necessary drugs without overordering. The challenge is to ensure that the system collects the data necessary to measure the depletion of inventory, so the nurses using the drugs can define their usage rate fairly accurately. This way, the nurses know how much of each drug they need to keep on hand and that the ordering system can accurately predict how long it takes to reorder and receive the necessary products. A system can be designed to collect and analyze this information to ensure that the proper quantity of each necessary drug is maintained in inventory.

As is true of any procedure designed to improve service to patients, the organization needs to assess the relationship between the value and the cost of the information before it establishes such a system. Because nurses are busy service providers and not accountants, they may not get around to gathering and organizing data on medical supplies often enough to justify the expense and sophistication of an online system. If data input is haphazard, the value of the information is low because it will be frequently out of date, and the expense of installing a sophisticated system is unwarranted.

Expert Systems

Expert systems seek to duplicate the decision process used by an expert who gathers information, organizes it in some way, applies a body of expertise to interpreting the information, and makes a decision. An expert system is built by finding out what information an expert uses, how that expert organizes it, and what decision rules that expert uses to make decisions based on the information.

Once these pieces of information are collected, usually through extensive interviewing of an expert or a group of experts, a series of decision rules can be written to duplicate the decision-making process of the expert. Healthcare journals frequently offer new illustrations of expert systems that assist clinicians in a wide variety of applications of these powerful systems. As clinicians face the same explosion of knowledge that all managers face, they will increasingly rely on expert systems to help sort through the volume of information to find the best solutions to healthcare problems.

Decisions Requiring Judgment

Expert systems can be developed to facilitate decision making in a wide variety of recurring situations that require expert judgment. For example, expert systems can schedule personnel to ensure proper staffing levels and keep track of hospital room inventory to ensure maximum use for each day's inventory of available rooms. Expert systems can be used whenever a straightforward algorithm or mathematical formula can calculate the best or optimal answer for a problem. In these types of expert systems, the optimal answer can be determined once the data are gathered and analyzed by the algorithm and expert judgment is applied.

The key to using expert systems is to find the right experts, identify the criteria they use in making decisions, program their decision rules in a logical sequence, and apply the program to problems that lend themselves to computerized analysis. This creates a category of decisions that can be made 24 hours a day for any person having access to the system. For example, a pharmacist wanting to find out about interactive effects of a newly prescribed medicine can call up the system from a remote terminal, at any time of day or night, and ask the system to investigate any possible interactions with the drugs the patient is taking.

Clinical decision support systems (CDSSs) are computer-based information systems containing thousands of treatment options for different diseases. They are designed to help in the diagnosis and treatment of illnesses. Some CDSSs simply collect, organize, and communicate data about patients to physicians, but others, such as the Cochrane Collaboration, actually use medical databases to suggest diagnoses and treatment regimens. Some CDSSs are expert systems that contain, first of all, a general knowledge base of medical information supplied by experts. Clinical information about particular patients is related to the information in the knowledge base. The computer then uses decision rules to draw conclusions and make recommendations to the attending physician.

Following are some examples of ways expert systems are used in healthcare:

- A computerized system accurately monitors the fetal heart rate during the birth process. A rule-based expert system uses heart-rate data to classify the situation as normal, stressed, indeterminate, or ominous.
- A smart pillbox monitors and reminds patients with human immunodeficiency virus (HIV) to stay on their drug treatment regimen. The pillbox is connected to a medical expert system that analyzes patient information and provides

Web-enabled reports and urgent outbound alerts to caregivers when patients miss medication or suffer declining health.

- An expert system can analyze hospital billings to spot irregularities in doctors' charges, classification of charges, and specification of charges.
- An expert system can detect and alert staff about adverse drug events such as allergies, unpredicted drug interactions, and dosage problems.

BayCare Health System in Tampa, Florida, and PeaceHealth system in Bellevue, Washington, are two examples of healthcare systems that have purchased TheraDoc's Expert System Platform, which combines real-time monitoring with an expert CDSS. Using the system's capabilities, these two organizations monitor hospital-acquired infections and adverse drug effects. The expert system allows the organizations to not only monitor these specific problem areas but also offer solutions (*Business Wire* 2008).

The existence of expert systems has far-reaching implications. As expert systems that are capable of providing up-to-date data and recommendations based on expert opinion become more widely available, physicians may become obligated to use them. Not to do so might leave them open to legal liability for not using state-of-the-art methods for diagnosis and treatment.

Artificial Intelligence

More advanced applications of expert systems open the way to the use of artificial intelligence (AI). AI is used in situations where some decision rules are available but they are incomplete because part of the decision process is unknown or too unpredictable to model accurately. AI programs are designed to allow the computer to learn from successes and failures by ensuring that all the decisions it makes have a feedback loop, which allows the result of implementing the decision to be fed back and tested against predetermined evaluative criteria to find out whether the decision was good or bad. If the outcome was good, the logic the decision process used is affirmed. If not, the feedback allows the computer to "learn" not to make the same mistake the next time it faces the same situation.

The simplest and classic illustration of AI is a chess-playing program. A computer can be programmed to behave like an expert chess player who knows all the rules and the traditional chess gambits. As it plays games against various opponents, however, the computer can also learn which moves lead to bad outcomes and which moves lead to good outcomes. Over time, this knowledge accumulates to improve the computer's decision-making capabilities just as accumulated knowledge improves the capability of a human expert.

Adding a learning capability moves an expert system's sophistication level up to that of an AI application. The use of AI is still limited because of the cost and time required to develop this learning capability and the cost of errors while the learning takes place, but even so, AI has a following: The Artificial Intelligence in Medicine Europe (AIME), which started in 1991, holds an annual meeting that offers a forum to expand the applications of this powerful decision tool in healthcare settings. From diagnosing congenital heart disease to scheduling patient tests to developing treatment protocols, AI can be a useful tool in absorbing the complex interdependencies of the human anatomic system and the volume of new science that advances the treatment of healthcare problems. AI never sleeps, learns continuously, and offers consistent expert advice, so some believe it may be the only way for the human mind to adapt to and incorporate the increasingly complex world of clinical knowledge.

Advantages and Disadvantages of Advanced Systems

As Exhibit 10.1 shows, there are good reasons to use these systems, such as the fact that they give users instantaneous access to a decision maker who makes quick, consistent decisions, which may be critical for an emergency department doctor seeking a quick consultation on a tricky diagnosis. These systems also have disadvantages. For example, the user cannot ask further questions if the problem or query is not quite what the model expects.

Customers have unique needs, and expert systems have to be designed from the customer's point of view if they are to be truly useful in problem solving within an organization. Because of the potential problems indicated in Exhibit 10.1, expert systems should not be used for trivial, unimportant, or infrequent decision situations; they are simply too expensive. Expert systems should not replace human decision makers in life-and-death situations either. They may, however, add greatly to healthcare quality by making medical expertise available at any time and any place to assist an attending physician.

PROBLEMS WITH INFORMATION SYSTEMS

No healthcare organization is likely to abandon its information system, but these systems can present potential and actual challenges, including (1) information overload, (2) overfocus on the numbers, (3) bad information, (4) no assurance

Exhibit 10.1 Advantages and Disadvantages of Advanced Information Systems

Advantages	Disadvantages
• Makes consistent and impartial decisions	• May make bad decisions if problem is not routine
• Makes decisions quickly	• Eliminates human participation in decisions
• Rapidly sorts through large amounts of information	• Assumes that experts will reveal decision-making secrets and rules
• Frees up experts from making routine decisions	• Some decision processes are too obscure to duplicate in expert systems
• Allows instantaneous 24-hour access to a decision maker	• May present legal issues regarding who owns decision rules
• Retains expertise forever	• Circumstances may change too quickly for the system to keep up
	• May frustrate users whose problems do not exactly fit system parameters

of security and confidentiality, and (5) difficulty of weighing the system's value against its cost.

Information Overload

Information systems are helpful and revolutionary but far from perfect. Too much information is as bad as not enough. Although sophisticated systems are designed to provide only the right information to the right person when that person needs it, many information systems provide a lot of raw data that users have to sort through until they can find the needed information. As these systems are being designed, planners ask users what information they need. Most users will ask for as much information as they can get, instead of only as much as they really need. Most people believe it is better to have too much information than not having enough, and the proof is that they have seen people disciplined or even sued for having too little information but never for having too much.

A second aspect of this issue is that, when asked, most people indicate that they use many different informational data sources, instead of mentioning the one or two they actually use. Not wanting to admit ignorance or own up to how little information they use, they ask for a lot and then get lost in the pile. Everyone has done a Google search only to be overwhelmed by the millions of sites that appear. Benchmark healthcare organizations collect and feed back a lot of information on customer satisfaction but must make sure the information is in a format that is accessible and useful.

Overfocus on the Numbers

Because computers excel in transmitting, organizing, and analyzing numbers, much computer information is in numeric form. Although this format helps data be converted into information accurately, it tends to focus attention on only those things that can be quantified or somehow expressed in numerical terms. Much of a healthcare manager's life revolves around subjective, qualitative information rather than quantitative data. The availability of numeric information creates an overemphasis in decision making on such information and an underemphasis on qualitative information. Many clinicians believe medicine is an art, so trying to determine what data should be processed to accurately represent the practice of the art is a difficult challenge.

Bad Information

Regarding data collection, the old saying that garbage in leads to garbage out is quite true. A sophisticated information system can quickly provide a lot of bad data to a lot of people; if bad data get into the organization's decision-making structure, the data will be plugged into multiple calculations used in many decision situations. What if the wrong financial information is submitted to Medicare, or the wrong lab result gets into the system? The results can be worse than garbage; they can be catastrophic.

No Assurance of Security and Confidentiality

How can the integrity of the database be maintained? This is an enormous challenge in healthcare. Information systems have to be protected so that one organization cannot access confidential or proprietary data from another and so that only authorized persons can gain access to patient information. Although it is still possible in many hospitals for anybody to walk into a hospital room and look at a patient's chart, the concern over computerized medical records has led to a wide and deep conversation about patient rights to privacy and how to protect that privacy in an age of digital records.

In this era of telemedicine and doctors working at a distance, connected to the information system by modem or computer terminal, protecting the integrity of the database from unauthorized or inappropriate access is an important concern. If hackers can get into the computers of the U.S. Department of Defense, as they have, then competitors or others may well be able to get into healthcare databases. Protecting against such unauthorized entry is a big problem and big expense for organizations. The problem exists even internally, as database managers need to ensure that unauthorized persons cannot obtain confidential patient data.

Acquisition of private healthcare data by unauthorized users is one problem; misuse of private information by authorized users is another. Hospitalized patients are often unaware that many employees look at their health records without permission. Upon discovering the easy accessibility of this information, some patients request for their records to be kept confidential and for a list of people who accessed their file to be kept.

Despite the passage of the Health Insurance Portability and Accountability Act (HIPAA) in 1996, many organizations continue to face increased pressure to profit from their patient health data. Because of HIPAA, hospitals ceased to ask patients which medical information they wanted shared and which they wanted private. Patients' access to their own records became impossible, yet the same information could be released to other entities, including providers, employers, government agencies, insurance companies, billing firms, transcription services, pharmacy benefit managers, pharmaceutical companies, data miners, and creditors (patientprivacyrights.org 2009). This situation may change if the consumer protection included in the Obama administration's stimulus package is enforced. This little-known provision prohibits the sale of personal health information, with exceptions for research and public health purposes. Also, this protection mandates organizations to inform consumers if their Social Security number or medical information is "hacked" or stolen (Freudenheim 2009).

Breach of Electronic Medical Records

News reports of privacy breaches related to electronic medical records appear regularly. In June 2008, Walter Reed Army Medical Center notified 1,000 patients of a privacy breach (Ottenheimer 2008). Just a few days earlier, the University of California at San Francisco had disclosed that it had notified more than 3,000 patients of a privacy breach in its pathology department. The *Wall Street Journal* reported that complaints of privacy breaches in the United States reached 23,896 for the period between April and November 2003 (Francis 2006).

Based on a 2006 study by the Markle Foundation, although a majority of Americans believe electronic data can improve care, 80 percent are very concerned about the risk of access without their authorization, including access related to marketing, identity theft, and fraud. The Association of American Physicians and Surgeons published a similar study in 2007, which found that 70 percent of patients asked doctors to "suppress information" because of privacy concerns—this means that doctors did not put information in patient records for fear that someone (e.g., an employer) would use the data against the patients. In addition, 50 percent believed control of their records was already lost (Ottenheimer 2008). Patients have a right to be concerned. During the course of a typical hospitalization, approximately 150 people are estimated to have access to a patient's medical record (Fried 2007), and medical identity theft has been made easier by the ability of criminals to hack into hospitals' online files (Faust 2007). Clearly, the security and privacy of information in the healthcare system is a growing concern to everyone involved in healthcare—regulators, healthcare organizations, and consumers alike.

Difficulty of Weighing Value Against Cost

Information is not free. Buying data terminals and computers, hiring programmers, running a wireless data network, and building an information system are hugely expensive. Yet many of the benefits of an information system are intangible. How does one measure the value of instantaneous access to a patient database so a patient can be greeted by name, the information necessary for excellent patient care is immediately available, and the patient's unique requirements can be identified in advance and supplied? And how does one measure the cost of problems, including fatalities, that an adequate information system might have avoided?

In *To Err Is Human: Building a Safer Health System,* the Institute of Medicine (IOM 2000) stunned the U.S. public by reporting that up to 98,000 people die each year from preventable medical errors. In *Crossing the Quality Chasm: A New Health System for the 21st Century,* the IOM (2001) said the industry's problems had increased. Still, not much progress has been made in applying advances in information technology to improve administrative and clinical processes (IOM 2001). A 2008 study by the Agency for Healthcare Research and Quality found that one of every ten patients who died within 90 days of surgery did so because of a preventable medical error. The study also found that preventable medical errors cost nearly $1.5 billion annually (Encinosa and Hellinger 2008). The Obama administration's emphasis on improving health information systems affirms how little progress has been made thus far.

Determining how much better a decision was because the manager or clinician had the right information available is usually impossible. Yet most organizations believe their systems are worth the cost. The problem is that when budget time comes and paybacks on investments are calculated, defending information system upgrades and improvements is difficult because evaluating the contribution of such a system is difficult. Still, companies can make estimates. About 85 percent of medical practice revenues come from insurance reimbursements, but the average time for processing claims is between 45 and 90 days. The assumption is that the cost savings of more efficient claims processing will exceed the cost of the required investments.

Cost of Learning the System

Top managers and physicians are the very people who need to learn how to use information technology, but they are often the very same people who are most uncomfortable and unfamiliar with it. Worse yet, given the problems in quantifying the value of the technology, these are the same people who make the decisions about buying the equipment, investing in the system, and getting trained to use it effectively. A lot of learning has to take place before those who are uneasy talking about MP3s, Twitter, and podcasts are totally comfortable using the new electronic information system.

Even though increasingly user-friendly software makes it easier for managers to learn and use the powerful technology, the challenge is that as soon as they master one technology, a newer and more powerful one will inevitably come along that they will need to learn as well. Busy managers, clinical staff, and others in the healthcare system cannot learn about information systems once and then forget about them. The rapid changes in what computers can do in managing information require all participants in the healthcare system to change as fast. This takes valuable time, which is a major challenge.

HEALTHCARE ORGANIZATIONS AS INFORMATION SYSTEMS

Perhaps the easiest way to understand how information ties the healthcare organization together is to consider the organization itself as a big information network. Everyone is a transmission point on the organizational network, gathering, sending, and processing information into a decision-friendly format. Those responsible for designing the organization as an information system must consider how all these network participants are linked together and what each participant's information needs are.

If an admitting clerk is responsible for taking a phone call from a family member inquiring whether a relative has been admitted and, if so, what that patient's medical status is, then the information system had better be designed to obtain and provide accurate information to the clerk when the phone rings. The system design will therefore require communication linkages, across all parts of the organization, that provide access to all information needed by the clerk so that the clerk can respond helpfully and accurately. Reengineering the organization and its information system to focus on the needs of patients and their families is a necessity in the present-day competitive healthcare marketplace.

The Primacy of Information

The logic of organizing around the flow of information changes the way jobs are organized, tasks are performed, operations are sequenced, and departmental units are organized. The organization should be designed in a way that responds to information requirements. Jobs and departments dealing with uncertain, ever-changing, and ambiguous situations require a lot of information from many sources to ensure that the managers responsible for decisions on those units can get all the information they need to make those decisions. Jobs or units that are relatively insulated from uncertainty, ambiguity, and changing circumstance may not require the same volume or quality of information; they can likely anticipate that whatever happened or was true yesterday will be pretty much the same today and tomorrow.

Organizational units facing uncertainty need to add the information capacity that will allow the necessary information to be gathered, or they must find ways to reduce the need for that information. Both strategies involve integrating the organizational design into the information system and vice versa.

Increasing Capacity

When the organization must increase its information-handling capacity, its system designers must look at all the ways information is transmitted across the organization. They will probably have to build an expert-level system with the capability to screen out unnecessary information while conveying necessary information. Furthermore, the system will have to create redundant sources of critical information.

Information a decision maker absolutely must not miss should be provided in more than one channel of communication to ensure that the end user has it when it is needed. That way, if one channel breaks down or fails, the information can be provided through another means.

A simple example is sending someone an e-mail, followed by a fax, followed by a mailed hard copy, with the same information in all three communications. Building in this redundancy obviously creates additional demands on the information system, and organizations should carefully consider what information is so important that it needs to be sent in more than one way.

Reducing Need

The organization can seek ways to reduce the need to handle information. One major way to do this is to create self-contained decision-making units that are empowered and enabled to make decisions about their areas of responsibility. By increasing the number of decisions made at the point where the information is generated, the use of information channels is reduced. This is the classic strategy of decentralized decision making or, in the more current literature, the trend toward individual or group empowerment.

The idea here is that with proper training in asking for job-related data and turning these data into information used for decision making, the individual employee or department can make many decisions that otherwise would have been routed up the administrative chain of command. The time and effort it takes to check with a supervisor or higher-level organizational unit can use up information channel capacity, but even worse for a healthcare organization, it also slows down the response to the problem. If a furious patient is complaining to an employee, that patient does not want to wait until someone upstairs gives approval for resolving a problem.

Everybody Online

The most effective strategy for increasing the information flow is to put everyone online with immediate and easy access to the relevant parts of the organization's database via an intranet. Increasingly, rather than sending masses of information through the communication channels, the trend is to put information on the intranet so any employee with a computer terminal and the appropriate access code can ask for it.

Most organizations now have e-mail capability that allows any employee to ask any manager or expert any relevant question electronically. The flow of information back and forth across all levels of the organization and even outside the organization is incredibly enhanced by this technique. The increasing involvement of healthcare organizations in regional and national information networks and their rich databases and informational resources means even more information is available to anyone who needs it, whenever they need it. Frontline employees now often have access to much of the same information their bosses have access to, and with proper education about organizational goals and training in decision making, they can make decisions of the same or better quality than their bosses could in previous eras.

Integrated Systems

The growth in interconnectivity has created an expanded ability to access useful information.

One example is the formation of Premier in 1996. Owned by more than 200 of the nation's leading not-for-profit hospitals, Premier's website claims that it operates "the nation's largest healthcare supply purchasing network, the most comprehensive repository of hospital clinical and financial information." (See www. premierinc.com.)

One of the more elaborate networks of information interconnectivity has been established in Oregon. The Oregon Community Health Information Network (OCHIN) provides administrative services to 21 member organizations in more than 100 locations, and it has more than 2,500 end users in private and public health centers in both rural and urban settings. OCHIN's stated goal is to provide quality health information and management services to the safety-net community. As a collaborative, OCHIN believes it can provide these services more efficiently and effectively than would be possible by individual organizations.

OCHIN was founded in 2000 as a department of CareOregon to address concerns about the impact of an information technology gap in the field of healthcare. The belief was that, if unchecked, this technology gap would leave families in poverty and with more expensive, less efficient, and less effective care than those with access to mainstream systems of care. The founders of OCHIN also envisioned an opportunity to secure significant gains in quality healthcare for populations who have tended to be most neglected by the healthcare system as a whole.

OCHIN leverages its size to purchase software that can make practice management and electronic medical records affordable for more safety-net clinics to implement and maintain. OCHIN seeks to subsidize the cost of the software through grants and foundations.

CONCLUSION

The impact that these information systems have on empowering frontline employees to do their jobs better, quicker, and cheaper is astonishing today and will grow even more so in the future. The implications of these changes for all staff, who are responsible for accurately transmitting information from one part of the healthcare system to another, are also important to consider in managing the organization. Technological trends will continue to have a profound effect on organizational design and frontline employee responsibilities, and healthcare organizations will need to ensure that information is accurate and that they are accountable for who uses it.

Electronic technology has changed and will continue to change the way organizations are structured and managed; it will also fundamentally change the nature and role of employees who are concerned with delivering high-quality healthcare experiences. The information systems of healthcare organizations should be designed to incorporate all the components of the healthcare experience. Such a total information system provides the needed information simultaneously to patients, family, management, patient-contact staff, and even external stakeholders when they need it and in a way they can use it. Achieving this end requires the system designer to pay close attention to the needs of users and their capabilities and willingness to use informatics to enhance the customer experience.

Service Strategies

1. Learn the unique informational needs of each internal and external customer, and satisfy them.
2. Find out the value of communicating information, and be aware of the cost of providing that information.
3. Make information available in a format that each customer expects, can use, and will use.
4. Ensure access to information to people who need it, and exclude access to those who do not.

5. Put organizational information online, but protect confidential data.
6. Ensure that the information system generates and feeds back information for those who need it.

Being nice to people is just 20 percent of providing good customer service.
The important part is designing systems that allow you to do the job right the first time.
—Carl Sewell, *Customers for Life*

CHAPTER 11

Delivering the Service

Service Principle:
Provide a seamless healthcare experience

ENSURING THAT ONLY well-trained, clinically competent, motivated, enthusiastic employees are serving patients is necessary, but it is not sufficient to produce an extraordinary patient experience. A healthcare organization must also ensure that the process by which the service is delivered is working as it should.

Healthcare managers often assume that the employee has made an error when a service problem arises in any part of the healthcare experience. But the reality is that frequently the fault lies in a poorly designed system that makes it difficult, if not impossible, to deliver the service with the excellence that the organization, the staff, and the patient want (Baker et al. 2008).

If you talk with nurses, admissions officers, and laboratory technicians, they will tell you how frustrated they become when the service systems cannot help them do the jobs they are hired, trained, and paid to do and want to do well. When the service delivery system fails, everyone loses. The patient is unhappy, the employee is frustrated, and the organization disappoints a patient and may lose all the revenues the patient's future business represents.

In this chapter, we address the following:

- How to properly design the service delivery system to make sure all aspects of the healthcare experience are provided as planned
- How to plan, measure, and improve the system as illustrated by examples that are applicable in real-world situations

- Techniques commonly used in the services sector and healthcare, such as blueprinting, fishbone analysis, Program Evaluation Review Technique/Critical Path Method (PERT/CPM), and simulations
- How an organization's design should be considered part of the service delivery system

Because the type of service will influence the design of the service delivery system (e.g., Sung-Eui 2005; Correa et al. 2007; Zomerdijk and Vries 2007), we will focus on a more general discussion of tools that can help design the best delivery system for healthcare applications.

CHECK THE SYSTEM FIRST

Kumar and colleagues (2008, 183) suggest "that practitioners should focus on process management to impact upon TSQ (technical service quality) rather than simply addressing service quality from a functional perspective." Moreover, "If companies have problems in maintaining service promises, there is a requirement to review the service delivery system: a system of interconnected processes which deliver value to the customers." Achieving patient satisfaction and avoiding problems in the healthcare experience can both be greatly affected by delivery system design (Prajogo 2006). Every healthcare organization should invest time and energy in studying and planning the entire system to get it right.

The total quality management (TQM) movement has taught organizational leaders two important lessons:

1. Everyone is responsible for delivering quality and monitoring the quality of the entire healthcare experience.
2. When a service failure occurs, the system must first be checked for problems before blame is passed down to people; after all, even systems of high-performing service organizations fail from time to time.

Consider the following example of a system failure and the outcome that resulted from employee involvement. After several doctors complained about their x-rays not being brought to the operating room in a timely manner and not having available x-ray technicians when needed, the chief operating officer (COO) of General Hospital decided to act using a nontraditional approach. The traditional managerial solution to the problem is to blame the staff. First, the section manager is loudly criticized for technical incompetence, poor supervisory skills, and other unsatisfactory outcomes brought about by the entire department. Then, the disciplined manager transfers the fault and criticizes or disciplines the technicians.

But the COO had a different problem-solving approach in mind. He organized a team of technicians and asked them to investigate the matter and to suggest ways to solve whatever problem they found. The team did exactly that. They found out that the cause of the problem was that not enough x-ray technicians were available in the hospital when the surgeons needed their expertise. This inadequate staffing level, the team discovered, resulted from a new manager's decision to change the hours of operation of the mobile x-ray unit. Some technicians served in both the in-hospital x-ray unit and the mobile unit.

Previously, the mobile unit had been out in the field only when no surgeries were scheduled, but a new supervisor had taken over the mobile unit, had been told to cut costs, and saw that costs could be cut by reducing the overtime hours worked by the driver of the mobile unit. That reduction forced the mobile unit to operate during some of the same hours surgeries were regularly scheduled.

As a result, technicians who used to be available for in-house x-ray work were now sometimes out in the field when their services were needed back at the hospital. Because a new manager followed orders and tried to save some money in the mobile x-ray unit, the rest of the system was disrupted. This cost-saving move irritated the doctors, slowed down the surgical procedures for patients, and drove up the costs of surgery because the operating rooms and surgical teams were tied up for longer periods. Solving a problem in one part of the service delivery system without thinking about its possible impact on the overall system created problems for another part.

Three lessons can be drawn from this example:

1. *Department managers often do not have enough time, information, or insight to figure out the best solutions by themselves.* These managers tend to find the simplest, quickest solution and rely on the traditional theory, addressing the problem by correcting personnel.
2. *Employees may have a better chance of finding the root causes of a problem than the manager does because they are more involved in the actual process of operating the system.* Not using the talents, intelligence, and job-related knowledge of employees is a waste of these human resources.
3. *Every problem should be addressed first from the perspective of the entire service delivery system.* Although one person may end up being the cause of a service failure, the fault is frequently in the system and not a person. Simply putting out one small fire ("we are spending too much money on overtime") without thinking about the system can cause big problems elsewhere.

Self-Correcting Systems

The goal of TQM is to use the people and the system designers to create a self-correcting system—an environment in which employees can override the system (or break the rules) to correct problems or failures. Employees in a self-correcting system are responsible for telling management where the system has failed so they can fix it together. Just as everyone is responsible for providing and maintaining quality, everyone is responsible for avoiding and fixing service failures. The sidebar illustrates two contrasting examples that highlight the importance of a self-correcting system.

Because the patient is always the ultimate judge of the quality and value of the healthcare experience, designers of the service delivery system must ensure that they fully consider the patient's point of view, not just the clinical employees' perspective. Although the system should be user-friendly for clinical employees, the system must also cater to the patient's needs, expectations, and capabilities. The service delivery should be smooth, seamless, easy, and transparent from the patient's point of view.

ANALYZE THE SYSTEM

Analyzing the service delivery system has three major components: planning, measuring or controlling, and improving. In the quality improvement literature, these components are known as "Juran's trilogy" or the "quality trilogy."

Any good delivery system must begin with careful planning, the first component. Years of experience in working with older people can give a new nursing home administrator a good head start in designing a comprehensive treatment, care, and recreation schedule. However, a careful analysis and detailing of every step in the entire service delivery process that provides comprehensive care and physical therapy for older people makes the difference between having it mostly right and reaching the level of excellence that the very best service organizations deliver.

The second component is measuring for control. You cannot manage what you do not measure, and this is especially true of service delivery systems. The service industry in general, and healthcare in particular, have lagged behind in understanding how to apply measurements to the largely intangible patient services. The need for measuring not only the clinical status but also the patient care status in every step of the service delivery system is critical in understanding where any service delivery problems are and how one can tell whether the attempted solutions are actually fixing the problem.

SIDEBAR

A man was on vacation in France when he had a sudden attack of gout. Having neglected to pack his medication, he sought medical care from a local doctor. He received treatment, paid the bill, and kept the receipt for later reimbursement from his insurance carrier. He did not call his carrier's 800 number for authorization; that number does not work in France.

When he arrived home, he sent the bill to his insurance carrier for processing. The processing clerk told him the bill could not be paid because the expenditure, although made for a covered ailment, had not been authorized. After several fruitless discussions and a brief phone conversation with a manager, he still could not get reimbursement. The rules did not allow reimbursement for a reimbursable but unauthorized expenditure.

The clerk and its system both failed the patient. The insurance carrier's procedures were not sufficiently flexible to handle the somewhat unusual request properly. The employee had been taught to follow the inadequate procedures to the letter, and the manager did not get sufficiently involved to find out what was really going on. If the insurance carrier's employees had been sufficiently empowered and motivated, the failure might have been avoided.

Contrast this clerk with the motivated, empowered assistant administrator in the following example. The hospital administrator told the assistant administrator to handle a particularly difficult Medicare case. An elderly woman frequently came to the hospital claiming illnesses and diseases that required her to be admitted. The billing clerk had noticed that a large number of claims for treating the woman were being sent to Medicare; the clerk alerted the hospital's management to the possibility that the organization would be audited if they did not "stop admitting this malingering patient." When the woman appeared again, requesting admission, the assistant administrator was given the task of convincing her that she should go home. After some discussion, the woman agreed to leave if the assistant administrator would take her home.

Because he knew the organization's philosophy was to do whatever was necessary to satisfy the patient, or at least try to, he agreed and drove her to her apartment. The apartment was filthy and showed signs that the old woman was unable to care for herself. The assistant administrator was deeply affected, so he arranged to fix the place up and clean it and volunteered to come back in a week to check on her.

When he arrived the next Friday afternoon, he found the place in worse condition than before. The power cords for the refrigerator, television, and lights had been cut, and the phone line had been snapped at the box. Upon the assistant administrator's questioning, the woman revealed that her drug-seeking nephew had trashed her place, as he did frequently, in search of money. The assistant administrator called the hospital and, even though the woman was not "sick," arranged for an ambulance to transport her back to the hospital so she would be safe until the police caught the nephew.

The empowered assistant administrator solved a problem by going beyond the regulations. If he had not made two trips to the woman's apartment and had not brought her back to the hospital, the problem would not have been solved: the woman would have continued to return to the hospital for unnecessary and costly medical treatment and the abuse would have continued. Through the assistant administrator, the system "healed itself" to achieve the organization's primary goal: patient satisfaction. The system failed once when it concluded that the woman was simply a malingerer who needed to be sent home, but it redeemed itself by giving the frontline administrator the autonomy to solve the patient's problems.

The points here are simple:

- Study your system in intimate detail.
- Design accurate early-warning measures

(Continued)

for each of the many possible failure points in both the clinical and nonclinical parts of the healthcare experience.

- Engage everyone in the organization in watching those measures.
- Empower employees to ignore policies and rules that impede customer service.
- Follow up on everything.

If failures occur repeatedly at certain points, change the system design. If the organization has a patient service guarantee, make sure the delivery system can meet and exceed patient expectations on that guarantee. Excellent healthcare managers know they must keep a careful eye on all the places where the system might fail, and they do their best to keep these failures from happening. All healthcare organizations should design systems that ensure success and avoid failure on the key drivers of an outstanding overall healthcare experience.

Saying to a floor nurse, "I want you to do a better job of satisfying patients because patients on your floor seem unhappy," is easy but probably useless. Explaining to a nurse exactly what level of excellence was achieved last month, what level is being achieved now, and what the measured target level is can be extremely helpful.

In the best circumstances, when the measures are clear, fair, and completely understood by the employees whose performance is being measured, employees are able to measure and manage themselves. If you teach employees what is important to their individual job success and then train them to measure how they are performing on those critical factors, you have the beginning of a self-managing workforce.

Ideally, the measures can permit employees to monitor their own delivery effectiveness while actually delivering the service. For example, if a nurse knows that the organizational standard for responding to a patient call is a maximum of three minutes, and a computerized device displays a running record of how many minutes it takes for the nurse to answer calls, she knows at all times where she stands in relation to the standard.

In addition to measuring employee performance, a good service delivery plan should include a way to measure how well the plan is being implemented at every step of the service delivery process and how well the overall plan is succeeding. The measures should trigger an analysis of exceptions or variations from the plan and should quantify every critical part of the healthcare experience and the total experience. Most patients respond to the healthcare experience as a whole. Patients usually know why they are satisfied by the healthcare experience if the clinical outcomes were exceptional—the heart transplant was a success, the malaria was cured, or the therapy led to recapturing a physical capability.

However, in routine encounters, such as annual checkups, patients are often unable to identify how any one part of the experience influences their determination of the experience's value and their sense of satisfaction. They can, however, give an overall impression of service quality that can trigger managerial investigation. If a patient is unhappy with a visit to the clinic, the clinic's managers will not know why until they carefully collect and analyze the data measuring patient perceptions of each step in the entire healthcare experience.

Management may not recognize that the dissatisfaction was caused by a long wait in x-ray, a rude doctor, or a dirty restroom. Knowing the components of the system and having the measures for each can trigger the necessary corrective actions. A well-designed service system will include a way to measure every critical part of the patient experience and the experience as a whole.

After measurements have been developed, the third component in the analysis of the service delivery system is improvement. Information about what is actually occurring drives system improvement: If you can identify the failures, you can figure out where to fix the system. Once the plan is clearly laid out and the results of implementing that plan are adequately measured to yield insights into how well the system is operating, both management and employees have the information needed to redesign the system or fix the problems and thus yield continuing improvement in the healthcare experience.

A major factor in improving the system is training staff to put customer service ahead of policies and procedures when the two conflict and rule breaking does not compromise patient safety or medical needs. Frontline employees are often the first to notice or be informed of system faults or failures. If they have been properly selected, trained, and motivated, they will report the need for system improvement.

For example, a nursing aide responsible for responding to patient call buttons, providing bed pans, and cleaning up was frustrated by the chronic understaffing that left him unable to respond promptly to patient needs. One day he noticed a predictable pattern: The call buttons began lighting up for bedpan requests at the same time food trays were delivered. He discovered that if he timed his visits to the rooms before food delivery, he could often be walking into the room to provide bed pans just as the patient was reaching for the call button. This nursing aide is an example of a dedicated, motivated, observant employee who improved the system by observing it.

The cycle of planning, measurement for control, and improvement should never stop. The plan lays out what you think your service delivery system should be doing, the control measures tell you if what you planned is in fact happening, and the commitment to improvement focuses everyone's attention on analyzing and fixing any problems and moving toward a flawless healthcare experience. The point is that the design of any service delivery system should incorporate all three elements.

SYSTEM PLANNING TECHNIQUES

The first step in a customer-driven approach to service delivery system design is planning out the steps and processes in the entire system. At this stage, a detailed description of the steps involved is developed. Managers of benchmark service organizations start their planning by surveying their potential patients to determine the key drivers of the experience from the customer's perspective. Once those key drivers are identified, the delivery system can be designed to ensure that patients' expectations regarding those drivers are met or exceeded.

If patient participation is included in the delivery system design, the plan should account for the possibility that the patient may not or cannot participate in treatment. For example, consider a professor who is used to having her healthcare needs met at the medical school and group practice affiliated with her university. She moves to another town, and her new primary care physician recommends that she visit a testing laboratory for certain tests. Accustomed to one-stop shopping for healthcare, the professor does not go to the laboratory and instead finds a new primary care physician who performs tests in the office. The first doctor's delivery system planning should have taken this possibility into account and included measurement of the key drivers of customer satisfaction with all parts of the delivery system.

Four basic techniques—blueprinting, fishbone analysis, PERT/CPM, and simulation—are commonly used to develop a detailed plan for delivering the healthcare experience. Managers can also use these techniques to focus on any aspect patient feedback indicates is a problem area. These techniques are especially useful because they can readily incorporate the measurements necessary for control and analysis of problems that may appear in the system.

Each technique has its own advantages, but all are premised on the idea that a detailed written plan leads to a better system for managing the people, organization, information, and production processes that deliver the total healthcare experience. If effort and care are devoted to the plan, failures should be minimized. If situations regularly get to the point where problem-solving and problem-recovery techniques are necessary, some patients will inevitably become so dissatisfied that they will not choose the provider again if they can help it.

Blueprinting

Detailing the delivery system through a blueprint or service process diagram has several immediate benefits to managers seeking a fail-safe delivery of their service. First, managers can better understand and study a diagram (in a flowchart form, for example) that delineates all parts of the system. Second, managers can easily use the diagram to show the plan to others.

Exhibit 11.1 is a simple flowchart of activities associated with a patient's visit to a physician office. All activities head toward and center on the patient's consultation with the doctor. Each activity related to the office visit must be successfully planned, designed, and managed if the healthcare experience is to succeed. Like most chains, the flowchart is only as strong as its weakest link. Although some activities are more important than others, each is a potential moment of truth that can affect the quality or value of the experience from the patient's perspective.

Employees must be trained and motivated to perform their responsibilities at each step on the flowchart. When a patient calls for an appointment, staff must answer the phone promptly, be courteous and friendly, and find the earliest mutually convenient appointment time. If a patient arrives by car and parks, the organization must make sure the parking area is clean and safe; if valet parking is provided, the patient must be given information about it ahead of time. As the first personal contact with the patient, the valet must be helpful and friendly.

When the patient arrives at the front desk, staff must extend a friendly welcome and explain what is going to happen and when. At sign-in, staff must provide all necessary paperwork, help patients fill it out, and explain the organization's billing policies and procedures. During any waits, staff must stay in touch with the patient, explain any undue delays, and provide estimates of how long the wait may extend.

Although the patient may not be present at most other points of activity on the chart, which usually involve different organizational units serving each other as "internal customers," those points must also be similarly managed. For example, if the report of the patient's lab work (upper right on the chart) is not completed promptly and inserted into the folder sent to the nurse, the doctor will not have the needed information at the consultation. Another consultation may have to be scheduled, and the patient will be inconvenienced.

Blueprinting is a more sophisticated form of flowcharting (Bitner, Ostrum, and Morgan 2008). In effect, a good blueprint displays and defines every component and activity not just of the delivery system but also of the entire healthcare experience, from the moment the patient sees the front door to the time the patient departs.

Exhibit 11.1 Flowchart of a Typical Patient Office Visit

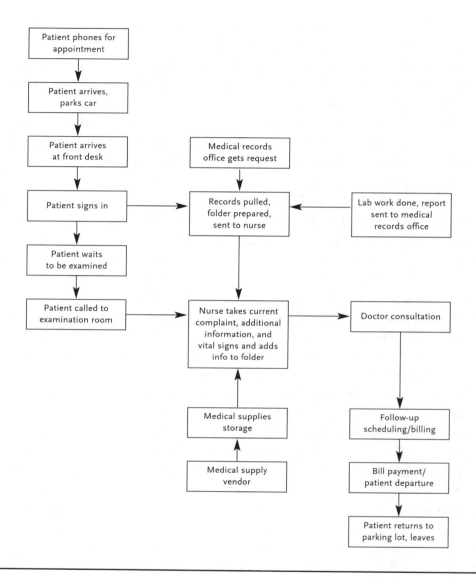

Every event that is scheduled to happen in between is laid out on a blueprint, as is every contingency that can be reasonably projected. The points at which service problems are most likely to occur can be identified, and early-warning mechanisms can be included.

The blueprint not only should present the activities and processes involved in providing the service, but it should also include the time it takes to complete each activity. If an excellent clinical visit is provided in 20 minutes, a patient may feel quite pleased; if it takes an hour, the patient may be satisfied; but if it takes two hours, the disappointed patient may never return. Finally, providing the service according to a well-designed blueprint will help the organization achieve its revenue goals while maximizing the patient-experience quality and value.

Exhibit 11.2 shows a simple blueprint of an elementary school nurse treating a playground injury. As diagrammed, the service begins with the nurse being told that a child needs attention on the playground. The nurse goes to the child, examines the wound, applies antiseptic, and dresses the wound.

The blueprint of the service also shows an arrow dropping from the application-of-antiseptic step to represent a potential area of failure where the nurse might forget to bring the antiseptic. If this happens, the next step shown is for the nurse to fix the problem by going to the office or supply room and then returning to the application-of-antiseptic step. The blueprint provides time estimates for each step so the total time of the service experience can be calculated. The blueprint also shows the line of visibility, which separates the events the patient can see from those that cannot be seen.

Work cycle times are calculated from carefully studying the process. The entire finished schematic shows the planned sequence of activities, shows the measures for each step in the cycle of service, and provides an easily communicated picture for analyzing the entire service cycle. The example in Exhibit 11.2 is simple and incomplete, but it is a good starting point. An excellent school nurse or the healthcare manager for a school system will want to extend this schematic to include certain events that happen before the nurse is summoned to treat a student.

The manager should start at the point where the overall strategy for student health was established in the first place. Doing so allows the manager to see all the other influences that have an impact on the student's total healthcare experience, including its many other intangible and tangible aspects. The simple example can be extended and completed by incorporating all the fine points of elementary school nursing care; the blueprint can go into even greater detail by breaking down each step into a detailed subroutine and by adding complementary services such as administering shots, conducting hearing and eyesight testing, and doing wellness counseling.

Other settings may require more elaborate blueprints. For instance, the need to treat hundreds of people a day in a large emergency department, serve dozens of people a day in a surgical center, or respond to countless phone calls on a health insurance information line may require service delivery steps to be broken down into highly specialized and routinized jobs to make the process as efficient as possible or to make the process work at all. The challenging

Exhibit 11.2 Blueprint for Nurse Treating Playground Injury

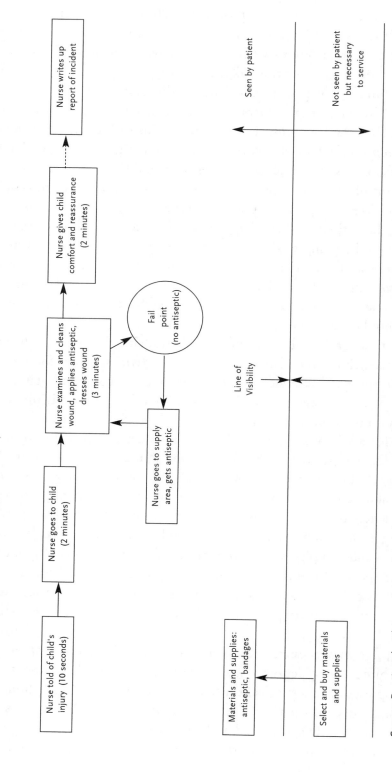

Source: Reprinted with permission from *The AMA Handbook of Marketing for the Service Industry*, published by the American Marketing Association, edited by C. A. Congram and M. L. Friedman, 1991.

question about such jobs is how to retain the human interaction component in the healthcare experience. The numbers of patients can be so large and the service contact may take place so rapidly that even the most personable professional will find it difficult to achieve a caring interaction with patients under the circumstances.

Fishbone Analysis

Fishbone analysis was developed by Kaoru Ishikawa of Tokyo University in 1953. It provides a way to concentrate on the problem area and generally involves the participation of the area's employees. Although a fishbone diagram analyzes the causes of faulty service outcomes, it can be considered a planning strategy because its results are often used to make major changes in the delivery system.

Exhibit 11.3 shows an application of this technique to a problem in the hypothetical General Hospital chain: Too many blood donors show up at the blood bank for their set appointment times and subsequently experience unreasonable delays. The problem (delayed blood donation) becomes the spine of the fish in Exhibit 11.3, which is derived from the classic Wyckoff (1984) study. The general resource areas within which problems might arise that can delay blood donation are attached as bones to the spine.

For example, "equipment" (which is a bone) is required to take blood promptly, so this resource area becomes a potential source of delay if, for example, the equipment is already in use or otherwise unavailable. All of the possible contributors to the equipment failure are also shown as bones attached to the main equipment bone. The potential contributors to resource failure are typically identified through group discussion with the employees involved, as they should know the reasons for treatment delays. General Hospital's employees use the fishbone diagram to identify the possible trouble spots.

The resources required for receiving blood donations can be categorized as equipment, personnel, material, procedures, and other. They are attached to the spine (problem). Within any one of these categories, a problem can arise that will cause the undesirable effect of unreasonable delays in serving blood donors. The potential problems associated with each resource will then be identified, listed, and prioritized by the employee group working on this problem. This analytical technique is known as Pareto analysis, which is used to assess the fishbone technique by arranging the potential causes of the problem in order of importance.

Exhibit 11.3 Fishbone Analysis: Delays at the General Hospital Blood Banks

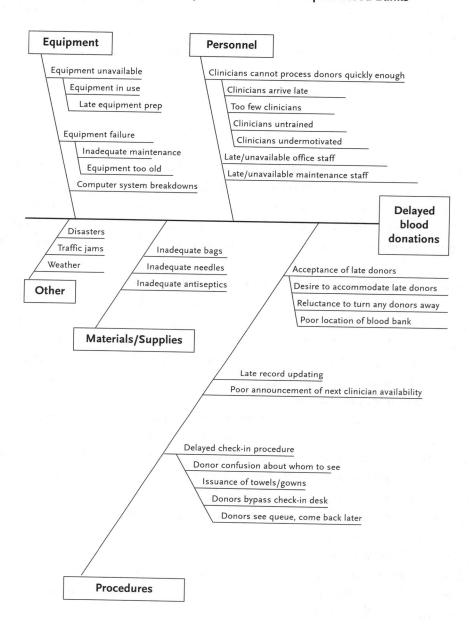

Source: Adapted with permission from *Cornell Hotel and Restaurant Administration Quarterly*, published by the American Marketing Association, D. Daryl Wyckoff, 1984, 25 (3): 158.

In Exhibit 11.4, the data representing the percentages of delayed service to blood donors associated with each cause are listed next to the cause in order of importance. The Pareto analysis revealed that about 90 percent of all service delays at General Hospital chains were caused by only 4 of the approximately 30 possible causes. The most frequent reason for delay at all hospitals combined was donors being late for their appointments, followed by too few clinicians, late record updating, and computer system breakdowns. General Hospital realized that it was giving immediate service to the donors who least deserved it: those who arrived late for their appointments to give blood.

The data can also be analyzed by individual hospitals in the General Hospital chain to see if the overall problems with blood donation are the same as those found in each individual hospital. As the data show, both the percentages and the reasons for delay at the Newark hospital are somewhat different from those seen at the other hospitals. The fourth most frequent factor at Newark, failure of old equipment, does not appear to be a problem for the Washington hospital, but computer breakdowns do. By arranging the information in this way, managers looking for causes of service delivery failures have an easily used analytical tool. For each potential failure point, they merely collect and arrange the data the fishbone categories tell them to gather.

Recognizing the problem is the first step in improving the service delivery system; knowing the causes is the first step in solving the problems.

Once the impact of late-arriving donors was identified, General Hospital decided it would no longer wait for donors who did not arrive on time. Although this solution seemed to contradict the hospital's desire to attract blood donors, and staff naturally wanted to accommodate late-arriving donors, the hospitals in the chain had clearly been denying timely service to the many donors who made sure to get to the center on time.

By setting up this fishbone analysis and comparing the survey data against the key factors, the hospital group was able to identify the problem and discover a solution that worked: Do not wait for anybody. Of course, that solution initially caused a customer-relations problem with late arrivals, but General Hospital decided that it was less serious than the problems that the late arrivals caused. As a matter of fact, when word got out that General Hospital was not going to wait anymore, fewer donors arrived late and the number of donors did not decline.

The individual parts of any delivery system can be broken down in the same way to discover the other factors—equipment, staff, procedures, material—that may contribute to a service problem. Once managers measure each factor's contribution to the problem, finding a solution is relatively straightforward.

Exhibit 11.4 Pareto Analysis of Delays at the General Hospital Blood Banks

Cause of Delay	Percentage of Incidence	Cumulative Percentage	Cause of Delay	Percentage of Incidence	Cumulative Percentage	Cause of Delay	Percentage of Incidence	Cumulative Percentage
Late donors	53.3	53.3	Late donors	23.1	23.1	Late donors	33.3	33.3
Too few clinicians	15	68.3	Late record updating	23.1	46.2	Too few clinicians	33.3	66.6
Late record updating	11.3	79.6	Too few clinicians	23.1	69.3	Computer breakdowns	19	85.6
Computer breakdowns	8.7	86.3	Old equipment failures	15.4	84.7	Late record updating	9.5	95.1

Source: Adapted with permission from Cornell Hotel and Restaurant Administration Quarterly, published by the American Marketing Association, D. Daryl Wyckoff, 1984, 25 (3): 158.

PERT/CPM

Say you want to build a backyard barbecue. You design the barbecue and then buy bricks and mortar. But once you go out to dig the foundation, you find you do not have a shovel and need to buy one. Finally, you start digging the foundation, and while you are doing so your neighbor tells you that you need permission from the neighborhood homeowners' association before you can build a structure of that size on your property.

The impediments to the process in this scenario are merely time wasters and annoyances to the barbecue builder, but these types of impediments can cause much bigger problems to a healthcare organization. Healthcare organizations cannot afford to start building a hospital or clinic and then find out in the middle of the process that it lacks material or permits to complete the project. When the planning and delivery of the service product involve different activities, and especially when those activities recur in a repeating cycle (like planning a heart transplant or rehabilitation therapy treatment), a helpful technique to use is PERT/CPM.

The PERT/CPM planning technique is frequently used in the construction industry and the military, but it has many applications in the healthcare industry as well. The PERT and CPM techniques are similar and thus have become merged into a single planning strategy. The combined PERT/CPM provides managers with a detailed, well-organized plan combined with a control-measurement process for analyzing how well the plan is being executed. PERT/CPM is useful in planning major projects such as building a new hospital, setting up a new healthcare insurance plan, or opening a new clinic. It is also useful in smaller projects such as planning a patient treatment or surgical procedure or installing a new magnetic resonance imaging (MRI) machine.

Using a PERT/CPM diagram like that seen in Exhibit 11.5 allows the healthcare manager to achieve several important objectives. First, the manager gains all the usual advantages of planning. Unforeseen events and activities can be identified, and how long something will take to do is readily estimated. Everyone involved in the project has an easily understood picture that shows all the pieces of the project, the sequence in which they are laid out and must be accomplished, the time estimates for finishing each project step, and the total time for completing the entire project. PERT/CPM can be used to plan any project involving lots of activities that have to be accomplished on time to meet a deadline.

PERT/CPM diagrams are simple to create. They consist of circles or bubbles that represent completed events and arrows that represent the activities that must be done before an event can be considered complete. The arrows connect the circles, and the arrow points to the particular event for which the activity is necessary.

Exhibit 11.5 PERT/CPM Diagram

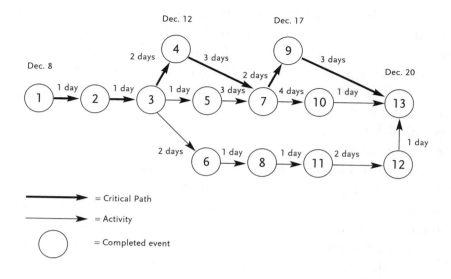

In Exhibit 11.5, for example, Event 1 must be completed before work can start on the activity that leads to the completion of Event 2, and the same is true of Events 2 and 3. Only after Event 3 is completed can work begin on the activities leading to Events 4, 5, and 6, which can be worked on independently of each other.

Three arrows point at Event 13, which signifies that Events 9, 10, and 12 must be completed before Event 13 can be completed. As the diagram shows, Events 9, 10, and 12 cannot be completed before prior activities and events are first completed. The critical path—the sequence of events that must occur on time if the project is to be completed on time—in the diagram will be explained in more detail later in the chapter. It has no slack time as the other two paths do.

As an example of how the PERT/CPM approach is used, consider the HMO plan for senior citizens that Universal HMO, Inc., wants to start in a new market. The final event in the sequence, the final circle on Universal's PERT/CPM diagram, will be "First day of HMO operation." One activity arrow leading up to that circle might be labeled "Hold three staff training sessions." But before those training sessions can be held, several other activities and events must take place: Universal HMO, Inc., must find a place to hold training, order training materials, hire and prepare a trainer, and hire the new HMO personnel. Some of those activities can be done simultaneously. Their completion might be indicated in the diagram by a circle labeled "Preparations for training sessions finished." Also included in the diagram are estimates of how long each activity will take. Summing the activity times will give Universal HMO, Inc., a pretty good estimate of how long it will take to have a trained HMO staff available.

Five steps are required to build a PERT/CPM network (Chase, Jacobs, and Aquilano 2006):

1. *Identify events and activities.* The manager defines all events that must occur, and all activities leading up to those events, for the project to be completed. The real fruits of the planning process occur at this step. By taking the time and making the effort, the manager can detail every activity in the project and uncover every step that must be taken.

2. *Determine the sequence of activities leading to the events.* The manager places defined activities and events in their proper sequence or the order in which they must be done. Developing the sequence may reveal previously undiscovered or unknown events that must be scheduled. If you are describing how to tie a shoelace, for example, you may forget Event 1—that you must first have a shoelace—unless you take the process step by step.

3. *Estimate times.* The manager estimates how much time each activity will take so that an expected time for completing each event and the entire project can be calculated. Managers frequently use a simple formula to arrive at a weighted-average time estimate for each activity:

Expected time = [Optimistic time + (4 × most likely time) + Pessimistic time] / 6.

4. *Create and diagram the network of activities.* The manager puts all pieces together into the total project diagram. As seen in Exhibit 11.6, each activity and event is set out in the diagrammed network along with the expected times.

5. *Identify the critical path.* The manager estimates the total time for completing the project and identifies the critical path—the sequence of activities that leaves no slack time—by summing up the activity times across the paths leading to the project completion. If these events do not happen on schedule, the project will not be finished on schedule. Other paths in the network may have a time difference between when the events must happen and when they are scheduled to happen based on the calculation of activity times. Say, Event 6 must happen on April 28 or the entire project will get behind schedule, but Event 6 is scheduled for completion on April 25, so the project manager has some slack time. Even if Event 6 takes five days to complete instead of two, the delay will not affect the project completion date. Slack time also represents

Exhibit 11.6 PERT/CPM Diagram for Starting an HMO

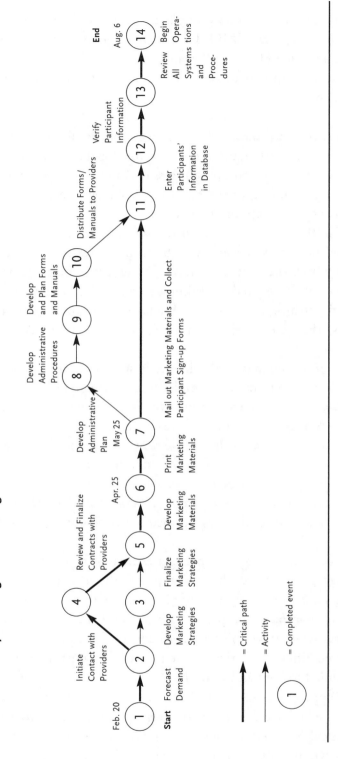

an opportunity to shift resources and attention away from events that finish earlier than they must and toward activities that need help.

The PERT/CPM diagram also provides a terrific visual of what is involved in the project. Using the diagram, the project manager can show everyone what the whole project looks like, what each person's part in the project is, when each activity needs to be done, which activities are critical, and which events precede and follow each person's job. Even more helpful is that the manager now has a complete model that can be used to test what might happen under a differing array of assumptions. What will happen, for example, if some of the pessimistic time estimates come true—that is, if whatever could go wrong, did go wrong (Prajogo 2006)?

Having the PERT/CPM diagram available also gives the manager an easy and quick way to substitute new numbers and revise the time schedule for total project completion if necessary. Obviously, every major project involves a lot of uncertainties. With this technique, however, the manager can plug in the uncertainties and refigure their impact on the project if they should occur (Chase, Jacobs, and Aquilano 2006).

Exhibit 11.6 represents the steps necessary to prepare for and begin offering a new HMO plan in a specific market. An HMO benefits manager followed the steps in building a PERT/CPM network to determine the activities, their sequence, and the time estimates. Then he set up the PERT/CPM diagram to show himself, the members of his organization, and the provider with whom his organization was contracting all the things that must happen to successfully introduce the HMO plan to this market. This diagram serves as a daily planning guide to the benefits manager and members and providers of the organization; it can be hung on the wall to show everyone what activities they need to accomplish each day.

A well-constructed and complete PERT/CPM diagram may be used repeatedly because new product or service introductions generally have the same events and follow the same sequence of activities. The same is true for building a new hospital, planning a new clinic, or planning a particular operation in a surgical theater.

A caveat is in order, however. The PERT/CPM process assumes that the activities leading to a project's completion are independent and can be clearly defined, but that is not always the case. The process also depends on the accuracy of the time estimates. Because these estimates are done by fallible human beings, they may be incorrect, and it does not take many incorrect time estimates to throw off an entire project.

Because the activities of healthcare organizations are often sequences or processes with a beginning and an end—from a brief clinical encounter to cleaning and preparing a room for the next day's patients—the possible applications of PERT/CPM to healthcare facilities and service situations are endless and surprisingly painless.

Simulations

Making changes in the healthcare environment is often difficult because of the many issues that must be considered, such as cost and the effect on patient satisfaction. The organization must ensure that any proposed change does not have a negative effect. A properly run simulation enables the organization to try out changes before implementing them, without running the risks associated with actually making the changes.

A simulation is an imitation of the real thing. It is done either through illustration on paper or a computer or through reenactments and scenario performances. Some simulations are big, like a computerized simulation of activities in a university health center, and some are small, like a role-playing exercise at a training session. Some simulations involve professional actors enacting a specific healthcare experience to show the observing employees and managers where problems can occur in service delivery. These simulations can reveal problems employees may not have thought about.

Simulations can also improvise patient-created problems to see if the system has safeguards to keep the patient from failing in the experience or, if a failure does occur, to keep the patient from irreparably harming the value and quality of the experience. Organizations can use all types of simulations when planning the service delivery system.

Computerized simulation techniques are the most sophisticated; they allow incredibly detailed simulation of the service delivery system and provide ways to measure and manipulate the system to see what might happen under different assumptions. Computers can also simulate behaviors of patients, with their infinite needs and ranges of behavior, on the receiving end of the system.

The unique challenge in patient care is that each patient is different. Because predicting how any one patient is going to behave within the service experience is almost impossible, the opportunities for system failures are tremendous. Simulating patient behavior allows a better comprehension of how that variability in patients affects the system's ability to deliver the service at the level expected. Across the entire healthcare experience, simulation can identify problems created by both the organization and the patient (Alvarez and Centeno 2000; Powers and Jack 2008; Pullman and Thompson 2003).

A good illustration of simulation is the recent trend for large urban hospitals to run computer simulations of their emergency departments. They gather data on arrival patterns and healthcare needs of patients at different times and days of the week and enter the data into the computer. The data may show that on a typical weekend evening, patients with trauma injuries begin arriving early in the evening and that the frequency and severity of traumas increase as the evening progresses. The data may also show that minor problems (e.g., cuts and bruises) increase during weekend days, when physician offices are normally closed.

The emergency department can use the data generated by the computerized simulation to predict the type of medical care required by time of day and day of week and the number of staff required to serve the predicted patient population efficiently and effectively. Moreover, the hospital can estimate patient bed requirements, medical equipment demand, optimal stocking of supplies, and even the number of meals consumed in the cafeteria.

Not every healthcare organization has the patient volume to justify or pay for the creation of a full-scale computer model to study its service delivery system in detail. Nonetheless, with the increasing availability of computer technology in smaller, more user-friendly software packages, even individual physicians can now economically create computerized simulations of their systems.

Already available to small healthcare organizations is the General Purpose Simulation System for Personal Computer (GPSS/PC) software. Such systems allow organizations to simulate portions of their delivery systems or an entire delivery system. For example, the GPSS/H simulation system allows a medical clinic to model appointment sequencing patterns to determine what is most effective in reducing patient waiting time, doctor idle time, and overtime without incurring any trade-offs.

CROSS-FUNCTIONAL ORGANIZATIONS

Thinking of the service delivery process as a system that requires the integrated, coordinated activity of people who work in different departments leads to reflection on how the overall organization is designed. Is it designed so that individual departments can perform their individual functions smoothly, or is it designed so that the overall service delivery system functions smoothly? Anyone who has ever worked in an organization where different functional areas never communicated with one another knows full well that the two designs are not the same.

One method of organizing people and groups to enable them to work temporarily across the boundaries or functional units in which organizations are traditionally structured is the cross-functional structure. This term is also used to refer to a group or project team overlaid on the traditional functional organizational structure and assigned to work on a task for a limited time. Traditional organizational forms are characterized by a single line of authority running from top to bottom: An admissions clerk reports to a supervisor, the supervisor reports to a manager, and so forth.

A cross-functional organization is characterized by multiple lines of authority: An operating nurse may report to more than one person, for example. In healthcare organizations, many situations arise that call for focusing everyone's clinical skills on solving a patient's problem or meeting a patient's expectation right at that moment. Examples might include a surgical team or patient safety team. Cross-functional structures, therefore, are especially useful in the healthcare industry, and in fact in any industry that is service driven.

Karl Albrecht (1988) tells a story about showing a group of hospital managers how the cycle of service appears from the patient's point of view. After an excited discussion in which they defined all the tasks necessary for delivering the hospital services needed by the patient, one manager suddenly said, "But no one is in charge." In other words, because of the way the typical hospital is organized, no one person is responsible for making sure service is smooth, seamless, and focused on the patient. Every department and every function is someone's responsibility, but no one is responsible for ensuring that all the subservices work together for the patient's benefit. This story, although 20 years old, is still relevant today. It may explain why patients are encouraged to bring along a family member or friend to a clinical service or visit.

In elaborating on this point, the manager stated:

> Our hospital is organized and managed by professional specialty—by functions like nursing, housekeeping, security, pharmacy, and so on. As a result, no single person or group is really accountable for the overall success and quality of the patient's experience. The orderlies are accountable for a part of the experience, the nurses for another, the lab technicians for another and so on. There are a lot of people accountable for a part of the service cycle but no one has personal accountability for an entire cycle of service. (Albrecht 1988)

More and more hospitals believe major change is needed to provide patients with a seamless service experience. Toward that end, many have reorganized their healthcare delivery systems to use cross-functional teams in delivering their services. A cross-functional team is a group staffed by a mix of specialists (i.e., physicians, nurses, nurse assistants, and so forth) formed to accomplish a specific objective. Team membership is usually assigned rather than voluntary. One example is the formation of a safety and security committee, an approach used by Sharp Healthcare, the 2007 Baldrige Award winner. The committee comprised members from various clinical disciplines, and its purpose was to identify safety and security concerns throughout the organization and to attend to them before they became problems or caused harm.

In healthcare, many such teams have involved the use of multiskilled health practitioners who are cross-trained to provide more than one function, often in more than one discipline. The combined functions can be found in a broad spectrum of health-related jobs ranging in complexity from the nonprofessional to the professional level and including both clinical and managerial functions. Research indicates that cross-functional teams have been successful in lowering costs, improving clinical quality, and enhancing patient satisfaction (Lemieux-Charles and McGuire 2006).

Lemieux-Charles and McGuire (2006) reviewed the literature on healthcare teams to determine the impact of team redesign on team effectiveness. The researchers found that the type and diversity of clinical expertise involved in team decision making largely accounts for improvements in patient care and organizational effectiveness. Collaboration, conflict resolution, participation, and cohesion are most likely to influence staff satisfaction and perceived team effectiveness.

Healthcare organizations use project teams, matrix structures, and other cross-functional forms. Because these forms generally involve people working under more than one line of authority, some traditional managers who believe strict lines of authority are important have problems working with cross-functional forms. On the other hand, crossing functional areas and focusing everyone on the patient can offer some important benefits. Exhibit 11.7 presents the advantages and disadvantages of these organizational forms.

CONCLUSION

Most service problems are caused by deficiencies in the service delivery system rather than individual staff members. Consequently, benchmark healthcare organizations analyze their delivery system from their customers' viewpoint, starting with their service expectations. There are many tools available for them to use to systematically and thoroughly investigate the service delivery system.

Exhibit 11.7 Advantages and Disadvantages of Cross-Functional Structures

Advantages

1. Create lateral communication channels that increase frequency of communication across functional areas in the organization
2. Increase quality and quantity of information up and down the vertical hierarchy
3. Increase flexibility in utilization of clinical expertise and capital resources
4. Increase individual motivation, job satisfaction, commitment, and personal development
5. Enable achievement of clinical excellence more easily

Disadvantages

1. Violate traditional "single line of authority" and "authority must be equal to responsibility" principles of organization
2. Lead to ambiguity about control of resources, responsibility for technical issues, and human resources management issues
3. Create organizational conflict between clinical and team managers
4. Create interpersonal conflict among individuals who must work together but have different backgrounds; clinical training; and perspectives on work, time horizons, and goals
5. Create loss of status, causing unit managers to think that their autonomy has been eroded
6. More costly for organization in terms of increased overhead and staff, more meetings, delayed decisions, and more information processing
7. More costly for individuals in terms of role ambiguity, conflict, and stress

Healthcare organizations should use whatever organizational design best enables every unit and every person to focus on the patient's needs, wants, and expectations. Although the organizational chart may show functional divisions with different people responsible for different things, such as maintenance, information systems, accounts receivables, nursing services, and so on, everyone in these excellent healthcare organizations knows that his or her real organizational function is ensuring that the healthcare experience meets or exceeds the patient's expectations.

Service Strategies

1. Check for system failure before blaming people.
2. Use detailed planning to prevent most service failures.
3. Plan for patient failures and how to recover from them.
4. Design the organization to ensure a seamless customer experience.
5. Use all available tools to break down the service experience into steps that can be studied.
6. Determine the cause of a service problem.
7. Identify and eliminate current policies, procedures, and rules that may impede customer service.
8. Train staff not to use policies, procedures, and rules as excuses for not providing customer service.
9. Monitor and maintain the quality of the service delivery system; everyone is responsible for avoiding service failures.
10. Design the service system so that the overall service delivery system, rather than the individual departments, functions smoothly.
11. Designate a staff position that will be responsible for the entire cycle of service.

Hurry up and wait.
—Old military saying

CHAPTER 12

Waiting for Healthcare Service

Service Principle:
Manage all parts of the wait

How LONG PEOPLE wait and how long they are willing to wait are fascinating subjects. A British Airways television commercial says people typically spend about 8 1/2 weeks waiting in lines during the first 30 years of their lives. Long waiting lists are also a standard feature of modern life. Some parents put their children on the waiting lists of exclusive preparatory schools before the children are even born. And if you want to ride your own raft down the Colorado River in the Grand Canyon, rather than ride in a concession operator's raft, you will have to add your name to a waiting list—at current use levels, you'll be taking your raft trip in about 14 years.

Waiting is a universal concern to all service organizations, but it can be critical in the healthcare industry. A poorly managed queue will not only cause dissatisfaction with the healthcare experience, but it may cause a medical catastrophe as well. Effective management of waiting lines requires an understanding of the mechanics and the psychology of creating well-designed queues. Building enough service capacity to handle the average patient demand is not the answer. The tremendous variation in patient care needs makes averages largely unrelated to the ebbs and flows of actual patient demand. Healthcare managers are especially challenged by the need to balance the healthcare organization's commitment to patient care and satisfaction with the huge costs of building and maintaining today's healthcare capacity.

In this chapter, we address the following:

- The importance of the wait
- Strategies for managing the reality and perception of the customer's wait

- The importance of understanding the organization's capacity to meet customer needs
- The psychology of waiting and wait lines

Overall, the key to managing the patient's wait effectively is to use both quantitative and psychological techniques in the appropriate combination to make waits, even long ones, acceptable to customers.

THE IMPORTANCE OF THE WAIT

Waiting time is the length of time customers wait to have their needs addressed. A closely related concept for patients is the opportunity cost of waiting, that is, the time and other opportunities the customers must sacrifice to obtain needed or desired health services. Waiting is routine in the admissions office, in the physician's waiting room, in examination or testing rooms, and on telephone lines as customers attempt to schedule appointments, acquire test results, or resolve reimbursement issues. All patients wait to receive test results or prognoses, to be seen by a physician or nurse, and to be told what to do or where to go.

Nobody likes to wait in line, yet almost every healthcare organization relies on waiting lines to adjust its fixed service capacity to the variable number of customers who want service. Managing the lines and how long customers have to wait is a major concern of any healthcare service organization or system that wishes to improve its customer satisfaction and capacity utilization levels (Wilicox et al. 2007). Research shows that managing time well is an important predictor of patient satisfaction.

For example, a study by Anderson, Camacho, and Balkrishnan (2007) showed that the amount of time spent with a physician is a strong predictor of patient satisfaction and can overcome patient concerns over time spent in a waiting room. The obvious implication of this is that healthcare providers need to manage the total time patients spend in the healthcare system. When mismanaged time leads to physicians spending less time with each patient coupled with those patients waiting longer in overly crowded waiting rooms, patients become dissatisfied.

As a result, some healthcare organizations are beginning to look more closely at the issue of waiting time. The National Health Service (NHS) in Great Britain, for example, has pledged to reduce waiting times for British hospitals (Joy and Jones 2005). Other research on the NHS examines the role of price as a method for altering wait times for appointments and during the actual visit. For example, prices could be set higher during peak periods and lower during other times to balance patient demand.

Canada has also instituted a Patient Wait Times Guarantee Trust, which promises funding for any provincial or territorial government that will implement a wait-time guarantee for at least one procedure selected from five priority areas: cancer care, heart care, cataract surgery, joint replacement, and diagnostic imaging (McMillan 2007).

In some respects waiting is an inevitable part of the healthcare experience because no organization can perfectly prepare itself to meet the needs of all customers instantly. In another respect the wait is a service failure. Even if the wait at the physician's office is no surprise and therefore meets the patient's expectations, the patient still does not like it. If patients tire of waiting, and if they are not too ill to do so, they may just leave. For a healthcare provider that operates in a competitive market, this can be a serious loss of present and future patient revenues (Weiss 2003). For a healthcare provider that faces litigation attorneys representing patients whose overly long waits led to subsequent medical problems, this can be a major financial cost.

What makes patients wait? Opportunity cost is the answer. High expectations explain the large numbers of patients willing to wait for appointments with famous surgeons, with respected dentists, or at well-known cancer clinics. The people waiting believe the quality or the uniqueness of the medical treatment will outweigh the costs of waiting, despite the full patient schedule and the numbers on a waiting list. In effect, each person makes an opportunity cost judgment. If the expected benefits of that particular service or treatment outweigh the costs of idly sitting in a reception area, the patient will wait. On the other hand, in a clinic for the indigent, the patients may have no opportunity costs to waiting as they have no other choice but to wait.

Waiting time is an unfortunate but expected part of the service process in healthcare. As a result, receiving patient service on time is rare. In spite of the pervasive use of appointments to balance healthcare capacity with patient demand, being served on time is an infrequent event. Even more frustrating to patients is the fact that although their time is respected in most other services, waits seem increasingly to be the rule and not the exception in healthcare. Even staff may begin to believe long waits are normal and to be expected and that customers should tolerate them.

Stephanie Sherman (1999) identified four primary reasons patients and physicians leave a healthcare organization; the most important is that waiting times are too long. Since Sherman's study, more research has shown that waiting continues to be a major source of patient dissatisfaction (e.g., Hill and Joonas 2005). Today's busy consumers demand and expect prompt service. When a customer defects because that expectation is not met, the healthcare organization may lose the revenue that customer represents for a lifetime. Even worse, further revenue may be lost from negative word of mouth, as each dissatisfied customer will tell others to avoid using that provider.

Emergency Department Waits

Emergency department (ED) patients are waiting even longer now to see a doctor, a potentially dangerous development as rising numbers of underinsured and uninsured Americans turn to EDs for medical care (Francis 2008). The median wait for adults rose from 22 minutes in 1997 to 30 minutes in 2004. Heart attack victims had a median wait time of 20 minutes in 2004, up 150 percent from 8 minutes in 1997. Black, Hispanic, and urban patients spend more time in waiting rooms than rural and white patients. An increase in the number of ED visits plus a decline in the number of EDs has contributed to the increased wait (*Healthcare Financial Management* 2008; Wilper et al. 2008).

Physician Waits

Press Ganey Associates, a healthcare consulting firm, reviewed more than 1.5 million patient surveys in 1,500 acute care hospitals across the country to determine patient satisfaction with waits. It found that patient satisfaction scores drop significantly with the amount of time spent in the ED, from 89.3 when patients are seen in under one hour to 77.7 when they have to wait more than four hours (Press Ganey 2007a). These data are supported by another Press Ganey report on individual physicians that shows a significant decline in patient satisfaction as both time spent waiting in the physician's office and in the exam room increases (Press Ganey 2007b).

A 1997 study by Press Ganey evaluated 25 physician practice qualities in terms of their relative need for improvement. Seven of the top ten areas identified as needing improvement were related to customer waiting. These findings are still relevant today:

1. Availability of doctor on phone
2. How promptly phone call was returned

3. Lack of phone access to service
4. Speed of the registration process
5. Ease of obtaining a desired date and time for appointment
6. Length of wait in the reception area
7. Waiting time to see the doctor

A 2007 Web-based cross-sectional survey of 5,030 patients who rated their physician found that longer waiting times were associated with lower levels of patient satisfaction (Anderson, Camacho, and Balkrishnan 2007). However, length of time spent with the physician was the strongest predictor of patient satisfaction. The decrease in satisfaction associated with long waiting times was substantially reduced if the physician spent five minutes or more with the patient. Alternatively, if the long wait was combined with a short physician visit, the negative impact of the long wait was increased.

An earlier study by Dansky and Miles (1997) found that the total time waiting for a physician was the most significant predictor of patient satisfaction; however, informing patients of how long their wait would be and making sure they were pleasantly occupied during the wait were also significant predictors of patient satisfaction. These results suggest that even if waiting times cannot be shortened, they may be managed more effectively to improve patient satisfaction. Letting patients know their expected waiting time enhances patient satisfaction (Anderson, Camacho, and Balkrishnan 2007).

Appointment/Treatment Waits

Reducing patient waiting times for appointments can have a significant impact on enhancing patient outcomes. Williams, Latta, and Conversano (2008) note that timely access to mental health services is critical to successful treatment of adults with severe and persistent mental illness. Waiting for weeks for a psychiatric appointment increases psychiatric hospitalizations and risk of suicide. However, many administrators of community mental health clinics assume that waiting for services is inevitable given the high demand. The study by Williams, Latta, and Conversano (2008) found that systematic changes in the service delivery system reduced wait times for a psychiatric appointment, the no-show rate, and psychiatric hospitalizations; these changes also improved staff morale and teamwork. These outcomes can be successfully achieved in settings other than the mental health field.

CAPACITY AND PSYCHOLOGY

Managing the wait has two major components. First, ensure that the appropriate capacity has been built into the service facility to minimize the wait for the anticipated number of customers arriving at the anticipated rate. Second, ensure that the waiting customers' psychological needs and expectations are met while they wait.

The capacity decision results from careful study of the expected demand pattern. Whether one is trying to determine how many copier machines to buy to serve a medical records department, how many treatment rooms to build in the ED, how many phone lines to run into the hotline for an AIDS (acquired immunodeficiency syndrome) counseling center, or how many beds to add to a hospital, the need to make an accurate capacity estimate is the same. Management must predict and attempt to manage the three factors that drive the capacity decision:

- How many people will arrive for the service,
- The rate at which people will arrive, and
- How long the service will take.

The capacity decision would be easy to make if the same number of people arrived for service each day, their arrivals were evenly spaced throughout the day, and serving each person took the same length of time. For example, a psychiatrist can plan to see eight patients per day, schedule them to arrive on the hour, serve each patient for 45 minutes, and use the remaining 15 minutes to write up notes on that patient and prepare for the next. That psychiatrist has an easy capacity decision: one service facility (an office) with one chair for the psychiatrist and one couch for the patient.

If the service is an ED, however, the healthcare provider knows approximately how long each type of treatment will take, but the management has to predict how many people will arrive for service at different times throughout each day of each week and what types of treatment they will need. For example, in Daytona, Florida, ED arrivals will be different in timing and type of injury during Bike Week than during the Daytona 500. Furthermore, if the service has a less definite beginning and ending time, like some types of hospital stays, both the average time taken to deliver the service and the number of persons arriving for service will have to be estimated or predicted. Several methods for making these predictions will be discussed later in this chapter.

Capacity designs can also affect perceptions of service quality. A doctor's waiting area that has too many seats will appear empty to patients. The scarcity of other patients may lead those who did come in and sit down to conclude that the clinical quality or medical expertise is not up to par. This assumption predisposes patients to expect a less-than-superb medical experience. Furthermore, they may feel foolish for choosing a doctor who is so obviously unpopular. The physician has two strikes against her, just because the office designer put in too many seats. From the physician's point of view, the excess capacity also has a serious disadvantage: it costs money! Unused chairs, extra space, and empty coat racks represent capital that presumably could have been better spent elsewhere. Excess capacity may result in extra personnel costs as well. On the other hand, too few seats can convey a totally different message: The doctor does not care about the patients and is disorganized.

In an ideal world, healthcare organizations will have the exact clinical staff and physical capacity required to serve each patient immediately. Consider a hospital ED where each patient arrives just when medical staff and equipment are available to provide the desired treatment. Patients want that kind of service, and organizations want to provide it. Both are frequently disappointed, however.

Organizational Options

Because people do not arrive at service facilities in neat, ordered patterns, they sometimes have to wait for service. When the organization sees that its waits for service are becoming unacceptably long, healthcare managers face several choices (Heskett, Sasser, and Hart 1990; Kreindler 2008).

Refuse to Serve Additional Customers
This choice is highly undesirable; after all, healthcare organizations exist to provide service. But sometimes prospective patients must be told, "We do not have any appointments available until next fall," or "You will have to seek care at another facility."

Add Capacity
Because this alternative is usually expensive, organizations do not choose it unless they believe the high demand will continue to cause long waits. Of course, certificate-of-need laws in various states also constrain if and when capacity can be added. The organization will be particularly hesitant to add capacity if the capacity of its design day (a design day is a theoretical service day, and capacity is designed for the number of patients seen on that day) is set at a high level.

Stop-gap measures for adding capacity temporarily are sometimes available: Employees can be asked to work overtime; a team approach can be used to reassign employees from their normal areas to help unclog a service bottleneck; temporary help can be hired; physical facilities, like trailers or portable buildings, can be rented; and so forth.

Manage Demand

Simply informing customers about busy and slack times may smooth out demand. Rather than being open to all patients at any time, healthcare providers typically use appointments to smooth out ebbs and flows of patient demand. Some providers offer inducements to encourage use of capacity at nonpeak demand times. Early-bird specials and discounts for off-peak use of wellness centers and health clubs are some examples.

Reservations or appointments are useful and help balance capacity utilization when staff and equipment are too expensive to sit idle, such as at hospitals, dental offices, and magnetic resonance imaging (MRI) clinics. Most healthcare organizations have the market stature to insist that their patients make appointments, and the opportunity cost to the patient for not receiving the specific service at the specific time from the specific provider is usually so great that the patient is willing to make an appointment. When the cancer specialist is the only one in the city able to treat a certain rare form of the disease, or the heart surgeon is the only one you trust to do the bypass, or you love the physician who has treated your family for 40 years, you will make an appointment and thereby help the provider organization efficiently manage its capacity.

Another way to manage demand is by shifting demand. A good example is shifting elective surgeries from weekday mornings to weekends. An obstetrician will frequently estimate the due dates of patients who are expected to have a typical delivery and then schedule cesarean sections around those times. This shifting of demand for obstetrical services allows the doctor's time and the hospital's surgical capacity to be more efficiently used. Although such events cannot be perfectly planned, this type of demand shift allows far better utilization of obstetrical services than would otherwise be possible.

LaGanga and Lawrence (2007) borrow an idea from the airline industry to manage demand. They suggest overbooking as a way to ensure that the existing capacity is fully used even though it may lead to longer waits when more than the estimated number of patients actually arrive. As with the airlines, overbooking has a downside; on the other hand, every healthcare provider should have a historical record of the percentage of patients that actually show up for appointments. This historical record should allow a fairly close estimate of how much overbooking can be done without distracting patient care or causing dissatisfaction.

Triage is often used to address excess demand. Under triage, to ensure that the most serious medical problems are treated first, patients are divided into three groups: (1) those who must be helped now, (2) those who can be helped later, and (3) those who cannot be helped at all, which is rare.

Some EDs and clinics have taken this concept to the next level. They have established fast-track systems that put patients with routine or noncritical healthcare problems in a separate queue. Instead of using the more expensive doctors, this queue may use paraprofessionals, lower-skilled nurses, and low-tech treatment rooms. The fast-track queue reduces the cost of treatment and increases the speed at which both lower-level and more acute medical needs are met. Following are other examples of triage:

- St. Joseph Hospital in Orange County, California, implemented an ED program called Rapid Assessment and Discharge in Triage (RADIT) to reduce patient waiting time and improve patient satisfaction. A roving RADIT team serves ED visitors who have nonurgent problems. After 6 months of this practice, ED patients were discharged in 97 minutes, on average, and 96 percent of RADIT patients rated the quality of service received as either good or excellent (Vega and McGuire 2007).
- Ruohonen, Neittaanmaki, and Teittinen (2006) present a simulated triage model developed for a hospital in Finland. The model tests different process scenarios, allocates resources, and performs activity-based cost analysis—tasks that when performed appropriately can result in operational efficiencies and thus higher patient satisfaction rates. Efficiency at this Finnish hospital increased by more than 25 percent (Ruohonen, Neittaanmaki, and Teittinen 2006).

Despite efforts to match supply with demand or to make the waiting experience as entertaining and comfortable as possible, the long waits can still be a concern to both the organization and the customer (Dickson, Ford, and Laval 2005). This is especially true where waits can have far-reaching effects on the organization's ability to meet its customers' expectations. (See Sidebar A for a virtual wait management strategy used outside the industry but is now being adopted in healthcare.)

Divert Patients While They Wait

At a minimum, waiting patients should be offered something else to do. The traditional diversion in a healthcare office is a stack of magazines or newspapers, though some organizations also provide television, instructional videos or videos that feature additional services available, aquariums, toys, crossword puzzle books, and computer games. Today, some freestanding retail medical clinics hand out beepers, similar to those used at chain restaurants, to give their waiting patients freedom

SIDEBAR A: THE VIRTUAL WAIT STRATEGY

At Disney, despite innovative efforts to reduce wait times, the long lines at the most popular attractions continued to be a major dissatisfier with guests. The availability of new technologies led Walt Disney World to develop the virtual queue concept. Instead of standing in line, guests would enter a virtual queue by registering their place in line with a computer and letting the computer save their place. Then, when the guests reached the front of the virtual line, they would be notified to return to the line and immediately enter the attraction.

The system is called Fastpass, and as a result of overwhelming guest response, it was expanded to all the Disney parks worldwide and is now used by more than 50 million guests per year. The system works as follows. When guests approach a Fastpass attraction, they insert their park admission ticket into a Fastpass turnstile, which places them in a virtual queue. Based on how many guests are in the virtual queue and the current processing capacity of the attraction, the computer estimates how long it will take for guests to reach the front of the line. This estimated time becomes their designated return time and is automatically printed on their Fastpass ticket. To provide guests with plenty of flexibility, they are assigned a 60-minute window of time during which they can return and enter the attraction with little or no wait. This 60-minute window was deemed necessary to provide guests with plenty of time to visit another attraction without having to worry about getting back late and missing their assigned time.

The virtual queue system provides many secondary benefits. Previously, during peak days many guests spent as much as three to four hours a day waiting in line for the most popular attractions, which severely limited the total number of attractions they could see. The use of Fastpass not only allowed guests to see more attractions during the day but also greatly increased the use of the park's secondary attractions. Another benefit was that guests used some of their freed up time to engage in other revenue-producing activities, such as dining and shopping. This provides significant benefits to guests and to Disney. Lower perceived wait times have led to higher customer satisfaction levels, and Disney officials have seen increased spending on food and merchandise per person in the parks (Dickson, Ford, and Laval 2005).

The virtual queue strategy is an innovative way of making the waiting line invisible. With heavy reliance on word-of-mouth advertising and repeat business, hospitals and healthcare organizations cannot afford to develop a reputation for long waiting lines and dissatisfied customers. But now virtual queues provide an exciting new strategy for creating satisfied customers in waiting line situations. The challenge that remains is to extend the virtual queue concept to any service settings where waiting lines cause customer dissatisfaction. Halifax Health Medical Center in Daytona Beach, Florida, has already adopted this strategy.

---

to move about the surrounding areas without losing their turn in line (Lethlean 2009). To give customers someplace to go and something to do while they wait, some hospitals have expanded their gift shops.

Improve Waiting Areas

Uncomfortable waiting areas can make a moderate wait seem excessively long. Many healthcare organizations give low priority to the quality of their waiting areas. Some still use plastic chairs with hard bucket seats connected by a steel rod. Seating with sufficient personal space, attractive designs, and some padding can make the wait more tolerable. Similarly, attractive colors and noise-dampening rugs and drapes can make a difference in how patients see the quality and value of the heathcare experience. If a wait is also uncomfortable because the office or examining room is too hot or too cold, too noisy or too quiet, too dark or too light, too open or too closed, too busily patterned or too bland, or too smelly, the patients notice and find their waits less tolerable. Healthcare organizations should find the ideal balance for each of these factors as they are important to patients.

Create and Implement Wait-Time Standards

An efficiently operating registration process should require only three to five minutes of patient time and should be conducted upon the arrival of each patient with no waiting. Office staff should return phone calls in 20 minutes or less, and physicians should return theirs in an hour. Physicians involved in surgery or emergency care may not always be able to meet this standard, but designated office staff can return the call for the physician to keep the communication channels open. Cell phones and e-mail make these performance standards easier to achieve. Staff should not only inform customers that service will be delayed but should also explain why the delay is occurring. E-mailed updates are also useful, and a website that allows patients to see where they are in a queue also makes the situation better.

Sherman (1999) says no healthcare customer should wait more than 15 minutes for anything without receiving an explanation for the delay, including an apology and an estimate of how long the customer will have to wait to receive the service. Apologies are always a welcome and often surprising option. When delays exceed or are predicted to exceed one hour, the option to reschedule the appointment should be offered, as should paid transportation, if needed. Exhibit 12.1 indicates a possible format for collecting data on patient waiting time.

To correct unacceptable waiting times, an organization should look first at the service delivery system (discussed in Chapter 11). Do patients wait for staff, equipment, test results, or some other reason? Systematically record how long all customers wait and what they are waiting for and periodically summarize these reports, disseminate the information to staff, and use it as a basis for staff discussions about reducing waiting time through system adjustments. The reports can even be used as metrics for performance improvement goals. The American Academy of Family Physicians and the American College of Physicians offer technical help for organizations seeking ways to better schedule patient flow and manage patient time.

Exhibit 12.1 Patient Record Data for Tracking Patient Waiting Times

| | Patient Names | |
	Jane Doe	Harry Smith
Date	2/23/09	2/23/09
Time of appointment	9:00 a.m.	2:30 p.m.
Time of arrival	8:55 a.m.	2:35 p.m.
Time of sign-in	9:00 a.m.	2:35 p.m.
Registration completed	9:05 a.m.	2:39 p.m.
Times of communication regarding appointment		
First	9:10 a.m.	—
Second	9:22 a.m.	—
Third	—	—
Time of exam-room entry	9:27 a.m.	2:50 p.m.
Time of first contact with clinician	9:32 a.m.	3:08 p.m.
Time of last contact with clinician	9:47 a.m.	3:17 p.m.
Time of checkout	9:50 a.m.	3:25 p.m.
Time of departure	9:54 a.m.	3:32 p.m.
Total elapsed time	59 minutes	57 minutes
Service	15 minutes	9 minutes
Waiting	44 minutes	48 minutes

Did the patient receive timely communication about delays? Yes   No

A second strategy is to focus staff attention on the consequences of waiting. Evidence indicates that reducing waits increases customer service, so allowing employees to see the actual wait times experienced by their patients and combining that with performance goal setting may be a powerful motivator to improve wait times. A study by Slowiak, Huitema, and Dickinson (2008) found that setting goals and giving employee feedback reduced wait times in a pharmacy by 20 percent and significantly improved customer satisfaction.

Calculate and Use the Design Day

Whether they realize it or not, or whether they do it consciously or not, all healthcare organizations use the design-day concept. Design-day capacity is a management decision that determines how much capacity will be provided to handle a predetermined amount of demand without compromising the healthcare experience. If demand is less than the design-day model, customers are satisfied but the facility and staff are underutilized. If demand exceeds the design-day capacity, some customers will be dissatisfied. Waiting lines may form on design days, but they will not be so long that customers perceive a decline in the quality or value of their healthcare experience.

Benchmark organizations know just how long waits can be and still remain within limits acceptable to patients. An ED, a walk-in clinic, a pharmacy, or an individual physician's practice might use a 15-minute maximum wait for any one part of the healthcare experience as its criterion. On the design day, the provider does not want anyone to wait longer than this maximum time because surveys have shown that customer perceptions of quality and value decline sharply with longer waits, and longer waits increase the likelihood that the patient will leave. Although 15 minutes is the maximum wait deemed acceptable in the design-day decision, seeing the physician, receiving lab results, or seeing a nurse can take longer than planned. However, based on the accumulated data, a design day that targets a 15-minute maximum wait may be the best balance between the costs of having too much capacity and the patient dissatisfaction of not having enough.

A truly patient-focused healthcare provider may set its design day at a very high level, say 80 to 90 percent—that is, supply will be adequate for demand on 80 to 90 percent of the days of the year—because it appreciates the fact that most patients have only limited time in which to get the necessary treatment and may have other healthcare provider choices besides waiting. A patient with a broken hip cannot wait four weeks for treatment and expect a good medical outcome, so the design-day level for the hospital orthopedic facility must be set at a higher level than, say, for the pharmacy. The same may be true for the ED because many ED patients must be treated quickly.

To provide a healthcare experience of high quality, the organization may set its design day high and build more capacity than might otherwise be practical. The cost of an unhappy or an untreated customer to a major clinic that relies on return visits must be carefully balanced against the costs of building capacity. Similarly, not having adequate capacity to serve the needs of the medical staff (another type of customer) or patient families (another type of customer) will lead to dissatisfied physicians and families looking elsewhere for care.

Calculate and Use the Capacity Day

Many organizations calculate and use a capacity day, which is the maximum number of customers allowed in a facility in a day or at one time. This number may be set by the fire marshal, based on accreditation standards, or based on the number of square feet each patient must have available. The state of California, for example, currently regulates minimum nurse staffing ratios in healthcare facilities, which constrains management's flexibility to modify the capacity day to reflect fluctuations in patient demand. Typically, however, the capacity day is set by the organization to represent a point beyond which overall patient or physician dissatisfaction with waits or delays in service is unacceptable.

Do Nothing

The organization can accept the fact that waits will lead to unhappy patients and hope they are not so unhappy that they vow never to return or are unable to find any alternatives so that they have no choice but to return when they need that organization's medical service. Although there are hospitals located in remote areas, free clinics, or highly regarded medical providers that are so good they can be indifferent to waits, this alternative is becoming less and less desirable in this increasingly competitive world with increasing numbers of healthcare options.

Choosing a Strategy

Organizations can use all of these options in some combination. For example, an ED might decide to turn patients away (if legally permitted), limit usage by diverting patients to other hospitals, build a new facility, expand present capacity, have an on-call staff group that can be summoned when needed, provide diversions for waiting patients with nonemergency needs, improve waiting areas, minimize waits, communicate regularly concerning the reasons for waits, or simply accept higher levels of customer dissatisfaction. Good customer satisfaction research can identify the best strategy. The goal is to find the strategy that ensures the greatest customer satisfaction with the lowest capital and staffing costs and allows both customers and the organization to satisfy their needs.

Baptist Health Care, for example, focused on reducing patient waiting time as part of its customer service program. Lower wait-time standards were established, records were kept for all patients, staff members were held accountable, and several other wait-reduction strategies were implemented. As a result, patient satisfaction scores increased significantly over time and the percentage of patients waiting more than two hours for service or leaving without treatment declined significantly (Studer 2008).

MANAGING THE REALITY OF THE WAIT

Few organizations in any industry have the luxury of adjusting capacity quickly or managing demand by getting customers to show up when the organization wants them to instead of when customers want or need to come. Like organizations in other industries, most healthcare organizations must rely on predicting and managing the inevitable waits that are created when patients arrive seeking treatment. The dilemma for the organization is that although adding staff or capacity costs more, it reduces the wait, which improves the patient-experience quality, patient satisfaction, and patient loyalty. On the other hand, reducing staff saves money but increases the wait, which decreases patient-experience quality, patient satisfaction, and patient loyalty.

How can a healthcare organization find the proper cost–benefit balance? The place to begin is using queuing theory, sometimes called waiting-line theory, and the mathematical solutions this technique offers (VanBerkel and Blake 2007).

Queuing or Waiting-Line Theory

A typical queuing-theory problem might be the following: If an average of five patients per hour arrive at an ED or a public health clinic with a single service provider, and if it takes the service provider an average of nine minutes to treat or attend to a patient, how long does the average patient wait? During an average hour, how many minutes will the service provider be treating patients and how many minutes will the provider be idle?

Most applications of waiting-line theory in the healthcare industry are based on the idea that people who cannot otherwise be scheduled do not arrive in neat patterns. The typical approach is to sample the arrival and the service requirement patterns of patients and use this information to simulate the distribution that best matches the reality for the particular organization's patients. Large clinics or EDs should actually count all of its patients over a period of time, or sample them over a longer period using some appropriate sampling methodology, and let the actual patient patterns represent the distribution of arrival rates and service requirements.

All healthcare providers, regardless of size, should collect these data as well as they can. In this era of inexpensive computer power and software, it should be relatively simple to collect and analyze arrival patterns (as illustrated in Exhibit 12.1) at any physician's office, walk-in clinic, or pharmacy.

All waiting lines have three characteristics that any model must include:

1. *Arrival pattern* is the number of patients arriving and the manner in which they are entering the waiting line. Arrivals can be scheduled, random (e.g., any patients entering an ED), in bulk (e.g., patients arriving after a natural disaster), or in some other distribution that is difficult to describe (e.g.,

patients coming in irregular intervals). Queue management is easiest when patient arrivals can be scheduled. Even if arrivals cannot be strictly scheduled, however, they can sometimes be controlled. For example, a dentist can set aside the first hour of each morning for all dental emergencies. If none show up, the dentist can focus on other practice-related tasks or paperwork.

2. *Queue discipline* is the manner in which arriving patients are served. Options are first-come, first-served; last-come, first-served; or some other set of service rules, such as severity of need. On the battlefield or in the ED, for example, the triage principle is often used. As another example, patients waiting to have their teeth cleaned will not usually object if a patient entering the dentist's office with a painfully swollen jaw is attended to first. Patients understand service rules based on need; they do not understand an implicit rule such as "Answer a phone call before serving the client or patient standing right in front of you."

3. *Time for service* is the amount of time to serve patients. The time boundaries of some healthcare services can be carefully managed, like an MRI or the time spent in the recovery room after a routine appendectomy, but the time required for many services is unpredictable. Some ED patients may suffer from severe wounds, while others may have trivial problems. Some patients want to be treated and then sent home, and others want lots of attention with a flu shot. The amount of time it takes to serve the needs of different patients is as unpredictable as the patients themselves. If the waiting-line model is going to be an aid in managing the wait, it must take this variation into account. Waiting-line theory can be applied to anything that waits in line for something to be done to it. An insurance report waiting to be properly filed or a meal waiting to be served is as queued up and in need of managing as the arriving customer at the ED reception desk.

Types of Queues

The first type of queue is the single-channel, single-phase queue (note: In the following discussion, "channel" refers to a service provider, and "phase" refers to a step in the service experience once it is underway)—one service provider, one step. This queue type is represented in the top illustration in Exhibit 12.2. For example, in a small clinic, a single physician practitioner provides single-phase service to patients, who come in, wait their turn, get treatment, and leave. In a larger, busier setting, patients might stand in any one of several single-channel, single-phase queues

Exhibit 12.2 Basic Queue Types

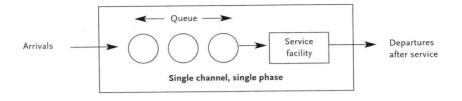

Single channel, single phase

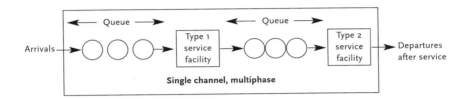

Single channel, multiphase

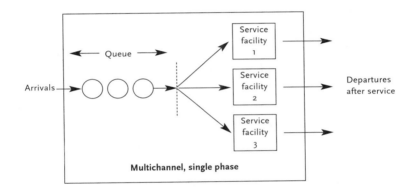

Multichannel, single phase

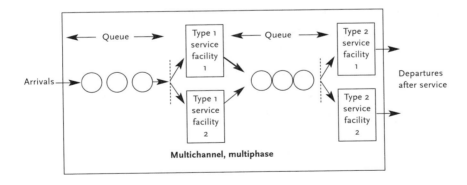

Multichannel, multiphase

to get a flu shot. The patient looks the lines over, chooses one, stands in it to wait for service, and eventually reaches the clinician who gives the shot. Highway toll plazas and McDonald's counters are examples of multiple servers at single-channel queues, but they still represent single-channel, single-phase queues because only one person can be served at a time.

The second type is the single-channel, multiphase queue—for example, a cafeteria line or a medical clinic. Essentially, this type is two or more single-channel, single-phase queues in sequence. The patient waits in one queue for service from a single service provider, then moves on to wait in another queue for another phase of service from another single service provider. At a typical clinic, patients queue up for the various phases. A patient requiring treatment may go to x-ray, then to hematology for a blood sample, and then to a waiting room for the physician.

The third type is the multichannel, single-phase queue in which the patient begins in a single line that then feeds into multiple channels or stations for service, each of which is staffed by a service provider. The patient waits to get to the front of the single line, then goes to the next available channel (service provider) for service. An example is an outpatient lab where everyone waits in a single queue. The queue discipline is to tell the next person in line to come to the next available phlebotomist, who in turn renders a single service (drawing a blood sample) in a single phase.

The Federal Personnel Office uses this method for incoming telephone calls. The automated system tells each caller how many callers are ahead, so the caller can decide whether to wait or call back later. The single phase of service is to have a phone call answered. The multiple channels for obtaining this service are the many operators handling calls. The queue is managed by having the next available operator handle the next caller waiting in line.

Many healthcare organizations find this method the most efficient way to manage their lines as it accounts well for the varying lengths of time it takes to serve different patients. Everyone has had the experience of choosing to stand in one of several available single-channel lines (at the movie theater refreshment stand or the hotel front desk, for example), only to watch all the other lines move much more quickly. The use of a multichannel, single-phase system eliminates this feeling of inequity or bad luck; everyone starts out in the same line.

The last type is the multichannel, multiphase queue system, which is the most complicated to manage. Essentially, it is two or more single-channel, single-phase queues in sequence, which is similar to the current check-in process at U.S. airports. The customer waits to get to the front of one line (check in), and then goes to the next available service provider. After receiving the first phase of service, the customer then gets in another line (security), waits to arrive at the front, and then goes to the next available service provider/channel to receive the next phase of service. In healthcare, a patient may wait in line to see the first available doctor of several on duty. Then the doctor may refer the patient to a lab where the patient waits in line to see the first available lab technician of several on duty.

A healthcare organization will often have numerous queues linked together in various combinations. For example, at a busy government clinic, patients may queue up outside the building before it opens in the morning, queue up at the cashier's office to pay a fee and take a number for consultation with a physician, queue up again in a waiting area for consultation, get in another queue for a specific diagnostic or treatment procedure, and then enter a final queue at the pharmacy if medication is needed.

Managing the wait times associated with single and multiple channels and phases is difficult, but it is critical for ensuring a satisfactory healthcare experience and maximizing the provider's capacity utilization.

Common sense suggests that the best queue type for an organization to use is the one that enables customers to begin receiving service as rapidly as possible. In actuality, the best queue type is the one that best meets patient needs, wants, and expectations. For example, they may prefer to stand in a certain type of line because they think they will be served faster, even if they will not in actuality. For these reasons, organizations must know not only what queue types are most efficient and cost effective but also which queues their customers prefer.

Simulation of Queues

Although a statistical distribution can be used to describe the arrival and service patterns of many standard queues, some situations cannot be described by any statistical distribution; only a simulation will yield the quality of data needed to explain and predict the reality of a particular queue. Here is how a simulation might work.

Take, for example, Aides, an extremely successful crisis help line for patients with AIDS. Aides has 20 telephone lines that, if fully staffed, require one person at each line (for a total of 20 people). If on an average day only 50 patients call in, then full staffing of all the lines is an obvious waste of money because the probability of more than 20 people calling at the same time is small. But if Aides opens only one phone line, most callers will hear a busy signal or be put on hold; they may get no counseling or help but will experience considerable frustration. What staffing level best balances the cost of staffing the phone lines against the cost of frustrated or lost patients?

Over several weeks the floor manager can monitor and record the flow of calls and length of time callers are on a line plus how many times callers receive a busy signal and hang up or are put on hold. If sufficient observations are made, the manager can create distributions that accurately approximate the number of callers, the arrival patterns of their calls, and the time spent asking questions or seeking help. With this information the manager can then simulate the telephone experiences of Aides clients to determine how to staff the phone lines appropriately at different times and on different days of the week. Following is a simple illustration of how that might be done.

In his office, the manager can conduct a Monte Carlo simulation by setting up two roulette wheels that appear in Exhibit 12.3. Spaces are allocated on the first wheel to represent, in percentage form, the time between calls. From the observations already made, the manager knows that 15 percent of the time there was no time (zero minutes) between calls—that is, calls arrived simultaneously. The time between calls was one minute 20 percent of the time, two minutes 25 percent of the time, three minutes 10 percent of the time, four minutes 10 percent of the time, five minutes 12 percent of the time, and six minutes 8 percent of the time. Spaces on the wheel are allocated to reflect these percentages. To simulate the arrival patterns of the phone calls, the manager merely spins the wheel and writes on a chart the arrival time noted in the section of the wheel when it stopped.

The second wheel in Exhibit 12.3 is, in similar fashion, portioned off to represent the observations about how long each caller was on the phone. This total includes the time to answer the call, diagnose the situation, and either refer the caller to some specialized service or listen to and counsel the caller. Because callers vary in their needs and desires, the time for service and the proportions on the wheel representing those times likewise vary. The observations might reveal that 5 percent of calls take one minute; 15 percent take two minutes; 20 percent take three minutes, 25 percent take four minutes, 15 percent take five minutes, 10 percent take six minutes, 5 percent take seven minutes, and 5 percent take eight minutes.

Now the manager can simulate phone demand by spinning the first wheel to randomly determine the time between customer calls and spinning the second wheel to determine how long each customer takes to be served once the phone is answered. By recording the numbers on a simple chart that notes the time between call arrivals, times for service, and the time callers were waiting, the entire day's activities can be simulated to determine the maximum, minimum, and average length of time callers waited for service plus the total waiting time for all callers.

The chart simulates a day's activities by beginning when the phone lines open and recording the calls throughout the day until the phone center closes. Running this simulation many times (typically more than 100 on a computerized model) allows Aides's management to draw some statistical conclusions about the length

Exhibit 12.3 Wheels Representing Time Between Calls and Time for Calls

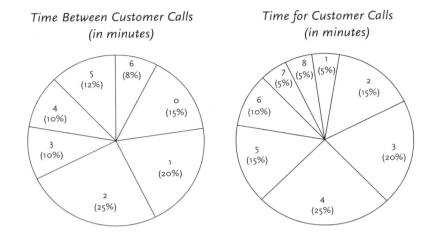

Time Between Customer Calls (in minutes)

Time for Customer Calls (in minutes)

of waiting time, counseling capacity utilization, and impact on waiting (and customer perception of the quality and value of the experience) that opening up more phone lines presents.

Although this is a fairly simple illustration, it shows the usefulness of mathematically determining the relationship between the service provider's capacity and the average waiting time for customers in a way that allows the healthcare organization to find the ideal balance between the two. This same technique can be used to determine the ideal number of monorails in a theme park, toll booths on a turnpike, beds on a hospital floor, servers and cooks in a restaurant, spaces in a parking lot, nurses in an ED, or any other application where an organization needs to balance the costs of providing capacity with the quality of the service experience.

Certain basic forces affect waiting lines, and they can be expressed mathematically. An explanation of the mathematics of waiting lines appears in Sidebar B.

Balancing Capacity and Demand

Determining the proper balance between supply and demand requires more than basic calculations. The AIDS hotline in the previous example has to gather more data about caller behaviors and expectations. If, say, management finds that clients hang up if they are put on hold for more than one minute, then a wait longer than one minute is unacceptable no matter what the remaining data might reveal. On the other hand, if the results show that callers are willing to wait because the help

SIDEBAR B: THE MATHEMATICS OF WAITING LINES

The mathematics are quite simple for a single-channel, single-phase line. An understanding of a few calculations will reveal much about how to manage customer waits. In the following example, we will use a single-channel line for a laboratory facility with one lab technician. We will calculate the average amount of time that a patient waits for service and remains in the system (time waiting plus time being served). In addition, we will determine the idle time of the technician. These figures will be useful to a healthcare manager wishing to control the waiting time for patients and to reduce the idle time for the technician.

These calculations for a single-channel, single-phase line can be done by hand. However, more complicated wait systems requiring more complex formulas should be (and can easily be) analyzed by computer. Standard spreadsheet products, such as Excel, have the capacity to perform a wait analysis.

The Hypothetical Laboratory has a simple waiting room and one technician. Ben Blake, the manager, has been observing the wait at the laboratory for several weeks. Not wanting patients to wait too long, but hesitant to incur the cost of hiring another technician, he wishes to calculate the average wait for his patients over a one-hour period. He also wants to know how much idle time the single technician will have during that hour. If the technician has substantial idle time, Mr. Blake would like for her to perform some routine tasks, such as fill out patient records and consult by phone with other technicians. He has compiled the following information for this one-hour period. For this example, we ignore variability and use averages to describe both arrival and service rates for the lab's patients.

- The average time it takes to treat a patient is four minutes; the technician can treat about 15 patients per hour. This is the service rate—the units of service provider capacity per time period.
- Ten patients are expected to arrive during the hour. This is the *arrival rate*.
- The formulas use the following symbols:
  l = arrival rate per hour (10)
  m = service rate per hour (15)

1. Average time a patient waits:
$Wq = l/m(l-m)$ $Wq = 10/15(15-10)$ $Wq = .133$ hours or 8 minutes
Wq means waiting time before being served. This calculation tells

(Continued)

Mr. Blake that the *average* wait for a patient is 8 minutes. If that wait time is unacceptable to him, he may have to add another technician.

2. Average time a patient spends in the system:
$T_s = 1/m-l$ $\qquad$ $T_s = 1/15-10$ $\qquad$ $T_s = .2$ hours or 12 minutes
This equation tells Mr. Blake that the average patient spends 12 minutes in the system, including both waiting time and service time.

3. Average number of patients waiting:
$L_q = l2/m(m-l)$ $\qquad$ $L_q = 102/15(15-10)$ $\qquad$ $L_q = 1.33$ patients
L_q means the average length of the queue, in number of patients. Knowing that only 1.33 patients are waiting at any one time, on average, reveals to Mr. Blake that the space available in the waiting area is sufficient.

4. Percentage of time the technician is busy:
$b = l/m$ $\qquad$ $b = 10/15$ $\qquad$ $b = 67\%$
The laboratory has one or more patients in it, either waiting or being served, 67 percent of the time, or about 40 minutes out of every hour, on average.

5. Probability that there are no patients in the laboratory at any given time:
$p = 1 - (l/m)$ $\qquad$ $p = 1 - (10/15)$ $\qquad$ $p = 33\%$
This is obviously the inverse of the previous formula. If the wait-plus-treatment system has someone in it about 40 minutes out of each hour, it is empty for the other 20 minutes. Mr. Blake can use this information to assign other tasks to the laboratory technician.

---

line is unique and they need assistance so badly, the help center might be able to let the phone queues grow without much adjustment. The essential feature of the calculation is to determine the point beyond which the length of the wait affects the quality of the client experience beyond the level acceptable to the client and the organization.

Once a decision has been made about capacity and demand balance, the organization has to plan for accommodating the inevitable waiting lines that uneven demand patterns create. Here the challenge is to manage the wait in such a way that the customer is satisfied with it. Two major dimensions are involved. The first is the way the waiting feels to the customer. The second is how to minimize the negative effects of the wait by managing the value of the experience to the customer. The organization wants each customer to conclude that the experience made the wait worthwhile.

A growing number of programs are helping doctors redesign their offices by fixing problems that have long frustrated patients, such as week-long delays to get appointments, hours spent in the waiting room on appointment days, too-brief visits with the doctor, and the near impossibility of getting the physician on the phone (Landro 2006b).

Programs that help doctors in solo and small group practices to work more efficiently heed lessons from other industries (Landro 2006b). One approach relies on calculations used by airlines, hotels, and restaurants to predict demand. The idea is that through better use of demand and capacity management strategies doctors can cut patient waits in much the same way restaurants seat diners and turn over tables efficiently. Other approaches involve relatively simple changes such as leaving afternoon appointments open for urgent visits, having patients fill out paperwork ahead of time online, or providing follow-up care through a phone call or an e-mail rather than taking up valuable office time. Kaiser Permanente has launched a program to help the 12,000 doctors who contract with its health plan to increase their efficiency by using a new electronic medical records system.

Weiss (2003) recommends the following practices for wait management:

- Do the math to make sure the schedule is not too tightly packed.
- Keep things moving during the day by having the right staff in the right place at the right time, appointing a patient-flow coordinator to keep things moving, not trying to do it all, setting aside time for returning phone calls and doing administrative tasks, allowing after-hours visits, and using modern technology.
- Provide continual communication to patients while they wait.
- Make sure the patient is provided with a variety of waiting room diversions, or perhaps include pagers as some restaurants provide so that the patient can leave the office for a while.

In many hospitals, ED patients are now able to check themselves in at computer kiosks (Stengle 2008). For instance, Parkland Memorial Hospital in Dallas, Texas, has three self-service computer kiosks, similar to those used by airport passengers and hotel guests. Patients spend about eight minutes at the kiosks using touch screens to enter their name, age, and other personal information and the ailments they would like to see addressed. A nurse monitors the screen to assess patient information, and those with chest pains, stroke symptoms, and other worrisome complaints take priority. The result is a shorter ED wait at Parkland.

Often, family members are left in waiting rooms with little or no information about the condition of their hospitalized loved ones. Creighton University Medical Center in Omaha, Nebraska, has addressed this problem by posting up-to-date patient information on an electronic screen in the waiting room. To protect patient identity, families are given a case number that represents their loved ones. (O'Connor 2007). In some hospitals, a color-coded system is used. Other hospitals have pagers that alert family members that they should go to the information desk. Such processes try to give family members information in real time.

THE PERCEPTION OF THE WAIT

Understanding what makes time fly or drag while a person is waiting is a fundamental concern in improving the quality of the patient wait. The research on the perception of waits has long supported the importance of managing this (DeMan et al. 2005; McKim et al. 2007). Mowen, Licata, and McPhail (1993), for example, studied the perception of waits in an ED and found that patients who received time estimates were more satisfied than those who did not. Healthcare managers must remember that everyone is different, that individual differences will influence how people feel about waiting in line, and that how people feel about the wait is at least as important as how long the wait actually is. Following are factors that influence customers' perceptions of a wait.

Occupied Time

As noted earlier, most line waits can be made to seem more enjoyable and less lengthy if people waiting can be distracted or diverted in some way. Many clinics and physician offices have gone beyond the traditional magazine rack by offering interactive video devices that help patients pass the time productively by learning something about their health. A cancer specialist might offer an interactive video that answers typical questions asked by new patients, or a dentist might feature a video describing a procedure to whiten teeth. A children's practice might offer toys in a play area, and a physician's waiting room might have a television showing CNN.

The Walt Disney Company is the master of managing time waits by providing diversion to its waiting guests. If the line for a particular attraction has become extraordinarily long, a strolling band, acrobats, or some other distraction is sent to entertain and occupy the guests. Although bands and acrobats might be inappropriate in a healthcare setting, pleasant diversions or distractions appropriate to the situation can be provided for customers.

Time Spent Waiting for a Service Versus Time Spent Receiving the Service

In many offices, before patients are examined by the doctor, they are interviewed by a nurse who listens to the medical complaint, gathers vital signs, and generally obtains information. By the time patients are actually seen by the doctor, they have already had considerable contact with a medical person, so the wait to see the doctor does not feel so long.

Another way to spend the wait time is to teach patients in line what they are supposed to do once they reach the treatment area. The education provided during the wait time can improve or enhance the service experience and, in that way, actually becomes part of the experience. Videos in an orthodontist's office can teach kids how to insert and remove their retainers before they actually get them. The orthodontist does not have to spend so much time teaching, and patients are engaged before being fitted for the device. Some organizations use a similar technique while placing callers on hold. Callers listen to a range of options in the phone menu, which helps them make the right choice. They may also be presented with recorded instructional material so they may be better informed when they talk to a real person. Most medical offices require patients to fill out lengthy medical history forms. These forms provide useful information, but they also give patients something to do, which reduces how long the wait feels.

Anxious Waits

To patients who are apprehensive about what will happen to them during an upcoming operation or about the results of a diagnostic procedure, the wait will seem endless. Communication geared to reducing anxiety during such waits is highly desirable. For most people, waiting to be discharged to go home is one of the longest waits they face. They are so anxious to leave that any time spent waiting is too long.

Uncertain Lengths of Wait

Providing a time estimate can help those waiting because they can see the end in sight. The wait before a scheduled appointment is bearable because the patient knows how long the wait will be, but once the appointment time is reached, in the patient's mind it is time to be served, and any time spent waiting after that will feel longer. One orthopedic hospital discovered that by having the nursing staff in the preoperative areas periodically check back with patients and update them on what was happening, patient satisfaction was significantly improved.

Unexplained Waits

When a patient does not know what is holding up the line or causing the delay, the wait feels longer. Effective managers keep people who are waiting informed, or they provide visual cues that explain the wait. For example, a longer-than-expected wait in a doctor's waiting room can be improved by explaining to those waiting that the doctor's schedule was interrupted by a serious emergency. On the other hand, effective managers of queues will ensure that unoccupied laboratory personnel or empty treatment rooms are kept out of the sight of waiting patients so that managers do not have to explain why their personnel are not serving patients or why their treatment rooms have no one in them while the waiting room is full.

Unfair Waits

If customers think the queue discipline is being consistently followed and fairly used, then the wait seems shorter than when they think people are being served out of sequence. Good organizations recognize this truth and manage their lines accordingly. At times, patients who are very sick or in some other special category require the line discipline to be broken. These patients can perhaps be brought in through another entrance so those waiting do not notice that the discipline has been interrupted. For example, the ambulance entrance to the ED is usually some distance from the walk-in entrance. This separation allows emergency patients to be served first and provides easy access for ambulances. Organizations that for one reason or another need to break the queue discipline must find some way to communicate a reason for the apparent unfairness that patients will accept, such as "Heart attack case coming through!" or "Abdominal gunshot wound!" People generally defer their own needs to accommodate other people's more immediate needs as long as they know why. For example, passengers needing assistance board planes first and nobody minds, drivers pull over to let emergency vehicles move past the traffic queue, and people seldom complain when a disabled person goes to the front of the line.

Solo Waits Versus Group Waits

Waiting by yourself feels longer than waiting with family or friends or even with people you do not know. Facilities that recognize this perceptual issue try to organize their waits in such a way that people are grouped with other people. Under this logic, a double line feels shorter than a single line, and a line structure that encourages people to interact feels shorter than one in which people are allowed to stay inside their own personal and highly individual spaces. In some waiting room areas, seating might be arranged to promote interaction and a sense of being part of a group.

Uncomfortable Waits

Finding a way to keep people comfortable while they wait for treatment is a managerial challenge. Besides the obvious methods, such as providing comfortable seats and air conditioning or heating, healthcare providers must take special care of those with special medical needs. For example, a seriously injured person is immediately given pain medication, and a comfortable bed is quickly found for the victim of a possible heart attack.

Uninteresting Waits

Because most people like to talk about themselves, they will be interested in conversing with someone who asks them questions. Having a nurse or a clinical assistant ask questions, take body measurements, and generally pay attention to the patient will make the wait time more interesting. Providing interactive games and other pleasant distractions may also make the wait more interesting.

Other Considerations

In all of these waiting situations, the customer's emotional state will have a significant impact on the wait for service. Different people react differently to anxiety, uncertainty, pain, and other perceived influences on the waiting time. If the waiting line is composed of people with diverse needs, the typical customer may drive the design of the line and the associated wait. Although managers must consider individual needs as much as possible in designing and managing waits, the queue for a large customer volume must be designed to accommodate the waiting expectations of a typical, average customer.

However, if the people in line are a more select clientele with identifiable features (e.g., big donors), then variability in treatment of the waiting customers should be planned to meet that group's expectations for an upscale level of service. Making the wait enjoyable or at least bearable is harder to do for a mass-market customer base than for a select, known clientele.

In all of these waiting situations, the contrast effect will also influence the perception of the wait. If a customer's first wait is comfortable, totally explained, and predictable, and the second wait is unpredictable, anxiety producing, and of uncertain length, the second wait will feel longer and less satisfying than the well-managed first wait. Similarly, if a customer has just had a long wait, a short one will feel even shorter in contrast. If the customer has just been in a waiting situation where employees were friendly and all staff were busy assisting customers, that wait will in retrospect seem shorter than a wait of identical length in which employees seem unfriendly and engaged in activities other than serving people who are waiting.

The key is to remember that the customer perceives the wait through his particular perspective despite the reality. If the objective data say the wait at your facility is not too long or the average wait at your organization is shorter than it is at a competitor's, those data do not matter to customers who think they have waited too long for your service. Customers have mental clocks that tell them when the wait is too long and when it is just right and extremely well managed. Managing the perception is as effective a technique as managing the actual waiting time, and if the organization is particularly good at managing perceptions, it can make even very long waits acceptable and tolerable to customers.

Perceived Value of Service

The more value the customer receives or expects to receive from the service, the more the customer will wait without complaining or being dissatisfied. Because the customer defines the value of services rendered, the perceived value of the service for which the customer is waiting must be managed. This strategy can be implemented before, during, or even after the service is performed.

Before receiving the service, waiting customers can be provided with information (or even with some other service) that will enhance the value of the service that motivated them to enter the queue in the first place. A health spa or wellness center, for example, can offer customers waiting in line healthy snacks or fruit or can play chamber music in the background. Such thoughtful touches not only distract and occupy the customer but also add value to the experiences that the spa and center are selling and for which the customer must wait.

During the performance of the service, its value (to the customer and as defined by the customer) can be enhanced over the customer's expectations by a number of strategies. The organization will want to use these strategies in any event, but if the service meets or exceeds expectations when the customer gets it, the wait will probably seem worthwhile. Besides providing customers with a service that is beyond their expectations in the first place, some subtle actions can enhance the value of the service experience. For example, some hospitals display their accreditation certificate, and some doctors display diplomas from medical schools to indicate the quality of their training. These touches tend to encourage the patient to think the medical treatment was worth the wait.

As a more direct response to the wait, the service provider can apologize for and explain any unusual factors that may have caused the wait. Apologizing adds a personal touch that may enhance the value of the experience for the customer. For example, a family physician extends his apologies to patients in the waiting room when he is running late on schedule. He says, "It never fails to bring smiles when I acknowledge that the patient's time is as important as mine" (Weiss 2003, 81).

Today, many healthcare organizations instruct their medical staff to apologize for inevitable waits, while other hospitals ask staff to act as patients so that they can understand what service waits feel like. Increasing their sensitivity to patient waits raises the possibility that staff will proactively engage the waiting patients and better manage their experience.

After the service, the value of the experience can sometimes be enhanced to make the customers feel better about having taken the time to wait in the first place. Although advertising is generally used to attract the attention of potential customers, people who have already purchased services are even more attentive to ads than those who have not. The ads reinforce their wisdom in not only purchasing the service but also waiting in line to do so. Ads seen ahead of time can also reduce the effects of the wait while it is in progress; by convincing customers that the experience will be worth the wait, they will wait more patiently. Some organizations have found that a follow-up phone call asking a customer for reactions to the service can enhance the value of the experience and reduce the negative effects of the wait.

CONCLUSION

Managing the customer's wait is a fundamental challenge for healthcare managers. Service cannot be stockpiled or inventoried, and the organization must find the right balance between having enough physical and personnel capacity to fill demand and having so much capacity that some healthcare services sit idle most of the time. In a perfect world, the flow of customers exactly matches the supply: When one patient leaves the facility, another walks in the door seeking medical care; when the physician finishes with one patient, another arrives; and so on across the entire range of services offered by healthcare organizations. In our less-than-perfect world, effective queue management can get patients into the medical setting and meet their time expectations to their satisfaction.

Service Strategies

1. Manage the wait; do not just let it happen.
2. Know how long customers are willing to wait without becoming dissatisfied.
3. Know the psychology of waits and manage waits to minimize customer dissatisfaction.
4. Use queuing or waiting-line models to understand how queues work.
5. Build in adequate capacity, and manage demand by calculating and implementing design days and capacity days.
6. Minimize the negative effects of the wait before, during, and after the healthcare experience.
7. Create and implement performance standards for waiting times.
8. To better balance capacity with demand, find out how much a dissatisfied customer costs the organization.

Standards—being able to specify what good, bad, and great service look like—
are prerequisites to asking people to deliver.
—Karl Albrecht and Ron Zemke

CHAPTER 13

Measuring the Quality
of the Healthcare Experience

Service Principle:
Measure the important things, and then pursue
the superb healthcare experience relentlessly

ALL CUSTOMERS EXPECT to have an outstanding experience every time. Even though they know perfection is elusive, they hope that whatever errors happen will not happen to them. All healthcare organizations face rising patient expectations and patients who are increasingly unwilling to settle for less than they think they are entitled to. Customer activism coupled with growing access to information have made service quality more important than ever as healthcare managers strive to identify and meet heightened patient expectations for their healthcare experiences.

Service quality has become an important competitive advantage in today's healthcare market (Berry 2009). Indeed, some evidence suggests that the process quality of providing healthcare (the how) is as important as the clinical quality (the what) (Marley, Collier, and Goldstein 2004). Because most patients are unable to accurately assess the quality of their clinical care, they rely on the quality of the processes they observe and the way they are treated to determine the quality of their patient experience (Otani, Kurz, and Harris 2005).

Consequently, the Malcolm Baldrige award for excellence in healthcare includes "focus on patients, other customers and markets" as one of the assessment factors. Research continues to suggest that the Baldrige criteria affect patient satisfaction (Goldstein and Schweikhart 2002; Naveh and Stern 2005). Healthcare providers that seek this prestigious award are paying more attention to both clinical quality in patient care and the process by which this care is delivered.

An obvious way of creating a flawless experience for tomorrow's patients is for the organization to know what errors are being made or what problems are occurring now. Therefore, measuring the quality of the healthcare experience is an increasingly important part of the leadership responsibility of the healthcare organization (Marley, Collier, and Goldstein 2004). Satisfied patients prefer to come back to the healthcare provider that met or exceeded their expectations for clinical and patient experience outcomes. Dissatisfied patients seek to go somewhere else when they have other healthcare options (Boshoff and Gray 2004; Rohini and Mahadevappa 2006).

The best time to find out about possible problems in the patient experience is before the patient leaves the healthcare facility, while the information is still fresh in the patient's mind. Finding out on the spot also gives the organization the opportunity to recover from problems before the patient leaves angry over some error or mistake that might have been corrected if someone had asked.

Accurately measuring what patients think about their experience in physical therapy, their overall hospital stay, or their experience in obtaining laboratory tests is a difficult challenge for healthcare organizations striving to achieve service excellence. Nevertheless, it must be done—preferably before the patient leaves—and it's best to do this consistently and carefully.

In this chapter, we address the following:

- How the patient perceives the quality of the healthcare experience
- How healthcare managers can see problems from the patient's perspective
- Measurement methods that show the organization where it needs to improve or change its service, setting, and delivery system to meet patient expectations

The critical challenge for healthcare managers is identifying and implementing the methods that best measure the quality of the experience from the patient's point of view. As we have stated throughout this book, the patient determines quality and value. Consequently, what is an acceptable experience for one patient might be a superb experience for another and a serious problem to a third.

The subjective nature of the quality and value of a healthcare experience makes identifying and implementing the appropriate measurement particularly difficult. No matter how well management or the medical staff plan a treatment, surgery, or therapy, the quality of the healthcare experience cannot be measured until the patient experiences it.

A variety of methods are available to measure the quality of the healthcare experience. These methods differ in cost, accuracy, and degree of patient inconvenience.

Measuring healthcare quality can have many organizational benefits, but as usual the benefits must be balanced against the costs of obtaining them.

In other words, the organization must balance the information needed and the extent and precision of the research expertise required to gather and interpret it against the availability of funding. As a rule, the more accurate and precise the information, the more expensive it is to acquire. Typically, organizations use both qualitative and quantitative methods. Each will be discussed in the sections that follow.

QUALITATIVE METHODS

Qualitative techniques are generally less expensive than quantitative methods. Exhibit 13.1 outlines the major qualitative techniques and their advantages and disadvantages. The qualitative techniques include management observation, employee feedback programs (e.g., work teams, quality circles), and focus groups.

Qualitative measures should have a quantitative component. Excellent healthcare managers seek to make quantitative even the most qualitative assessments by systematically recording what they observe or hear. If a manager encounters an angry patient with a complaint, the manager should have a record that four previous angry patients said the same thing. This systematic approach allows even the most qualitative assessment process to take on many of the beneficial features of the most quantitatively precise process.

Management Observation

The simplest and least expensive technique for assessing quality is to encourage managers to keep their eyes open, especially to the interactions between staff and patients and other customers, and to talk to employees and patients. This technique has been called "management by walking around," or MBWA. Some healthcare organizations, borrowing a term from the restaurant industry, call it "walking the front," which means observing what is happening firsthand, looking for problems or inefficiencies, talking to patients and staff to assess their reactions, finding solutions to any patient problems encountered, and sharing with staff any information that might enable them to improve the healthcare experience. More recently, other healthcare experts have borrowed the term "rounding" from the clinical side to describe this managerial technique. Indeed, Studer (2008) is so convinced of the

Exhibit 13.1 Advantages and Disadvantages of Various Qualitative Techniques for Measuring Patient Service Quality

Management Techniques	Advantages	Disadvantages
Management observation	• Management knows business, policies, and procedures • No inconvenience to patient • Opportunity to recover from service failure • Opportunity to obtain detailed patient feedback • Opportunity to identify service delivery problems • Minimal incremental cost for data gathering	• Management presence may influence service providers • Lacks statistical validity and reliability • Objective observation requires specialized training • Employees disinclined to report problems they created • Management may be unfamiliar with processes and customers
Employee feedback programs	• Employees have knowledge of service delivery obstacles • Patients volunteer service experience information to employees • No inconvenience to patients • Opportunity to recover from service failure • Opportunity to collect detailed patient feedback • Minimal incremental cost for data gathering and documentation	• Objective observation requires specialized training • Employees not inclined to report problems they created
Work teams and quality circles	• Develops employee awareness of management's strong commitment to service quality • Develops an understanding and appreciation of how each employee can directly influence service quality	• Employees may wish to avoid responsibilites of empowerment • Team may not act cohesively and work together • Necessary communication among team members takes large amount of time

(Continued)

Exhibit 13.1 (continued)

	Strengths	Weaknesses
Work teams and quality circles (con't)	• Through empowerment, improves employee morale, productivity, efficiency, effectiveness, and patient satisfaction • Team working together conveys confidence and competence to patients	
Focus groups	• Opportunity to collect detailed patient feedback • Opportunity to recover from service failure • Qualitative analysis helps to focus managers on problem areas • Other problems may surface during discussions • Suggests that facility is interested in patients' opinions of service quality	• May only identify symptoms and not core service delivery problems • Feedback limited to small group of customers • Recollection of specific service encounter details may be lost • One group member may dominate or bias discussion • Inconvenience necessitates incentives for participation • High cost of properly trained focus group leader • Information may be withheld due to fear of disapproval by others • May not be representative sample of the patient population
Service guarantees	• Provides feedback on service failures in significant areas • Enhances both measurement and marketing	• Self-selected sample of patients not statistically representative • Some patients may take advantage of organization

Source: Adapted with permission from R. C. Ford, S. A. Bach, and M. D. Fottler, "Methods of Measuring Patient Satisfaction in Health Care Organizations," 22 (2), page 77, © 1997, Aspen Publishers, Inc.

merits of this tool that he devotes two chapters in his book to rounding—one on rounding with employees and one on rounding with customers.

Managers know their own healthcare operation and its goals, capabilities, and healthcare quality standards. They know, at least from the managerial perspective, when staff members are delivering a high-quality experience.

Managerial observations do not inconvenience patients or staff, and they often permit immediate correction of patient-service problems. Everyone, including patients, appreciates being asked by a manager what he or she thought of the experience. Asking is strong evidence that the organization cares about service quality and is committed to helping employees deliver it.

Furthermore, managerial observation gives supervisors the opportunity to recognize, reinforce, and reward an excellent employee and coach an employee who might not be delivering the service as it should be delivered. It also provides a teaching opportunity where a supervisor who observes a service problem can model the way to fix it. Moreover, when managers walk the front to act as coaches and not as spies, their presence has a favorable influence on employee attitudes and performance as well as on patient satisfaction.

Relying only on managerial observation for assessing service quality has its downsides, however. Some managers may not have enough experience or training to fully understand what they are observing; they may have biases that influence their objectivity; they may not know how to effectively coach an employee or handle a distraught customer; or they may be too busy with paperwork or unwilling to make the time to actively observe.

Also, when employees know managers are observing the service delivery process, they invariably perform it differently. In addition, although management observation may ensure the quality of the experience for a particular patient, even the most energetic manager cannot watch every patient–employee interaction. An unobserved patient's reactions to an unobserved experience remain unknown to the manager.

Training healthcare managers in how to observe employee–patient interactions, measure these interactions against quality standards, and coach providers and employees can eliminate or at least reduce personal bias. Managers may think they have no time to observe interactions, but they could be wrong when they review their own time usage. Unobtrusive observational techniques, random observations, and video cameras can diminish employee awareness that the boss is watching.

For example, many organizations tell their telephone operators and callers that all phone conversations "may be monitored for training purposes" to eliminate the observation bias by making it uncertain when management is actually listening in. The operators know someone may always be listening, so they do the job by the book. Some larger companies use managers from one location to observe employees at another location for the same reason. The increasing use of video monitoring to enhance security has had the unintended but beneficial consequence of encouraging employees to think of themselves as being under constant supervision. For obvious ethical reasons, employees and customers should be alerted that they may be monitored.

Employee Feedback

Employee feedback should supplement management observation. Employees can provide input on such issues as cumbersome organizational policies and control procedures, managerial reporting structures, or other processes that inhibit effective healthcare service delivery. They know firsthand about organizational impediments that prevent them from delivering high-quality service (Gupta 2008).

In fact, a study by the authors (Fottler et al. 2006) found that a focus group of employees identified the same problems with more detail than a customer focus group. This raises the possibility of using employee focus groups as a less expensive alternative to customer focus groups or even employee surveys for discovering issues and concerns in the healthcare organization that interfere with patient service quality. The study concluded that employees know what is wrong with the patient experience and are glad to tell when management asks.

Employee work teams and quality service circles are other sources of feedback. Such techniques foster an understanding and appreciation of how each employee can directly influence service quality. Employee awareness of management's strong commitment to healthcare quality is affirmed when work teams are asked to review all aspects of the customer service experience. Use of work teams requires the organization to invest in employee training and to allow team members the time to meet. This step sends two important messages: (1) Management trusts employees' ability to find and fix problems, and (2) the organization is truly committed to service if it spends precious resources on providing it.

Another employee feedback process is the patient ombudsman position. The ombudsman is responsible for seeking out patients to hear their concerns and reporting these problems to someone who can address them, if the ombudsman does not have the ability to fix them. Generally, the ombudsman is viewed as a resourceful, friendly, trustworthy employee to whom customers can air out their grievances without fear of repercussions. Typically, the ombudsman reports directly to a senior manager who oversees patient satisfaction efforts.

For example, in one hospital, the "cheer bringer," who previously delivered cards and flowers to patients, was given the ombudsman role after management realized that the hospital had no formal complaint procedure. Inpatients were not likely to complain about the staff as they feared retaliation or mistreatment. With her new ombudsman role, the cheer bringer went around asking patients of their concerns. Because the cheer bringer was already a well-liked and trusted staff member, she was the ideal person to approach patients about their complaints.

Focus Groups

Focus groups provide in-depth information on how patients and other customers view the service they receive. Typically, a focus group of six to ten persons gathers with a facilitator for several hours to discuss real or imagined problems and to make suggestions. Many service organizations routinely invite customers to participate in focus groups. These invitations show customers that the company cares enough about their reactions to ask them to participate, and customers appreciate the dollars, complimentary dinner, or other expression of appreciation that typically compensates them for their time.

One reason organizations use focus groups is to supplement survey results, which often fail to produce information that is useful for program improvement because the information is not discriminating or comprehensive enough (Berry 2009). Surveys only tell management what the survey measures and not necessarily what is really important to the patient. Surveys may only ask for satisfaction ratings about areas that are not key drivers of customer (patient and staff) satisfaction.

Surveys generally are limited to asking about what happened in the past and not about what the patient desires in the future. In addition, surveys rely on patients' memories of experiences they are frequently eager to forget. Finally, surveys may too narrowly frame the range of possible responses, which could result in overestimating satisfaction (Fottler et al. 2006).

Patient focus groups can provide valuable feedback about what patients expect, and they are particularly effective in identifying factors patients find important or missing (Fottler et al. 2006). Because focus group questions are open ended and amplification is invited, participants' experiences, opinions, expectations, and suggestions are likely to be richer in content and context than survey data.

Service Guarantees

The service guarantee method is based on a given customer's subjective perception of whether an aspect of the service was or was not completely satisfactory. Promises such as "satisfaction guaranteed or your money back; no questions asked" and "satisfaction guaranteed or get 50 percent off your next purchase" have worked well across the service industry. A longitudinal study by Hays and Hill (2006) found that service guarantees have a positive, long-term effect on both employee motivation and customer intention to return. This study strongly supports using a service guarantee to improve customer loyalty and to increase employee motivation.

JetBlue is one organization that provides a service guarantee, and that guarantee is spelled out in its customer bill of rights (Airoldi 2007):

- JetBlue compensates customers if, as a result of JetBlue's decisions, an airplane takes more than 30 minutes to reach the gate after it lands.
- For arrival delays, customers receive vouchers applicable to the purchase of future flights: $25 for delays of up to 1 hour, $100 for delays of 1 to 2 hours, the cost of a one-way ticket identical to the one purchased for a 2- to 4-hour delay, and the cost of a roundtrip ticket for delays of more than 4 hours.
- JetBlue gives customers a $100 voucher for departure delays of 3 hours and a voucher for a new trip after 4 hours. People are removed from the airplane after delays of 5 hours.
- JetBlue provides customers with $1,000 in cash, rather than the $400 the federal government requires, if they are ever denied boarding.

By contrast, such guarantees and patient bills of rights are quite rare in healthcare. According to one classic study, the average business spends six times more money on marketing to potential new customers than it does working to keep the customers it has (Sherman and Sherman 1998, 164). Some evidence suggests that acquiring new customers is cheaper than retaining current ones, but some healthcare insiders argue for the exact opposite (East, Hammond, and Gendall 2006).

Healthcare facilities focus their marketing programs on recruiting new customers, yet they typically offer no quality or satisfaction guarantees to their current or prospective customers to assure them of the excellence of their healthcare service. So why do healthcare organizations not offer guarantees that are similar to those offered by other service businesses? They should be able to at least guarantee that staff will answer the phone in a reasonable period of time, patient paperwork will be minimized, food will equal restaurant quality, wait times at discharge and clinical locations will be minimal, all facilities will be clean, and staff members will be friendly and respectful.

According to Fabien (2005), service guarantees provide a number of important advantages to organizations, including organizational learning. If a company has a strong and well-understood service guarantee that is invoked by its customers, everyone in that organization learns about the service delivery system. Similarly, Hart (1988) lists several important benefits of a service guarantee:

- It forces everyone to think about the service from the customer's point of view because the customer decides whether or not to invoke it.
- It pinpoints where the service failed because the customer must give the reason for invoking the guarantee, and that reason then becomes measurement data on the service delivery system. A patient complaint is a good thing for a healthcare organization that hopes to be perfect. Guarantees are an incentive to get customers to complain if their expectations (and the guarantee's terms) have not been met, and these complaints then help the organization to fix whatever is wrong before other customers have problems.
- It gets everyone to focus quickly on the problem at hand because the costs of making good on guarantees can be quite large. Once a customer has to invoke the guarantee, the cost of the lost revenue forces management to direct its attention at correcting the problem.
- It enhances the likelihood of recovery from a service problem because the patient is encouraged to demand instant recovery, instead of writing a complaint letter and taking the business to a competitor.
- It sends a strong message to employees and customers alike that the organization takes its healthcare quality seriously and will stand behind it.

Sidebar A provides classic service guarantee criteria from Hart (1988).

QUANTITATIVE METHODS

Although qualitative methods for assessing service quality have their benefits, good organizations are even more interested in measuring what patients themselves (and sometimes their families) think about their experiences in some quantitative format. Patients are typically willing to tell healthcare providers what they liked or did not like about their experience. Studer (2008) stresses the importance of this. A large body of literature describes a variety of techniques to gather patient satisfaction and perceptions of service quality data (e.g., National Quality Forum 2005; Ford, Bach, and Fottler 1997). Techniques to collect data directly from patients vary in cost, convenience, objectivity, and statistical validity.

Exhibit 13.2 provides an overview of patient-sourced quantitative methods and shows the advantages and disadvantages of each technique.

CRITERIA FOR A SERVICE GUARANTEE

1. *Unconditional.* The more asterisks or conditions attached to the bottom of the page and the more fine print, the less credible the guarantee will seem to employees and customers. Few or no conditions should be required to use the guarantee.

2. *Easy to understand and communicate.* The more complicated the guarantee is, the less likely anyone will believe or use it.

3. *Focused on the customer's needs.* The guarantee should solve the customer's problems, not fit the organization's needs.

4. *Clear on defining the standard for healthcare quality.* If you are going to guarantee it, you better deliver it the way you are supposed to.

5. *Meaningful to the customer and the organization.* If invoking the guarantee only partially solves the customer's problem or is of little consequence to the organization, neither the customer nor the service people will value the guarantee.

6. *Easy to use.* Invoking the guarantee and receiving its benefits should be painless for the patient. The harder a guarantee is to use, the less credible it will be, and the less likely it will help identify serious service problems.

7. *A declaration of trust.* This trust extends to the customers you are trusting to use it only when they have a legitimate complaint and the employees you are trusting to correct the customer's problem quickly, fairly, and effectively without giving away the whole organization.

8. *Credible or believable by the customer.* If customers do not believe you will really make good, then they will not use the guarantee.

Source: Adapted by permission of *Harvard Business Review* from "The Power of Unconditional Service Guarantees," by C. W. L. Hart, 66 (4): 54–62. Copyright © 1988 by the Harvard Business School of Publishing Corporation; all rights reserved.

Performance Standards

Outstanding organizations develop quantitative performance standards and measurements so that employees can monitor their own actions. Some standards are used throughout the industry—for example, 3 minutes to respond to a Code Blue, 20 minutes for breakfast trays to be served after arriving on the floor, and 5 minutes for a room call light to be answered.

Most standards are specific to the organizations that create them and are designed to meet or beat the competition and to meet patient expectations. Emergency departments define how many minutes it should take for a newly arrived patient to be triaged. If it has not happened in, say, 5 minutes, then the healthcare quality standard has not been met. Nurses may use a measure of the number of

Exhibit 13.2 Advantages and Disadvantages of Various Quantitative Techniques for Measuring Patient Service Quality

Management Techniques	Advantages	Disadvantages
Comment cards	• Suggests that facility is interested in patients' opinions of service quality • Opportunity to recover from service failure • Minimal incremental cost for data gathering • Moderate cost	• Self-selected sample of patients not statistically representative • Comments generally reflect extreme patient dissatisfaction or extreme satisfaction
Mail surveys	• Ability to gather representative and valid samples of targeted patients • Opportunity to recover from service failure • Patients can reflect on their service experience • Suggests that facility is interested in patients' opinions of service quality • Allows comparisons of patient satifaction by department and patient demographics	• Recollection of specific service encounter details may be lost • Other service experiences may bias responses because of time lag • Inconvenience necessitates incentives for participants • Cost to gather representative sample may be high • Potential problems with the wording of questions
On-site personal interviews	• Opportunity to collect detailed patient feedback • Opportunity to recover from service failure • Ability to gather representative and valid sample of targeted patients • Suggests that facility is interested in patients' opinions of service quality	• May not be representative sample of patients • Other service experiences may bias responses • Respondents tend to give socially desirable responses • Inconvenience necessitates incentives for participants • Cost moderate to high

(Continued)

Exhibit 13.2 (continued)

Telephone interviews	• Opportunity to collect detailed patient feedback • Ability to gather representative and valid sample of targeted patients • Opportunity to recover from service failure • Suggests that facility is interested in patients' opinions of service quality	• Individuals tend to find telephone calls intrusive • Difficult to contact people at work; inconvenient at home • Costs of skilled interviewers and valid instrument are high • May not generate a representative cross-section of patients
Mystery shoppers	• Consistent and unbiased feedback • Can focus on specific situations • No inconvenience to patient • Opportunity to collect detailed customer feedback • Allows measurement of training program effectiveness	• Snapshot of isolated encounters may be statistically invalid • Cost moderate to high • Not applicable to all clinical areas (e.g., surgery) • Ethical concerns

Source: Adapted with permission from R. C. Ford, S. A. Bach, and M. D. Fottler, "Methods of Measuring Patient Satisfaction in Health Care Organizations," 22 (2), page 81, © 1997, Aspen Publishers, Inc.

rings for answering a patient call. If a nurse has not responded to the call within a certain number of rings, the quality standard has not been met.

These are examples of the types of standards that can be developed, measured, and used as ways to ensure that the healthcare experience is delivered as it should be. In his classic work *Quality Is Free*, quality expert Phillip Crosby (1978) notes that the price of not conforming to a quality standard can be calculated as the cost to fix errors and failures that result from not meeting quality standards in the first place. Some organizations may think that determining the cost of not answering the phone within three rings is impossible, but healthcare experts are convinced otherwise (e.g., Studer 2008).

To prevent customer service problems, an organization's own performance standards should exceed those of all but the most demanding patients. If they do, the organization's internal control measures may sometimes show that a standard has not been met, even if patients seem satisfied and no one complains. When that happens, some organizations in the service industry actually apologize.

Patients will remember healthcare organizations that behave this way as much as they remember other service organizations that have learned the power of the apology. Healthcare executives may fear that offering apologies may lead to a lawsuit, because an apology may seem like an admission of liability, but benchmark healthcare organizations have learned how to gain the benefits of offering apologies without admitting liability.

Comment Cards

Comment cards are the cheapest and easiest to use of all data-collection methods. If properly designed, they are easy to tally and analyze. These advantages make them attractive for gathering patient satisfaction data, especially for smaller organizations that cannot afford a quality assessment staff or consultants. Comment cards rely on voluntary patient participation and involve patients rating the quality of the healthcare experience by responding to a few simple questions on a conveniently available form, typically a postcard. Patients deposit the form in a box placed near the healthcare facility exit, return it directly to the service provider, or mail it to the organization's office.

Following are six reasons to use comment cards (Szwarc 2005):

1. To identify the particular needs and concerns of each major customer group
2. To be able to quickly and accurately assess the impact of service improvements from the customers' point of view

3. To speed up the feedback cycle, so customer input is gathered quickly
4. To have an easy method for getting candid feedback from customers
5. To supplement anecdotal feedback with quantitative data
6. To have a systematic way to find problems when you are implementing service improvements

To develop a useful comment card, a healthcare organization should identify its customers for particular services, study these customers, and find out what is important to them in terms of service. Once these expectations have been determined, comment-card questions are developed. If studies reveal that patients expect a friendly greeting, prompt attention, and detailed information about the treatment procedure when they visit a physician's office, the office's comment card will ask patients about those elements of the healthcare experience. If an organization tries to differentiate itself from similar organizations in some particular way, that differentiating factor may also appear on the comment card, so that the organization can gauge the success of its differentiation strategy.

Comment cards give an indication of whether the organization is meeting the general expectations of the customers who take the time to fill them out. Written comments about long call-response waits, lines at the reception desk, or housekeeping problems reveal the strengths and weaknesses of the service delivery system, the personnel and their training, and the service itself.

Positive comments can also provide management with the opportunity to recognize employee excellence. This recognition reinforces the behaviors that lead to good patient service and creates role models and stories about how to provide outstanding service that other employees can use in shaping their own behavior in their jobs. Negative comments can be used in training, without mentioning specific employees, to illustrate behaviors that caused negative healthcare experiences. Using comment cards in these ways allows managers to train employees in how to provide excellent patient service through the voices of the patients themselves.

Comments accumulated from cards may be plotted as numerical values on bar graphs and charts that visually display how patients perceived their experience. The plots will suggest whether service problems are occurring occasionally and randomly, or whether overall service quality might be deteriorating. Although patient comments and their visual representations are interesting and helpful to management, the information is not statistically valid because, for one, the random-sample requirement of most statistical techniques is not met.

The greatest disadvantage of comment cards is that many customers ignore them and do not fill them out, so the cards received are not likely to be a true general picture of the customers' perceptions. Typically, only 5 percent of customers return comment cards, and they are usually either very satisfied or very dissatisfied. It is difficult to know what percentage of the delighted total or the dissatisfied total these responses represent. When the other 95 percent of customers say nothing, the healthcare organization cannot determine if they were happy, unhappy, or merely indifferent. Research shows that a large percentage of dissatisfied customers fill out no cards, leave quietly, and never return.

Another major disadvantage of comment cards, and in fact of many methods for acquiring feedback, is that the time lag between patient response and managerial review prevents on-the-spot correction of service gaps and problems. Once the moment of truth has passed and the angry or disappointed patient leaves after expressing negative responses on a comment card, the opportunity to recapture that patient's future business or loyalty is diminished.

Even worse, negative word-of-mouth advertising generated by dissatisfied patients cannot be corrected. Any time patients are asked to provide negative feedback, they must be assured that their identity will not be revealed to prevent any kind of recriminations.

Surveys

Formal survey methods can obtain patient feedback about healthcare quality and value. Although surveying is more expensive than the methods already discussed, surveys can offer statistically valid, reliable, and useful measures of patient opinion that the other methods cannot. Surveys can range in sophistication, precision, validity, reliability, complexity, cost, and difficulty of administration.

Mail Surveys
Well-developed mail surveys, sent to an appropriate and willing sample, can provide valid information concerning patient satisfaction. Organizations can use mail surveys to their benefit, but many uncontrollable factors can influence patient responses to a mail survey. Inaccurate and incomplete mailing lists or simple lack of interest in commenting can produce a response rate too small to provide useful information. In addition, the time lag between the experience and survey response can blur a patient's memory of details.

Mail surveys are usually used to generate reports that tend to be upwardly biased. The subtleties of the healthcare experience and patient perceptions cannot be fully expressed numerically. Also, averages may not be sufficiently informative. If some patients remember an experience as terrific and give it a high rating, while others rate it as terrible, the numerical average will suggest that, on the average, patient expectations were met.

The nature of medical treatment may also make interpretation of the ratings difficult. If the operation was a success but the patient died, it would not matter to the surveyed survivors that the rest of the patient's experience was above expectations. Finally, formal mail survey techniques are expensive because they require proper questionnaire development, validation, and data analysis.

SERVQUAL

Several measures of service quality are available (see, for example, Castle 2007; Gupta 2008; Marley, Collier, and Goldstein 2004). One well-accepted survey technique is SERVQUAL (short for service quality), developed by Parasuraman and his associates (Parasuraman, Zeithaml, and Berry 1988). SERVQUAL, which has been extensively researched to validate its psychometric properties, seeks to measure the way customers perceive the quality of service experiences in five categories:

1. *Reliability*: The organization's ability to perform the desired service dependably, accurately, and consistently
2. *Responsiveness*: The organization's willingness to provide prompt service and help customers
3. *Assurance*: The employees' knowledge, courtesy, and ability to convey trust
4. *Empathy*: The employees' ability to provide care and individualized attention to customers
5. *Tangibles*: The organization's physical facilities and equipment and appearance of personnel

SERVQUAL also asks respondents to rate the relative importance of the five areas, so organizations can make sure they understand what matters most to customers. In each area, SERVQUAL asks customers what they expected and what they actually experienced to identify service gaps at which organizations should direct attention.

The SERVQUAL index was developed for the retail and other service industries. Ramsaran-Fowdar (2005) studied the SERVQUAL measures and identified additional service dimensions relevant to healthcare, including core medical outcomes (e.g., patient education, physician referral contacts) and professionalism (e.g., knowledgeable and skilled support staff).

SERVQUAL has been widely used in healthcare organizations (Rohini and Mahadevappa 2006; Pakdil and Harwood 2005) with varying results (Dagger, Sweeney, and Johnson 2007; Ramsaran-Fowdar 2005). An adaptation of the SERVQUAL survey instrument, intended to evaluate service quality at Hallmark Hospital, is presented in Exhibit 13.3.

Exhibit 13.3 SERVQUAL Application to Healthcare: Measuring Customer Perceptions of Healthcare Quality at Hallmark Hospital

DIRECTIONS: Listed below are five features pertaining to Hallmark Hospital and the services it offers. We would like to know how important each of these features is to *you* when you evaluate a hospital's quality. Please allocate a total of 100 points among the five features *according to how important each feature is to you*—the more important a feature is to you, the more points you should allocate to it. Please ensure that the points you allocate to the five features add up to 100.

1. The appearance of the hospital's physical facilities, equipment, and personnel
    _____ points
2. The ability of the hospital to perform the promised service dependably and accurately
    _____ points
3. The willingness of the hospital to help customers and provide prompt service
    _____ points
4. The knowledge and courtesy of the hospital's employees and their ability to convey trust and confidence
    _____ points
5. The caring, individualized attention the hospital provides to its customers
    _____ points

DIRECTIONS: Based on your experience with hospitals, please think about the kind of hospital at which you would prefer to receive healthcare. Please show the extent to which you think such a hospital would possess the feature described by each statement below. If you feel a feature is *not at all essential* for excellent hospitals such as the one you have in mind, circle "1" for *Strongly Disagree*. If you feel a feature is *absolutely essential* for excellent hospitals, circle "7" for *Strongly Agree*. If your feelings are less strong, circle one of the numbers in the middle. There are no right or wrong answers. All we are interested in is a number that truly reflects your feelings regarding hospitals that would deliver excellent service quality.

[The 22 survey items for this section are the same as those in the next section, but without any reference to Hallmark Hospital.]

(Continued)

Exhibit 13.3 (continued)

DIRECTIONS: The following set of statements relates to your feelings about the service at Hallmark Hospital. For each statement, please show the extent to which you believe Hallmark Hospital has the feature described by each statement below. Once again, circling "1" means that you *Strongly Disagree* that Hallmark Hospital has that feature, and circling "7" means that you *Strongly Agree*. You may circle any of the numbers in the middle that show how strong your feelings are. There are no right or wrong answers. All we are interested in is a number that best shows your perceptions about the service at Hallmark Hospital.

[On the instrument itself, the five category labels (Tangibles, etc.) will be omitted.]

TANGIBLES
P1. Hallmark Hospital has modern-looking equipment
P2. Hallmark Hospital's physical facilities are visually appealing
P3. Hallmark Hospital's employees are neat-appearing
P4. Materials associated with the service are clean and sanitary at Hallmark Hospital

RELIABILITY
P5. When Hallmark Hospital promises to do something by a certain time, it does so
P6. When you have a problem, Hallmark Hospital shows sincere interest in solving it
P7. Hallmark Hospital performs the service right the first time
P8. Hallmark Hospital provides its services in the way it promises to do so
P9. Hallmark Hospital insists on error-free service performance

RESPONSIVENESS
P10. Employees of Hallmark Hospital tell you exactly when healthcare services will be performed
P11. Employees of Hallmark Hospital give you prompt healthcare service
P12. Employees of Hallmark Hospital are always willing to help you
P13. Employees of Hallmark Hospital are never too busy to respond to your requests

Exhibit 13.3 (continued)

ASSURANCE

P14. The behavior of Hallmark Hospital employees instills confidence in customers

P15. You feel safe in going to Hallmark Hospital and doing business with them

P16. Employees of Hallmark Hospital are consistently courteous to you

P17. Employees of Hallmark Hospital have the knowledge to answer your questions

EMPATHY

P18. Hallmark Hospital gives you individual attention

P19. Hallmark Hospital has visiting hours convenient to all its customers

P20. Hallmark Hospital has employees who give you personal attention

P21. Hallmark Hospital has your best interests at heart

P22. Employees of Hallmark Hospital try to learn your specific needs

Source: Adapted with permission from "SERVQUAL: A Multiple-Item Scale for Measuring Consumer Perception of Service Quality," by A. Parasuraman, V. A. Zeithaml, and L. L. Berry. 1988. *Journal of Retailing* 64 (1): 38–40.

The SERVQUAL instrument reflects a point we have made throughout: the importance of the patient-contact staff to healthcare quality. Although tangibles refer primarily to the setting and to the physical elements of the delivery system, and reliability reflects a combination of organizational delivery system design and service provider ability, the remaining three elements—responsiveness, assurance, and empathy—are almost exclusively the responsibility of the patient-contact employees.

Internal Customer Metrics

Healthcare organizations too often overlook internal customers when they assess external customers. Many units within traditional full-service healthcare facilities provide service functions for other internal units in addition to services for patients and external physicians or as stand-alone functions (i.e., human resources, training, and payroll). These internal service providers are often thought of as overhead activities rather than service providers with customers. As a result, many healthcare executives pay little attention to these activities.

One hospital developed and implemented an internal customer survey instrument (Smith et al. 2007). This process included (1) an initial baseline survey of service managers concerning their satisfaction with internal nursing services, (2) feedback to service-area managers regarding the survey results, (3) an interim survey to determine improvement, and (4) a resurvey two years later to determine effectiveness of the implemented changes. In general, the scores in the initial survey were highly positive. Of the 15 areas, 13 received favorable composite scores and 11 received mean scores stronger than the "agree" category of 3.0.

After reviewing the results of the initial survey, senior nurse managers used the results as a baseline for service improvement. The service-area nurse managers picked three specific problems identified in the survey and then developed and implemented plans to address those problems. Most of the nurse managers then solicited staff input on these action plans. After two years, the satisfaction levels of the customers (users of nursing services) showed that all 15 service areas were received favorably and 14 of the 15 areas had mean scores greater than 3.0.

Researcher Ben Schneider has developed another widely used questionnaire that seeks to assess the degree to which employees perceive a climate of service. In a number of published studies, Schneider and colleagues have found a consistent relationship between employee assessments of a positive service climate and customers' perceptions of the positive service experience (Schneider, Macey, and Young 2006; Schneider and White 2004). Clearly, a link exists between the employee propensity to deliver excellent customer service and the actual delivery of service quality.

Structured Personal Interviews

Face-to-face patient interviews provide rich information when trained interviewers, who are able to detect nuances in responses to open-ended questions, have the opportunity to probe patients for details about their experiences. Interviewing can uncover previously unknown problems or new twists to a known problem that cannot be uncovered in a preprinted questionnaire or reflected well in numerical data.

However, personal interviews are costly: Interviewers must be hired and trained, interview instruments must be custom designed, and inconvenienced patients must be compensated for participating. Without incentives, most patients see little personal benefit from participating in a patient interview unless they are either very satisfied or very dissatisfied. Finally, the most desirable time to interview patients and/or their families is at the conclusion of the healthcare experience. Getting their attention and cooperation when they are anxious to leave is a challenge.

Another patient-interview approach is to employ consultants or employees (called "lobby lizards" in the hotel business) to ask randomly selected patients their opinions on several key service issues. In a healthcare facility, the person conducting the customer interviews is typically a manager or another patient-contact employee. For example, a billing clerk may have the best opportunity to question patients about their experience as they are leaving the clinic, office, or hospital and making their payment. Because patients may not always be motivated to tell the whole truth, a systematic interview should pose questions that are professionally developed and validated to help ensure that the information gathered is useful, accurate, and sufficient.

As mentioned earlier, one advantage of acquiring immediate feedback is that it may allow prompt recovery from service problems. Staff training should therefore include appropriate service-recovery techniques, as research confirms that the organization benefits greatly from soliciting and fairly resolving patient complaints. Because service-quality information derived directly from the patient is highly believable to staff and management, it motivates a serious consideration of the problems the patients identified.

Critical Incidents

Another important survey tool is the critical incident technique. Through interviews or paper-and-pencil surveys, customers are asked to identify and evaluate numerous moments—classified as dissatisfiers, neutral, or satisfiers—in their interactions with the organization. The survey lets the organization know which moments are critical to customer satisfaction, and the critical dissatisfiers can be traced back to their root causes and rectified. The Malcolm Baldrige report of Mercy Health System, for example, discusses the importance of the organization's "critical moments of service." These events are considered key to providing patient satisfaction and are monitored closely and updated often.

Knowing which incidents in the hospital stay are critical to patients allows the organization to concentrate on making them smooth and seamless (Mercy Health System 2007). In healthcare, the critical incidents tend to be related to customer expectations (discussed earlier) such as patients' concerns about personalized care, prompt attention, staff respect, physician and staff competence, a clean environment, privacy, and clear information. Information related to these critical incidents will generate usable information for service improvement.

Telephone and Web-Based Surveys

Telephone interviews are another useful method for assessing customer perceptions of service. A review of the Malcolm Baldrige award winners reveals a common use of these surveys. Many use commercial providers like Press Ganey or Gallup to gather this information, and others, such as Sharp HealthCare and Mercy Health System, collect these data monthly. Many healthcare facilities use telephone surveys to follow up with patients a week after the service was provided rather than having them complete a written survey at the time of the service. More recently, healthcare organizations have started sending patients e-mails with hot links to an Internet survey as a less expensive and less intrusive substitute for telephone surveys.

Although telephone interviews or Web surveys eliminate the inconvenience of gathering information while patients are still in the healthcare facility, they present other challenges. Survey methods rely on retrospective information that can be blurred by the passage of time. If the service received was too brief or insignificant for patients to recall accurately, or if patients have no special motivation to participate, the information they provide is likely to be unreliable or incomplete.

In addition, in this age of intense e-mail and telephone solicitations, customers often regard telephone and Web-based surveys as intrusions on their time and violations of their privacy. Annoyed respondents feeling resentment toward the organization for calling them at home are likely to bias the data.

Red Lobster and Steak & Ale avoid some of these difficulties by building into their customer meal-checks system a code that prints an 800 telephone number for every *nth* customer to call; the automated response system then asks customers to press touchtone buttons to answer questions about their experience at the restaurant. In return for participation, the restaurant offers coupons for free desserts or two entrees for the price of one on the customer's next visit. Healthcare providers can adopt this strategy by inviting patients to participate in a survey. Participants' names are then entered into a raffle to win health-related enticements such as free family passes to a gym or multiplex.

Because telephone interviews conducted by a trained interviewer are expensive, Web-based surveys are preferred. When data analysis and expert interpretation are included, the total cost for a statistically valid telephone survey can be high, whereas many Web-based tools offer automatic data analysis and are far less expensive.

Mystery Shoppers

Mystery shoppers provide management with an objective snapshot of the health-care experience. While posing as patients, these trained observers methodically sample the service and its delivery, take note of the environment, and then compile a systematic and detailed report of their experience. They can "sample" the admissions process or an overnight stay at a hospital or a routine checkup at a freestanding clinic.

Mystery shopper reports generally include numerical ratings of many aspects of an experience. These ratings then allow organizations to compare results before and after an improvement is instituted. Mystery shoppers may also be directed to observe competitors in the market, gathering information about the competition's quality level, program/service offerings, facilities, staff performance, and prices. Organizations may hire a commercial service, a consultant, an actor, or even a staff member to conduct a mystery-shopper visit (Buckley and Larkin 2007).

Generally, employees know that their organization uses mystery shoppers, but they do not know who the shoppers are or when they will appear. Because these visits are unannounced, employees cannot prepare or dress up their performance. Shoppers can be instructed to show up at random times during various shifts to assess differences in quality and value on different floors, conditions, employees, and managers (Van der Wiele, Hesselink, and van Iwaarden 2005).

One of the most important benefits of a mystery shopper program is that it produces information that can assist managers in identifying performance deficiencies that call for employee coaching. Employees may discount or feel antagonistic and defensive about supervisory feedback, making them reluctant to express their need for coaching or to follow through on manager-recommended improvements. Mystery-shopper observations spell out these needs, enabling the manager to use the customer's voice to coach employees.

An article in the *Wall Street Journal* reports that mystery shoppers in healthcare may make various inquiries over the phone, go to a doctor's office or an emergency department for a checkup, or even fake symptoms (Wang 2006). Generally, they pose as uninsured patients. Mystery patient reports lead to improvements, ranging from placing signage throughout the facility to training staff to empathize better with patients.

Mystery shoppers test the staff's ability to respond to anticipated service problems and service delivery failures. For example, shoppers can create a problem or intensify a situation by asking certain questions or requesting unique services to assess employee responses under pressure. The *Wall Street Journal* article reports one shopper's experience when she asked for an extra pillow: The nurse told her to send her husband to the dollar store to buy one. Mystery shoppers can also gauge the effectiveness of a particular training program by shopping at a healthcare organization before and after the training (Wang 2006).

The main disadvantage of a mystery shopper is the small size of the sample from which the shopper generates reports. Because anyone can have a bad day or a bad shift, a mystery shopper may base conclusions on unusual or atypical experiences. One or two observations are not a statistically valid sample of anything, but hiring enough mystery shoppers to yield a valid sample is impractical and expensive.

Further, the unique preferences, biases, or expectations of individual shoppers can unduly influence a report. Well-trained shoppers with specific information about the organization's service standards, instructions on what to observe, and guidelines for evaluating the experience avoid this pitfall.

However, a healthcare mystery shopper can only sample so many aspects of the healthcare experience. A mystery shopper cannot go through a surgical procedure, for example. Two other negatives are that the staff are spending time on a patient who is not really in need of medical service and that seeking treatment that is not needed may be unethical.

PUBLIC METRICS

One of the fastest-growing trends in measuring patient quality are those metrics provided by governmental or external organizations. For example, the University of Michigan's American Customer Satisfaction Index (ACSI) includes several categories for healthcare. Interestingly, of the services ACSI measures, ambulatory care scores the highest, with an 81 rating out of a possible 100. In Great Britain, the National Health Commission publishes an assessment of healthcare providers that uses patient assessment of their satisfaction for nearly 10 percent of the total score.

As mentioned in Chapter 10, many websites can help healthcare consumers gauge the service quality of hospitals, nursing homes, long-term care providers, and other organizations; see, for example, www.hospitalcompare.hhs.gov or www.leapfroggroup.org. *Consumer Reports* rates the service quality of hospitals by state, assessing aspects as how well doctors communicate and how attentive the staff are. Magazines, such as *U.S. News and World Report*, rank healthcare organizations on the basis of customer feedback and reported clinical outcomes.

Finally, many regional and state organizations and governments collect and make available data on various healthcare providers, from hospitals to long-term care and nursing home facilities to individual physicians. The point is that a wide variety of metrics can be used, and healthcare managers should be aware of those that can provide feedback metrics to staff and serve as benchmarks against which the organization's performance levels can be consistently and accurately assessed.

DETERMINING THE MEASURE THAT FITS

What gets measured gets managed and hopefully improved, but determining which measure is most appropriate to use is another challenge. A major hospital in a for-profit chain, for example, may require more elaborate and expensive strategies to measure feedback because poor service can harm the reputation and bottom line of the hospital, the chain with which the hospital is affiliated, and the livelihood of countless employees up and down the line.

The value to this hospital of finding and correcting service problems so that it can deliver the healthcare quality its patients expect is tremendous. Failing to meet patient expectations will quickly make it and everything affiliated with it uncompetitive in a dynamic marketplace. On the other hand, the office of a small independent physician who has a well-established reputation for providing superb clinical treatment in a caring manner may learn just as much from asking patients about their experience without incurring the expense of sophisticated quality assessment methods.

Costs and level of expertise used to gather data vary also. An important question to ask is who should collect data: employees, consultants, or a professional survey research organization. Using staff members is the least expensive alternative, but they also have the least expertise in customer service research and may lack the communication skills to interview effectively. Consultants and survey organizations cost more, but they are better able to gather and interpret more detailed, sophisticated statistical data using more sophisticated techniques. For example, employee surveyors cannot measure eye-pupil dilation, but professionals can.

Regardless of the evaluation technique selected to measure healthcare quality, one thing is certain: Patients evaluate service every time it is delivered, and they form distinct opinions about its quality and value. All healthcare organizations that aspire to excellence must constantly assess the quality of their healthcare experience through their patients' eyes. Most patients and their families are happy to tell what they thought about their experience if they are asked in the right way at the right time. Telephone surveyors calling on Friday night during dinner time will get the turndown they deserve, but a comment card left in a patient room to be turned in upon discharge will get far better attention. Healthcare managers striving for excellence need to ask the right questions at the right time, of the right mix of patients, to obtain the information necessary to ensure service that meets and exceeds patient expectations.

Irrespective of whether qualitative or quantitative assessment methods are used or which particular methods are used alone or in combination, follow-up is crucial. If internal or external customers provide data to organizations that they perceive to be unresponsive to their input, the quantity and quality of future input will be limited. Why provide new data if old data are ignored? Not collecting customer information is better than collecting and ignoring the information. Follow-up should include communicating to staff clear and accurate economic measures of loss from the defection of one customer, setting service standards based on customer expectations, eliminating substandard performance and performers, and communicating with both patients and staff about how their input has led to service improvements (Albrecht and Zemke 2002).

CONCLUSION

Numerous methods are available for measuring the degree to which service excellence is achieved. Each healthcare organization needs to assess which methods will work best for its own situation. Each organization also needs to determine whether to gather data using its own resources or contract the function to an outside group. The degree of sophistication required and the organization's internal resources will drive this decision.

Regardless of whether the organization uses qualitative or quantitative measures (or both) or internal or external resources to generate the data, the purpose of collecting data on service quality should be to enhance customer service. Once baseline information is established, the organization can focus on setting performance standards for a few critical areas at a time and spend several months achieving service excellence. Staff will not be overwhelmed, managers will be able to monitor a manageable number of critical areas, and everyone will be able to learn together and support each other in the process. Once the original areas are improved, the organization can take on additional areas.

A major challenge is how to achieve and maintain continuous improvement. One approach is to celebrate individual and group success in achieving service excellence. Staff need and want to be appreciated for their achievements and contributions. Among the more successful celebration methods are mentions in newsletters, posting positive letters about employees on bulletin boards, sharing stories of excellent service at staff meetings, and sending thank you notes. Every meeting should be viewed as an opportunity to teach, positively reinforce, and celebrate successes in achieving customer satisfaction. This process should be continuous.

Service Strategies

1. Focus on the quality and outcomes of both clinical service and customer service.
2. Be aware that if you do not measure it, you cannot manage it; if you do not manage it, you cannot improve it.
3. Use the best combination of qualitative and quantitative methods to measure customer satisfaction.
4. Balance the value of service information obtained from patients with the cost of obtaining it.
5. Recognize the strengths and weaknesses of the available assessment techniques.
6. Offer service guarantees.
7. Assess the quality of service for both internal and external customers.
8. Follow up on implementation of service improvement ideas generated from all quality assessment methods.
9. Get better or get beaten in the competitive healthcare marketplace.
10. Maintain momentum for customer service by continually using positive reinforcement and celebrating successes.

Those who enter to buy, support me. Those who come to flatter, please me.
Those who complain, teach how I may please others so that more will come.
Only those hurt me who are displeased but do not complain.
—Marshall Field, department store magnate

CHAPTER 14

Fixing Healthcare Service Failures

Service Principle:
Eliminate all sources of disappointment positively and quickly

EVERY CUSTOMER ASSUMES that the service she pays for will, at the least, meet her expectations. For example, a patient who makes an appointment for a lab test expects the appointment will be kept when she arrives and the test will be done properly. If the initial expectations are met, the patient is satisfied. If the initial expectations are exceeded, the patient is delighted and willing to return when the need arises. Exceeding patient expectations creates "apostles" and "evangelists"—happy customers who spread positive word of mouth to their family, friends, and associates about the excellent total healthcare experience they received. Such favorable words reinforce the provider organization's public image and reputation.

What happens, however, if the patient's initial expectations go unmet? For example, when the patient arrives for his scheduled appointment, the receptionist informs him that he needs to reschedule because the doctor cancelled her appointments for the day or a machine or equipment is malfunctioning. This patient will feel dissatisfied at best, and at worst, the patient will turn into an angry "avenger"—an unhappy customer who bad-mouths the organization to family, friends, and anyone else who will listen. A typical dissatisfied patient may tell eight to ten people about the problem he encountered, but an avenger will likely create a website to share his disappointment with millions of people.

Service failures, like clinical errors, are inevitable. Many healthcare organizations do plan well for clinical problems, but they do not anticipate service problems with the same care. They incorrectly assume or hope that the service will be available as promised, the setting and delivery system will function as designed, and the staff will perform as they were trained—consistently, every time.

Well-managed organizations, however, work hard to identify, plan for, and prevent all types of service failures, and they understand that these problems vary in frequency, timing, and severity. Not meeting patient expectations can occur any time during a single healthcare experience or across multiple experiences with the same organization. Because first impressions are so important, a problem that takes place early in the process will weigh more heavily on the patient's mind than a problem that occurs later. Big errors count more than little ones.

Customers have more tolerance for poor service than for poor service recovery (Michel, Bowen, and Johnston 2008). If a customer experiences a second failure of the same service, no recovery strategy can work well; in all likelihood, that customer will be lost forever. Furthermore, Michel, Bowen, and Johnston (2008) suggest that a customer is most annoyed and angered not by her dissatisfaction with the service but by her belief that the system that caused the failure remains unchanged and thus will lead to more failure. In other words, customers are turned off by an organization that is so indifferent to its service quality that it does not make the effort to learn from its mistakes.

Learning from failures is more important than simply fixing problems because learning results in process improvements. Improvements, in turn, have a direct impact on the bottom line, as they reduce costs of service errors, boost employee efficiency and morale, and increase customer satisfaction. Although many hospitals have instituted procedures for handling patient complaints in response to accreditation requirements, they do not formally track or capture complaints for learning and improvement purposes (Donnelly and Strife 2006).

In this chapter, we address the following:

- The importance of finding and fixing service failures
- The reasons such failures occur
- Strategies for service recovery and service failure prevention

Ultimately, if the organization neglects to respond to a service problem, it fails twice, not once: First, it did not meet the most basic customer expectation; second, it did not resolve, quickly and appropriately, the problem caused by the first.

ELEMENTS OF A SERVICE FAILURE

Despite the best-laid plans, service failure is a reality in all organizations. Complex organizations function as a system, with interdependent and tightly intertwined parts. One mistake in one part will affect the rest of the system, and the tighter the intertwining of these parts, the more susceptible the whole system is to disaster. The difference between an excellent and a poor service organization, however, is that the best one works hard not only to remedy failures but also to prevent them from occurring at all. Service failures occur for two reasons: human error and system error, which are discussed in the following section.

Sources

Providers can fall short of a patient's expectations at any point in the healthcare experience. The product, setting, or delivery system may be inadequate or inappropriate, or the staff may perform or behave poorly.

For example, if the patient's teeth do not look as white as she expected when she walks out of the dentist's office, she will be dissatisfied and a service failure could result. Similarly, if the patient's lab test takes several hours to complete, instead of the one-hour time frame he was promised, he will deem the experience a failure. The environment or setting can also cause service failures. If the patient thinks the ambient temperature is too cold, the smell of antiseptic too strong, the exam or waiting rooms too dirty, or the parking lot too dark and too far away, she will feel unhappy about these failures. Certainly, staff can bring about service failures if they are unfriendly or rude, poorly trained or inexperienced, and not forthcoming with information or misinformed. The service product, setting, delivery system, and staff must be carefully managed to minimize the likelihood of a service failure.

Magid and colleagues (2009) illustrate some organizations' failure in managing their services. These researchers surveyed 3,562 emergency medicine clinicians in 65 hospitals. The majority of the respondents said their emergency department (ED) lacks sufficient space in which to deliver patient care, and one-third said the number of patients who presented in the ED consistently exceeds their capacity to provide safe care. On the staffing front, two-thirds reported that the number of nursing staff is insufficient to handle patient loads during busy periods, and 40 percent said they do not have enough doctors to handle patient loads when the ED gets busy.

Taylor, Wolfe, and Cameron (2002) looked at the same ED issues but from the patient perspective. These researchers found 1,141 problems were related to patient treatment, including inadequate treatment and diagnosis; 1,079 problems were related to communication, including poor staff attitude, discourtesy, and rudeness; and 407 problems related to delay in treatment (Taylor, Wolfe, and Cameron 2002).

Patient's Role

Service failures come in different degrees, ranging from catastrophies (which make the newspaper headlines) to minor slipups (which happen behind the scenes and patients never know about). Along this continuum are an infinite number of mistakes. Because the patient defines the quality of the service experience, the patient also defines the nature and severity of each service failure. Two patients dissatisfied about the same failure can have different degrees of unhappiness—one can be "very unhappy," while the other can be "mildly unhappy."

Sometimes, the organization's product, setting, delivery system, or staff may not be the cause of the disappointment; the patient may be at the root of the problem. For example, a plastic surgeon performs a facelift as expected and requested by the patient, but the patient may still deem the operation a failure simply because she does not like the way her new face looks. The patient who ignores warning signs or fills out forms incorrectly also contributes to service failures. Other examples include patients who act belligerently toward staff and other patients and those who sabotage their own care by refusing to take their medication or follow their doctors' orders. These service failures are not initiated by the organization and are often beyond its capability to manage, but the organization must still anticipate, address, and prevent them as well as possible.

It is human nature to attribute successes to ourselves and problems to others. Thus, patients often point their fingers at someone else when a service failure occurs. Organizations that want to keep patient-caused problems from destroying the patient's healthcare experience and his feeling of goodwill toward the enterprise develop and use certain strategies (such as the following) designed to help the patient recover from the failures he created without making him feel foolish or blamed:

- Distribute a heart-healthy or calorie-restricted menu to patients who refuse to abide by dietary orders.
- Provide clear, simple care instructions to family members about the patient's care.
- Offer assistance with filling out forms.
- Make warning and directional signs bigger, bolder, and in languages understood by the primary service population (e.g., English, Spanish, Chinese, Polish, Arabic).

Customer Defection

Patients want an active, interested, positive attitude from their providers. They will not buy into television, print, Internet, or billboard ads that tout the excellence of an organization if they have experienced the opposite.

Customer defection—leaving one provider for another—can be prevented by ensuring that the total healthcare experience is excellent in the first place and, if a service failure occurs, by immediately putting a solid service recovery plan to work. According to Reichheld and Sasser (1990), just a 5 percent reduction in customer defection rate can raise profits by 25 to 85 percent. Clark and Malone (2005) suggest a similar increase in profits and customer retention as a result of successfully addressing customer complaints.

Usually, a service recovery effort yields one of three outcomes:

1. The problem is fixed, and the formerly unhappy patient is now happy.
2. The problem is not fixed, and the formerly unhappy patient remains unhappy.
3. The problem is fixed but not satisfactorily or completely, and the formerly unhappy patient has made concessions with the organization and is now "neutral"—neither happy nor unhappy.

As described earlier, happy patients may become "apostles" or "evangelists," while unhappy patients may turn into "avengers." "Neutral" patients, on the other hand, may forget the whole experience and, as a result, the organization as well.

In extreme cases, such as medical catastrophes, neutralizing the unhappy patient may be the best outcome the organization can reach. For example, if a patient develops an infection after a successful operation, all the organization can do to neutralize the patient's level of dissatisfaction is to ensure that all aspects of the hospitalization is as patient-centered and error-free as humanly possible. Here, the goal is to somehow offset the adverse event with service excellence. Even if that goal is achieved, the patient will still leave feeling neutral and will likely defect to another provider the next time around.

Furthermore, neutral customers are influenced by other factors. A recent study of insurance providers indicates that a patient's switching behavior (or customer defection) is primarily a function of three factors (QMS Partners 2009):

1. Name recognition or lack thereof
2. Stability of the provider
3. Efficiency with which billing complaints are handled

The third factor implies that healthcare consumers highly value the way they are treated by the organization's employees. A service failure in the people part of the healthcare experience can make the difference between customer loyalty and customer defection.

The Impact of Evangelists and Avengers

According to Sherman and Sherman (1998), 1 avenger tells his unfortunate experience to at least 12 people. Each of those 12 then shares the story to 5 or more people. On average, an avenger has an audience of about 72 people. Furthermore, if 8 avengers each spreads the disappointing news to 12 others, each of whom in turn tells 5 of their associates, then 576 people hear the negative word of mouth that only 8 patients actually experienced. A simpler calculation is this: Each dissatisfied customer sends out, verbally or in writing, about 70 negative messages.

Conversely, evangelists do not talk about their positive experience as widely as avengers do. Evangelists share their good stories to approximately 6 other people (Hart, Heskett, and Sasser 1990).

DISSATISFIED CUSTOMER'S RESPONSES

Unhappy patients react in one or a combination of three ways: never return, complain, and bad-mouth the organization.

Never Return

A dissatisfied patient vows to never return to the same provider. This is the worst customer reaction for an organization because it also means the angry patient will tell others about the negative experience. In this situation, the organization loses not only the current business of this patient but also the future business of all the people the patient can influence. Service recovery should be especially focused on this group of unhappy customers.

Complain

Benchmark organizations encourage patients and other customers to complain, and they thank them for it. A complaint should be viewed as an opportunity, not a challenge, because it gives the organization a chance to refine the system and make customers happy. Patients who complain either verbally or in writing allow employees and managers to fix the problem before the problem and the dissatisfaction are shared with others.

Organizations may also teach patients to complain, if necessary, as detailed complaints function as feedback that can be measured and monitored over time. Complaining patients are less likely to defect to another provider and to bad-mouth the organization than those who do not express their dissatisfaction to the organization. Making sure no customer leaves unhappy is obviously advantageous to any organization. The best way to ensure this is to seek out patient complaints before they leave the hospital, clinic, or office.

The results of a landmark study conducted by the Technical Assistance Research Program (TARP 1986) for the U.S. Office of Consumer Affairs strongly suggested that customers who complain are more loyal than those who do not and that having complaints satisfactorily resolved increased the customers' brand loyalty. These customers were happier with the organization after experiencing bad service than before because the dissatisfaction led to improvement. Research conducted on the relationship between customer loyalty and complaints since this TARP study has confirmed these findings from more than two decades ago.

Bad-Mouth the Organization

If the negative experience is costly—financially and/or personally—the patient is more likely to spread the bad word. The greater the cost to the patient, the greater the motivation to tell. People who hear such negative stories will be discouraged to patronize the same provider, if given a choice.

Angry customers (avengers) who used to be limited to writing letters to corporate headquarters or the Better Business Bureau, putting up signs in their yard, or painting "lemon" on the car now have a more powerful tool: the Internet. For a minimal fee, anyone with Internet access can create a website or a blog to tell the world about an offending company and also invite others to share their stories of poor treatment. In this day of instant and global communication, a "bad-mouther" can spread the message to millions of people; the same is true of evangelists.

Word of mouth is important for several reasons. Friends, family, colleagues, and other associates tend to be more credible sources than impersonal testimonials (Lake 2009). When a friend reports that a certain physician is cold and uncaring, you no longer believe or are at least wary of the advertisements that promote the "warm and personal touch" of that physician. Personal accounts, either good or bad, from friends and family are also more vivid, more convincing, and more compelling than any paid commercial advertising.

Dollar Value of Customer Dissatisfaction

Customer defection and negative word of mouth create an expensive problem for the organization. Over time, the loss of revenue from a patient who opts never to return and from potential customers who listened to the unhappy patient's bad-mouthing is tremendous. Because that dollar value is so high, hardly any effort to fix a service failure is too extreme.

Consider these numbers that illustrate the point. Suppose the average person is admitted into the hospital three times over her lifetime, and the average hospital bill for one stay is $15,000. For Patient A, who vowed never to return to and has bad-mouthed the hospital, the lifetime revenue loss sustained by the hospital is $45,000. If Patient A is married and has two children, the lifetime family revenue loss rises to $180,000. If the bad-mouthing damage is calculated (Patient A tells 12 others, according to calculations by Sherman and Sherman [1998]), the lifetime loss could reach $540,000 ($45,000 × 12) at a minimum.

A similar type of calculation can be done for a managed care organization that lost a multiyear contract with one dissatisfied employer that represents 300 covered lives. Let's assume annual premiums of $3,000 per enrollee over a five-year contract. The cost of this loss is $4.5 million (300 × $15,000 = $4.5 million). Similarly, a physician's defection from a hospital, assuming he brought in 2 admissions per week for 45 weeks a year, will result in a $1.35 million loss (90 × $15,000 = $1.35 million).

To make these figures meaningful to employees, the financial loss can be calculated at the department level—that is, what dollar amount is associated with the defection of one nurse? Such calculations can also lead to some surprisingly large numbers for even a small business. To show how a dentist might come up with numbers like these, assume that the dentist's satisfied patients come in for treatment twice a year and spend an average of $150 each time. The total value of each satisfied biannual patient's business for the next five years is $1,500. Conversely, positive word of mouth from happy patients can bring in enormous numbers in potential revenues.

The point of this exercise is simple: The long-term cost of patient defection and negative word of mouth is usually much more than the expense of correcting a service failure—immediately and appropriately.

SERVICE RECOVERY

An organization's attempt at service recovery can make a positive or negative impression on the patient who experienced a service failure (Berry 2009). A small problem can turn big if the effort is half-hearted, misguided, or too little too late. A big problem minimized or eliminated, on the other hand, becomes a great example of customer service that must be shared with the rest of the organization.

In addition, the way an organization responds to complaints and service failures, whether well or poorly, communicates how committed it is to patient satisfaction. Similarly, the way an organization seeks complaints and service failures sends a loud message about what it truly believes in. Compare the following hypothetical organizations.

Hospital A is defensive about patient complaints and keeps them secret (although employees usually hear about them anyway), resolves problems as cheaply and quietly as possible, and seeks people to blame for the complaints. Hospital B, on the other hand, aggressively looks for and fixes service failures, disseminates findings about complaints and failures throughout the organization, makes quick and fair adjustments and improvements, and seeks solutions rather than scapegoats.

Which of the two organizations provides better customer service?

Some companies claim strong financial benefits from successful complaint resolution. According to Sherman and Sherman (1998), even if a service failure occurs, about 70 percent of the patients affected will continue to do business with the provider if their issues are resolved eventually; that percentage jumps up to 95 if the issues are resolved on the spot. This finding translates into large sums of money over the lifetime of these patients and their families and friends. Such data motivate benchmark healthcare organizations to engage their frontline employees in handling service complaints and problems. These organizations empower employees to address the failures quickly and in whatever way they see fit, without manager authorization or approval. Hart, Heskett, and Sasser (1990) agree: "The surest way to recover from service mishaps is for workers on the front line to identify and solve the customer's problem."

Complaints and Other Service Failure Data

Most organizations generally obtain and study only a fraction of the service failure data collected from customers, employees, and managers. Even when managers agree that customer feedback is essential, often that information does not flow from the division that gathers and addresses it into the rest of the organization

(Michel, Bowen, and Johnston 2008). Also, "most firms fail to document and categorize complaints adequately," which makes it more difficult to learn from mistakes (Tax and Brown 1998).

Research indicates that the more negative feedback a customer service department collects, the more isolated that department becomes because it does not want to be seen as a source of friction. Some service recovery units soak up customer complaints and problems with no expectation of feeding this information back to the organization. Other organizations actually impede service recovery by rewarding low complaint rates and then assuming that a decline in the number of complaints signifies an improvement in customer satisfaction.

Employee attitudes (positive or negative) about management spill over to the way they treat patients and other customers. Positive attitudes result when employees believe that management provides them with the means and the support to handle service failures. When employees believe otherwise, they tend to think they are being treated unfairly and display passive and maladaptive behaviors that can sabotage customer service. At organizations that reward low complaint rates or punish/blame employees for service failures, employees may send dissatisfied customers away instead of keeping them by apologizing and addressing the issue, which employees most likely created.

SERVICE RECOVERY STRATEGIES

Berry (2009) argues that the organization should always apologize for service failures, but an apology alone is seldom sufficient. Three major strategies are available for dealing with service failures:

1. *Proactive or preventive strategies* for identifying problems before they happen; these strategies are built into the design of the service, employee training, and the delivery system
2. *Process strategies* for monitoring the critical moments of the service delivery
3. *Outcome strategies* for seeking out problems after the service experience has happened

Preventive Strategies

Preventing problems is easier and less costly than recovering from them. Proactive strategies are designed to identify and fix any trouble spots before they become a service failure.

Forecasting and Managing Demand

If a statistical prediction of patient demand on a particular day indicates that the hospital will be full, then a preventive strategy is to schedule full staff on each shift, make extra supplies available, and prepare departments for full capacity. The same strategies could work for a physician practice that is anticipating a lot of patient visits on a given day. An appointment system may help manage the expectation of patients, and sufficient staff and supplies can be made available.

If the organization plans poorly, and patients have to wait longer than they feel is appropriate, their perception of the overall quality of their service experience declines rapidly, and a service failure results. Keeping the wait time short avoids this type of failure.

If demand can be forecasted for a longer period, then other proactive strategies can be implemented. For example, if demand in two years is expected to increase by 20 percent, new capacity should be built, new employees should be hired and trained, and inventories should be increased to prevent the occurrence of long waits, unavailable supplies, or insufficient and untrained staff. Even if major steps (hiring more staff, building new capacity) cannot be taken because of limited resources, employees may be trained to cope with demand surges. Just as hospitals run disaster drills with fire-and-rescue teams, so too can hospitals and clinics train their healthcare workers and give them practice exercises to handle unexpected increases in demand.

Quality Teams, Training, and Simulation

The popular use of quality teams is another preventive strategy. Get staff who are directly involved in the service experience together, and ask them to identify problems they have seen or heard about and to suggest strategies for preventing those problems. Adequate training of frontline employees before they even begin to serve patients is also a preventive measure. Any highly reliable organization ensures that its frontline staff know exactly what customers need, want, and expect from the total experience and are motivated to do whatever it takes to meet (at a minimum) and exceed those customer factors, every time.

Another preventive/proactive approach is to use analytical models, such as those discussed in chapters 11 and 12, to simulate all or part of the delivery system or the service recovery process. Once a model is created that represents a wide variety of patient–provider interactions, the manager and staff can analyze each situation to determine areas of service failures. On a simpler level, role playing and structured scenario simulations can help employees evaluate all types of service problems and learn effective recovery strategies.

Michel, Bowen, and Johnston (2008) suggest creating and communicating a service logic that explains how everything fits together. This should be a kind of mission statement or a summary of how and why the business provides its services. It should integrate the perspectives of all three groups—customers, employees, and managers:

- What is the customer trying to accomplish and why?
- How is the service produced and why?
- What are employees doing to provide the service and why?

This statement should include a detailed study of internal operations, map out how the organization responds to customer complaints, and describe how that information is used to improve the service recovery process. Similar mapping should detail every step of customer experiences, highlighting customer thoughts, reactions, and emotions.

Performance Standards

Performance standards are tools that not only help employees do their job during the service experience but also guide employees and the organization in evaluating the performance afterward. Employees and their managers can also use these standards to monitor how well or poorly they have performed over time.

Some standards are purely preventive because they can be met before patients enter the door. For example, if a clinic can reliably predict the number of patients who will come in on a given day of the week, that forecast can be used as a basis or standard for the quantity of medical supplies to prepare and order. If the prediction is correct, the service failure of not having enough supplies on hand should not occur.

Other preventive performance standards should be set for the following:

- Number of training hours required for staff annually
- Number of equipment to be purchased
- Number of examining tables to be set up
- Level of supply inventory

Performance standards also help patients understand the level of service they can expect. Examples of such standards include "We will try to resolve problems of types A, B, and C within two hours," "We will try to resolve problems of types D, E, and F within one week," or "If you leave a message on our help-desk voicemail, we will call you back within one hour."

Many customers of the Ritz-Carlton Hotel know, for example, that phone calls are supposed to be answered within three rings and that after a customer registers a complaint, a Ritz employee is supposed to make a follow-up call within 20 minutes. Similarly, hospital nurses in many facilities are aware that the patient call bell is supposed to be answered within 30 seconds.

JetBlue provides an excellent example of service recovery reinforced by a service guarantee. After snowstorms left some JetBlue customers stranded for many hours on planes that were not equipped to provide food, water, and other creature comforts, JetBlue engaged its customers in a dialogue about what went wrong and how the airline might fix it. The CEO also instituted a service guarantee to indicate the service standards it would implement in the future and the steps it was taking to support that guarantee (Lane 2007). As a result, most JetBlue customers continue to patronize the airline.

Poka-Yokes

To avoid wrong-side surgery, sometimes called bilateral confusion or symmetry failure, the National Academy of Orthopedic Surgeons has urged its physician members to sign their names on the spot to be cut. Surgical patients often write in felt-tipped marker "I hurt here" with an arrow pointing to an elbow or "yes" on one knee and "no" on the other. These doctors and patients, probably without knowing the term, are using "poka-yokes."

The poka-yoke is a proactive strategy that aims to keep service as flawless as possible. Conceived by the late Shigeo Shingo, an industrial engineer at Toyota and a quality improvement leader in Japan, poka-yoke makes service quality easy to deliver and service problems difficult to incur because it requires the inspection of the system for possible problems and the development of simple means to prevent or point out those mistakes. For example, a surgeon's tray and a mechanic's wrench-set box often have a unique indentation for each item to ensure that no instrument is left in a patient or no wrench is left in an engine. Another example is the identification bands hospitals use to ensure that the right patient gets the right treatment. Shingo called these problem-preventing devices or procedures "poka-yokes" (POH-kah-YOH-kay), which means "mistake proofing" or "avoid mistakes" in Japanese.

Shingo distinguished three types of inspection:

1. Successive inspection, where the next person checks the quality and accuracy of the previous person's work
2. Self-inspection, where people check their own work
3. Source inspection, where potential mistakes are located at their source and fixed before they can become service errors. Poka-yokes are used mainly to prevent source mistakes.

An example of successive inspection is when an orderly checks a patient's chart to ensure that it corresponds with the instruction about where the patient should be transported. An example of self-inspection is when an attending nurse compares the prepared drug against the patient's chart before administering the drug. An example of source inspection is when a surgical nurse examines the prepared medical supplies (e.g., surgical tools, bandages) to ensure that sufficient kinds and quantities of the items are available.

Poka-yokes are either "warnings that signal the existence of a problem or controls that stop production until the problem is resolved" (Chase and Stuart 1994). A warning poka-yoke could be a light that flashes when a patient's blood pressure is too low, signaling the nurse to adjust the drip before the patient goes into shock. A control poka-yoke could be a device that turns an x-ray machine off whenever the roentgen level is too high. Warning and control poka-yokes can be further divided into three types: contact, fixed values, and motion step.

Contact poka-yokes monitor an item's physical characteristics to determine if it is right or meets a predefined specification. Some pharmacies, for example, prepare standard quantities of drugs to ensure the dosage is correct before the medicine is distributed. *Fixed-values poka-yokes* deal with established quantities. For example, surgical teams use prepackaged surgical supplies so that they know exactly how many bandages, surgical tools, and so forth are available for use. When the surgery is completed, the team can count every item to make sure nothing has been left in the patient. *Motion-step poka-yokes* are useful in processes where one error-prone step must be completed correctly before the next step can take place. A simple example is the start button on the x-ray machine. The button is outside the exposure area so that technicians cannot take the x-ray until they leave the room and are protected.

All poka-yokes should be simple, easy to use, and inexpensive. Something can go wrong at any point in service delivery, and the poka-yoke method encourages managers to think first about what might go wrong.

Process Strategies

Process strategies for finding service failures monitor the delivery while it is taking place. The idea is to design mechanisms into the delivery system that will catch and fix problems before they affect the quality of the healthcare experience; blood pressure and heart monitors are examples of such mechanisms. The advantage of process controls is that they can catch errors as they happen, enabling immediate correction.

Process performance standards provide employees with objective measures with which to monitor their own performance while they are doing their job. One example is specifying how long a patient has to wait in the emergency department before receiving attention. Other illustrations include the number of times per hour that a nurse must check on an intensive care patient or the number of patients waiting for service before a cross-trained staff member steps in to reduce the waiting time at peak demand. These are all process-related measures that allow the staff to minimize errors or catch them while the healthcare experience is underway.

An important part of any process strategy is to get unhappy patients to complain during the healthcare experience. This is a more difficult challenge than one might think: Although some patients are comfortable with complaining, most are not. Most patients are either unwilling to take the time, believe no one cares or will do anything about their complaints, or are too angry or too disappointed to say anything.

Research on complaint behavior has identified strategies for encouraging patients to complain (Michel, Bowen, and Johnston 2008):

- *Solicit complaints.* Because many service failures are caused by provider errors, all personnel should be trained to solicit complaints about their own performance. This is not an easy task for providers, as they may see mistakes are punished while catching errors is rewarded, and most people do not want to admit their mistakes or feel criticized for them. Thus, the organization must design a complaint strategy that accommodates its staff's perception about complaints.
- *Read a patient's body language for clues on her dissatisfaction.* This observation can yield information that might otherwise go unmentioned. Frontline staff or direct caregivers should be trained to watch and recognize body language and to be receptive and sympathetic once the complaints are verbalized. Patients must perceive these employees as being interested and concerned about their well-being and opinions. Otherwise, patients will feel wary and will choose not to say anything.
- *Empower staff.* Provide employees with the freedom to address complaints and service failures on their own, as much as the organization's business strategy allows. Autonomy encourages staff to do what is right for the customer, and that prevents service failures from happening in the first place. For example, Ritz-Carlton authorizes front-desk personnel to credit unhappy customers up to $2,000 without asking approval from a supervisor.

Outcome Strategies

Outcome strategies identify service problems after they have occurred so that problems can be fixed and future problems can be prevented. The most basic outcome strategy is simply to ask the patient, "How is everything going today?" Other more systematic illustrations include (1) providing toll-free or 800 phone numbers for use by former patients who want to report their dissatisfaction and (2) asking patients to fill out a brief questionnaire when they pay their bills.

Organizations must make unequivocally clear to patients that they care to know about any service failures that patients have encountered. What influences a patient's decision to seek redress for a problem or to let it go is her perception of whether the organization will do something about it. Even patients who are reluctant to complain are more likely to do so if they think something will be done about the problem (Davidson 2007). Customers often do not want a payoff; they simply want a resolution, an apology, and the reassurance that the problem will not happen again to them or to others.

The more the organization depends on repeat business and recommendations from past patients through word-of-mouth reputation, the more critical it is that the complaints of its customers are acknowledged and acted on. Some healthcare organizations report their complaint investigations back to those patients who made the complaint in detail, including information on what people were affected and what systems were changed. In that way, the organization shows it is responsive to the patient's complaint and gives the complainant a sense of participation in the organization, which may positively enhance loyalty and increase repeat visits. If the complaint identifies a flaw the organization can correct, and if knowledge of the correction provides the patient with a sense of satisfaction for reporting a complaint that was important and acted on, a true win–win situation results.

Some numerical measures that organizations collect as a matter of normal procedure can point to real and potential service problems. Total staffing or nurse staffing per patient day is an example. Although it is used primarily to keep track of costs, staffing varies by department, floor, or shift. If one shift is significantly below the norm, this may indicate possible service problems.

Healthcare organizations should also collect meaningful measures of employee performance as it relates to service recovery. Positive reinforcement and incentives should be offered for solving problems, but this requires a good system for measuring customer satisfaction. Salary increases and promotions could then be linked to an employee's achievements in these areas. Likewise, there should be disincentives for poor handling of customer complaints.

On the positive side, organizations should spotlight employee successes in customer service using available media such as in-house publications, the intranet, and bulletin boards. Such success stories may also be shared during customer service or culture trainings. Rewards and recognition should flow to heroes in service recovery, including those who helped to develop systems for handling complaints or provided extraordinarily helpful treatment after a service failure (Michel, Bowen, and Johnston 2008).

Consumers in the healthcare industry are reluctant to complain because they fear they may receive lower service quality if and when the need for future care arises (Fottler et al. 2006). Fewer than half of the patients who have a negative experience with a hospital actively try to change the unsatisfactory situation. This suggests that written complaints only reflect a small portion of total complaints (Berry and Seltman 2008).

Employee-Driven Strategies

Employees, especially direct or frontline providers, should be trained to handle service failures and to creatively solve problems as they occur. Scenarios, game playing, videotaping, and role playing are good strategies for developing employees' service recovery skills. Just as umpires can be trained to recognize balls and strikes, healthcare personnel can be trained to recognize and fix service errors.

Do Something Quickly

The basic service recovery principle is to do something positive and to do it quickly. Strive for on-the-spot service recovery. Capturing the many benefits of quick recovery is one major reason benchmark service organizations empower their frontline employees to exercise discretion in correcting errors. Employees of one service organization carry a card on which the following three principles of service recovery are written:

1. Any employee who receives a customer complaint "owns" the complaint.
2. React quickly to correct the problem immediately. Follow up with a telephone call within 20 minutes to verify that the problem has been resolved to the customer's satisfaction. Do everything you possibly can to never lose a customer.
3. Every employee is empowered to resolve the problem and to prevent a repeat occurrence.

Many times, customers will log complaints with the nearest employee they can find, so organizations benefit from asking employees to attempt to capture the complaint as soon as possible. The physician or staff member who initially receives a complaint should complete a patient complaint form, and staff members who receive the complaint should immediately refer the patient to management personnel. Even if a manager is not immediately available, the staff member should complete the form and begin to take action because complaints must be captured as soon as possible.

Other suggestions for service recovery include the following (Grugal 2002):

- Ask patients the critical question, "What can I do to make this right?"
- Evaluate the complaint to identify significant dissatisfiers.
- Write down the specifics.
- Communicate and interact in a pleasant manner.

Management must empower employees with the necessary authority, responsibility, and incentives to act quickly after a problem occurs. The higher the cost of the problem to the patient in terms of money, personal reputation, or safety, the more vital it is for the organization to train the healthcare staff to recognize and deal with the service problem promptly, sympathetically, and effectively. Of course, empowering staff to resolve problems will not be sufficient if recovery mechanisms are not in place. If the rest of the system is in chaos, empowering the front line will not do much good.

A quick reaction to service problems has numerous benefits:

1. It reduces the overall expense of correcting a wrong.
2. It keeps and creates goodwill between the organization and patients and their family.
3. It generates positive word of mouth that could lead to repeat business or referral and recommendation.
4. It strengthens the message that customers are valued.
5. It encourages employees to commit to providing high-quality service consistently.

Address Root Problems

A necessary further step in any service recovery strategy is that employees should inform their managers about any system failures they encounter, even if they have already initiated successful recovery procedures. If they do not report the failure, the problem may recur elsewhere in the organization.

Collecting these data enables management to move beyond reacting to complaints and on to determining the root causes and preventing them from happening. Cause-and-effect diagrams might focus staff's attention on those areas that need the greatest improvements.

The reactions of frontline workers to service failures caused by the system have significant implications for customer satisfaction. The common reaction is simply to remove the obstacle or solve the problem and to continue patient care. But an empowered staff should also be offered incentives for removing the root cause of the problem to prevent future recurrences.

For example, a nurse may find that her newest patient was not served lunch. Assuming that it was an oversight, she might call food service and order the lunch for the patient. This might solve the immediate problem, but if the underlying cause was that admissions failed to advise food service of the new patient's arrival, the same problem will occur in the future because the root cause was not addressed.

The best service organizations encourage staff members to address both the immediate service failure (the symptom) and the root cause. This is facilitated by including problem resolution as an explicit part of the staff's jobs, allowing enough time to address the problem, encouraging communication between staff, dedicating proper attention to problems, and giving incentives/rewards to those who engage in this type of "extra" work.

Apologize and Let the Customer Vent

All healthcare personnel should be trained to apologize, ask the patients about the problem, and listen in a way that gives patients the opportunity to blow off steam. Considerable research indicates that allowing customers the opportunity to vent to someone with authority (e.g., manager, supervisor, vice president) is an important step in retaining their patronage (Heskett, Sasser, and Hart 1990).

This strategy is more effective when it is followed up with an acknowledgment, a thank you, and a tangible reward, even if it is small (Berry 2009). The tangible reward could take the form of a meal voucher at the hospital cafeteria, and the acknowledgment could take the form of an apology and thank you letter from the CEO.

Patients' Evaluation of the Recovery Efforts

Patients who have suffered a service failure and lodged a complaint want action. Procedural fairness refers to whether or not the patient believes organizational procedures for listening to the patient's side and handling service problems are fair or merely a procedural hassle full of red tape. Customers also want an easy process for correcting problems. They think that if the organization failed them, it is only fair that the organization makes it easy for them to receive a just settlement.

Interactive fairness refers to the customer's feeling of being treated with respect and courtesy and being given the opportunity to express the complaint fully. If she has a complaint that the service provider is rude, indifferent, or uncaring, and the manager cannot be found, the customer will feel unfairly treated. Common sense suggests that a customer who is encouraged to complain, treated with respect and courtesy, and given a fair settlement is more likely to return than a customer who is given a fair settlement that is offered with reluctance and discourtesy.

Distributive fairness, or outcome fairness, is the third test patients apply to an organization's attempts to recover from problems. What did the organization actually give to the unhappy patient as compensation for the problem? If the patient complains about a rude housekeeper and gets only a sincere apology because that is all hospital policy calls for, the patient will feel unfairly treated; somehow "we're sorry" may not be enough in the patient's judgment to compensate for the rude treatment.

Once again, it all comes down to meeting the patient's expectations. The issue is difficult because each patient is different. Finding the satisfactory compensation may involve methodical trial and error on the organization's part. Some research indicates that customers feel more fairly treated when organizations offer a variety of options as compensation for service problems (Berry 2009; Tax and Brown 1998). For example, a physician can offer a patient the choice of an immediate appointment (if desired) or can offer to fill the patient's prescription for free.

In sum, investing time, money, staff, and effort into service recovery is just plain good business.

CHARACTERISTICS OF A GOOD RECOVERY STRATEGY

In their classic study, Hart, Heskett, and Sasser (1990) believe service recovery strategies should satisfy several criteria. More specifically, service recovery strategies should be as follows:

- Ensure that the problem is addressed in some positive way. Even if the situation is a total disaster, the recovery strategy should ensure that the patient's problem is addressed and, to the extent possible, fixed.
- Be communicated clearly to the employees charged with responding to patient dissatisfaction. Employees must know that the organization expects them to find and resolve patient problems as part of their jobs.
- Be easy for the patient to find and use. They should be flexible enough to accommodate the different types of problems and the different expectations that patients have.
- Always recognize that because the patient defines the quality of the service experience, the patient also defines its problems and the adequacy of the recovery strategies.

A strategy that does not make some improvement in the situation for the complaining patient is worse than useless because the organization makes it plain that it cannot or will not recover from a problem even when informed of it. The work of Hart, Heskett, and Sasser (1990) suggests that most recovery strategies are in serious need of improvement. More than half of organizational efforts they identified that respond to consumer complaints actually reinforce negative reactions to the service. In trying to make things better, organizations too often make them worse.

One reason that patients view many recovery strategies as inadequate is that the strategies do not really take into account all of the costs to the patient. Did the doctor miss an appointment? Schedule another one. Is there a busy signal on the telephone line for hospital information? Interject a recorded apology. The organization may think the relationship is back where it started, but for the patient many costs are associated with service problems, and effective organizations will try to identify them and include some recognition of them in selecting the appropriate service recovery. After all, the fact that the test results were not delivered by the promised date is not the patient's fault, so why should the patient have to suffer additional mental stress waiting for results? Why should the patient lose more work time as a result of a provider-cancelled appointment?

Patients clearly think that when a healthcare problem occurs, organizations need to do more than simply make it right by replacing it or doing it over again. The high numbers of malpractice suits substantiate that point. For example, if the excessively long wait beyond the appointed time causes the patient to miss half a day's salary, then the recovery strategy should include not only an apology but also some compensation for the patient's loss of income as well. Outstanding healthcare organizations systematically consider how to compensate patients for economic and noneconomic losses and take extra effort to ensure that dissatisfied patients have not only their time and financial losses addressed in a recovery effort but also their ego and esteem needs.

Even when the patients themselves make mistakes, good healthcare organizations help to correct them with sensitivity. They make sure patients leave feeling good about their overall experience and appreciating how the organization's staff helped them redeem themselves. Imagine how depressed you would feel if you came back to the hospital parking lot after a long day of visiting a terminally ill family member only to find that you have lost your car keys and are locked out of your car. You tell the parking attendant, and half an hour later a locksmith hands you a new set of keys, no charge!

Even though car key problems are not its fault, a customer-oriented organization believes the customer needs to be wrong with dignity. It knows that customers who are angry at themselves may transfer some of that anger to the organization. To overcome this very human tendency, customer-focused organizations find ways to fix problems so that angry, frustrated people leave feeling good because a bad experience has not been allowed to overshadow or cancel out all the good. By providing this high level of customer service, the healthcare organization earns the gratitude and future patronage of patients and enhances its reputation when patients and their families tell external and internal customers' stories of these service successes.

Matching the Recovery Strategy to the Problem

The best recovery efforts are those that address the customer's problem. For example, suppose a patient tried to contact her physician by phone (as instructed) on a certain day and time, was put on hold, and ended up leaving a message asking the physician to return her call. If the return call was never made, a communications problem undoubtedly occurred, but the result for the patient is that the physician appears to be uncaring. An appropriate recovery effort might be to provide the patient with the physician's personal cell phone number.

Categorizing the severity and causes of service problems might be a useful way to show the type of recovery strategy a healthcare organization should select. In Exhibit 14.1, the vertical axis represents the severity of the problem, ranging from low to high, and the horizontal axis divides service problems into those caused by the organization and those caused by the patient. When severity is high and it is

Exhibit 14.1 Matching the Recovery Strategy to the Failure

		Organization	Patient
Severity of Failure	*Relatively Severe*	Red-carpet treatment and apology	Provide help to the extent possible and apologize
	Relatively Mild	Apologize and fix/replace/repeat	Apologize and extend sympathy

Cause of Failure

the organization's fault (e.g., when a service failure occurs that totally alienates the patient), the proper response is the red-carpet treatment. The organization needs to bend over backward to apologize, communicate empathy and caring, and address the patient's problem, because it will take an outstanding recovery effort to overcome the patient's negative feeling.

The two types of situations in Exhibit 14.1 where the patient caused the problem provide terrific opportunities for the organization to make patients feel positive about the experience, even though the patients caused the problem. In a low-severity situation, a sincere apology is sufficient and will make the patient think the organization is taking some of the responsibility for a situation that was clearly not its fault. Indeed, some organizations will do even more, if the cost to make a patient feel better is not substantial. Hospitals will often change meals if patients say they do not want them, even when the records show the meals were just what the patients ordered. The wrong meal may not be the hospital's fault, but the patient feels good that the organization will not make patients pay for their own mistakes.

The upper-right box represents situations where the problem is relatively severe and the patient or some external force created the problem. These are opportunities for the organization to be a hero and provide an unforgettable experience for the patient. For example, if the patient is late for an appointment because she got delayed in traffic and arrived when the physician is busy with the next patient, the receiving nurse can come out and promise that the physician will see the late patient next.

CONCLUSION

Service recovery rules can and should be developed for staff. For example, an employee should be given permission to spend a specific sum to correct a service problem. If the cost is beyond the limit an employee is allowed to spend, the staff member should contact her supervisor to discuss other alternatives or to seek approval for the expense. In this way, staff are empowered to fix the problem on their own without any bureaucratic delay that could cause an unhappy customer to defect.

In addition, staff should be trained on what to do and say to a patient in the event of a service failure. Employees must be told that they will not be criticized for "overserving" customers, that risk taking and innovative approaches to please customers are encouraged, and that service failures and recovery are monitored. The latter requires installing a system for collecting detailed information on customer dissatisfaction and defection. Gathering such information should involve frontline staff, as they are intimately familiar with the service problems that take place and thus can help the organization determine the root causes and prevent them from happening.

Learning from failures is more important than fixing problems. It is crucial to address the system and process problems that cause the failure in the first place.

Service Strategies

1. Realize that service-failure prevention is superior to and less costly than service-failure recovery.
2. Encourage patients to complain; a complaint is a gift.
3. Train and empower your staff to find and fix problems.
4. Train your staff to listen to dissatisfied customers with empathy, and then record the service problem and its resolution.
5. Find a solution the customer believes to be fair, and help patients fix service failures they caused.
6. Remember that unhappy patients tell twice as many people about their dissatisfaction than happy patients tell others about their excellent experience.
7. Find out and share with employees how much a dissatisfied patient costs the organization to illustrate the importance of service recovery.
8. Address the root causes of service failure.

A good leader is best when the people barely know he leads. A good leader
talks little but when the work is done, the aim is fulfilled,
all others will say, "We did this ourselves."
—Lao-tzu, Chinese philosopher

CHAPTER 15

Leading the Way to Healthcare Service Excellence

Service Principle:
Lead others to provide a superb healthcare experience

PROVIDING AN EXCELLENT healthcare experience is simple. Study your patients and other customers to find out what they really need, want, and expect, and then provide those and maybe even a little bit more. Healthcare managers committed to providing a superb total healthcare experience do not stop studying their customers, using all available scientific tools.

Because no two customers are alike and their personal preferences and conditions change, this process of discovery is never complete.

The service product, the service environment, and the service delivery system must change or evolve along with and to complement the customers. The information from this continuous study is used to shape the decisions on strategy, staffing, and systems.

This chapter brings together the book's important concepts to help the healthcare manager achieve service excellence. In this chapter, we address the following:

- A model of service excellence in healthcare
- Our view of healthcare in the future and the leader's role

Again, we emphasize that service excellence is insufficient by itself in meeting patient needs, wants, and expectations. Excellent clinical service that successfully addresses the patients' health concerns is the prerequisite to service excellence.

A SERVICE EXCELLENCE MODEL

Exhibit 15.1 presents a conceptual framework for achieving service excellence that shows the impact of service excellence on a healthcare organization. The box on the left outlines some of the major environmental trends currently affecting or expected to affect organizations. Some of these may impede and others may potentially help the efforts of organizations to enhance customer service. Among the most significant of these environmental trends are consumer-driven healthcare, a shortage of primary care providers, and potential health insurance reform.

The external environmental and other factors noted in Exhibit 15.1 affect the structures, processes, and outcomes of healthcare organizations. Among these effects are increased incentives for organizations to develop more customer-focused strategies, staffing, and systems. If successful, such strategies, staffing, and systems should enhance patient satisfaction in the short run (Platonova, Kennedy, and Shewchuk 2008). If sustained over the long run, this customer-focused approach will improve customer loyalty to the organization (Garman, Garcia, and Hargreaves 2004; Platonova, Kennedy, and Shewchuk 2008). Similarly, it will increase the probability that the patient will return for service and recommend the organization to others (Platonova, Kennedy, and Shewchuk 2008).

More organizations are realizing that patient loyalty and retention are paramount issues (Bendapudi et al. 2006). The feedback loop (as shown in Exhibit 15.1) indicates that a customer's intention to return to and recommend an organization are associated with increased revenue and reduced resource demands, which positively affect the organization's structure, process, and outcomes (Evanschitzky and Wunderlich 2006; Platonova, Kennedy, and Shewchuk 2008). The process is continuous because more resources enable the organization to enhance its service product, environment, and delivery system.

External Environmental Changes

Healthcare Reform and Consumer-Driven Healthcare

The Obama administration puts a high priority on health insurance reform, highlighting that an estimated 45 million Americans are uninsured. Hospitals, insurers, government officials, managed care providers, corporations, and academicians have also proposed a wide variety of reforms, most of which do not give a high priority to consumer choice.

One exception is Regina Herzlinger (2007b), who advocates for a consumer-driven healthcare system in her book *Who Killed Healthcare?* Herzlinger proposes the following:

Exhibit 15.1 Service Excellence Process and Associated Outcomes

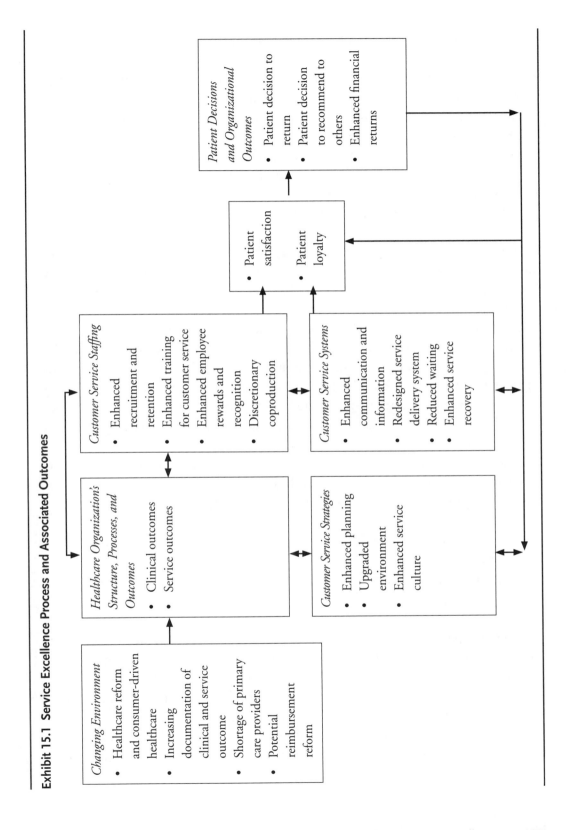

- Consumers tailor their own healthcare coverage in a national insurance market.
- Everyone must buy insurance, and the federal government maintains strict oversight to ensure price and coverage fairness.
- Small, disease-specific hospitals care for patients who do not need all the services offered by medical centers.
- A national database contains the prices and outcomes for procedures at every hospital and clinic so that consumers can make informed choices.
- Individuals get generous tax breaks to buy their own insurance, and subsidies are provided for those with low incomes.

In other words, Herzlinger asks, "Why can't healthcare be run like the retail sector?" (Arnst 2008). If hospitals, insurers, and doctors all had to compete in the open market for patient customers, she believes innovation would flourish, prices would drop, and quality would improve.

Herzlinger does not want anyone but consumers managing health benefits. Given that the average consumer is able to choose between 240 makes and models of cars, why can't they do the same when it comes to their health? In other words, regardless of who pays for the health benefits, Herzlinger would like consumers to have a wide range of options regarding the selection of providers. That decision would be buttressed by widespread information on prices, clinical quality, and service quality.

For those who believe government agents, employers, and private insurance companies are best suited to make healthcare decisions, consumer-driven healthcare is anathema. They are united by two common beliefs (Kapp 2007):

1. Patients are not able to act as intelligent consumers when it comes to healthcare.
2. Consumer-driven healthcare will result in loss of their money, power, or control.

These people prefer a top-down command-and-control approach to healthcare reform that will not emphasize customer choice and service as primary goals. They would limit consumer choices to the "best options" as defined by "experts" in the field. Such a limitation will likely reduce consumers' perception of the overall quality of the services received.

For those who respect consumers' ability to make choices, however, healthcare reform represents a tremendous opportunity; that is, if the reform that passes ends up to be centered on choice and service excellence. In addition, it should reward providers who achieve excellent clinical and customer service outcomes. However, if the special interests in the healthcare industry (e.g., insurers, pharmaceutical companies) sabotage a consumer-oriented reform and enhance the command-and-control approach, the average American may experience a less responsive and more bureaucratic healthcare system in the future (Kapp 2007).

In 2007, the federal government began posting patient satisfaction scores for hospitals (see HCAHPS [Hospital Consumer Assessment of Healthcare Providers and Systems] on www.hcahpsonline.org). The HCAHPS and state governments' posting of hospital prices and quality measures (including patient satisfaction) give consumers greater transparency in healthcare practices and outcomes, regardless of the outcome of the proposed healthcare reform. Consumers have been increasingly considering customer service, price, ease of access, clinical quality, and ethics of the provider in assessing their healthcare options, regardless of whether or not healthcare reform is characterized as consumer driven (Bodnar 2007).

In other words, clearly, the healthcare reform debate has touched on many issues paramount to consumers, including who will pay for services, how providers and insurers will be held accountable, and how quality and choices will be managed. Final answers to these questions have not yet been determined; however, the 2009 reform will have a major impact on the quality of customer service experienced in the future.

Increased Documentation of Clinical and Service Outcomes

As customer service information becomes readily available to providers, employers, insurers, and consumers, performance-based reimbursements will likely increase along with the importance of customer service. In addition, stakeholders will consider ease of access, clinical quality, and effectiveness of treatment in evaluating the value of a provider. As calls for public accountability and data transparency intensify, the concepts and principles discussed in this book can help organizations make adjustments to improve their overall service and quality performance. Ignoring service excellence will be costly to an organization's bottom line.

The retail clinic trend may also enhance the documentation of clinical and service outcomes (Fottler and Malvey 2010). Advances in technology will boost the transparency, low cost, and easy access to services offered by retail clinics, allowing these clinics to make public the service and clinical outcomes they have achieved. Eventually, such clinics may begin to offer specialty services as well. Wal-Mart and other major retailers would not be entering this field if consumers were satisfied with the access, quality, and prices available to them in the current healthcare system.

Shortage of Primary Care Providers

In 2008, the Physician Foundation commissioned a survey of every primary care doctor in the United States, and the results suggest that primary care doctors are an endangered breed (Rubin 2008). More than three of four respondents said they believed the United States is facing a shortage of primary care physicians. Moreover, this perception of a shortage could grow more critical, as half of the respondents said they planned to reduce their patient load or stop practicing within the next three years. More than half of the respondents said they would not recommend that young people pursue careers in medicine because of "red tape" and "payment issues." These results indicate that the healthcare system tends to undervalue what primary care doctors do.

To keep up with service demands over the next decade, the United States must add 40,000 physicians to its current pool of practicing providers, or else the country will face a soaring backlog (Associated Press 2009). The current shortage in all physician specialties is expected to worsen. A study by the Association of American Medical Colleges found that the rate of first-year enrollees in U.S. medical schools has declined steadily since 1980, and if this pattern continues, the country will have about 159,000 fewer doctors than it needs by 2025 (Associated Press 2009).

The survey results are relevant to the concept of service excellence in healthcare because primary care physicians are often the first provider a patient sees. Research shows that a sustained relationship with a primary care physician, as well as the resulting comprehensiveness of care, organizational accessibility, and coordination of care, is associated with higher levels of patient satisfaction (Donahue, Ashkin, and Pathman 2005; Saultz and Albedaiwi 2004) and better treatment outcomes (Parchman and Burge 2004). If primary care physicians are overworked and understaffed, patients will have long waits for appointments, and time spent with the physician will be minimal. The shortage of primary care providers is exacerbated by the fact that a shortage of nurses and allied health professionals, such as physical therapists, is ongoing.

This shortage of primary care physicians is a problem that must be addressed because it is difficult to imagine high levels of service excellence without them. Federal subsidies for the education of primary care physicians as well as other health professionals appears to be a necessary prerequisite for achieving long-term service excellence.

Potential Reimbursement Reform

Under the current reimbursement system, physicians are reimbursed for procedures but not for such activities as e-mail and phone communication, listening to patients, coordinating care for patients, and so on (Szabo 2007). All of these activities are related to customer satisfaction, so changes in reimbursement that recognize the importance of these activities for enhancing the healthcare experience of patients is overdue. Whether it will occur under a command-and-control healthcare reform or a consumer-driven reform remains to be seen.

For example, physicians agree that patients with chronic conditions, such as cancer, deserve coordinated care provided by a team of healthcare professionals. However, most doctors do not have time for group consultations, are not used to working in teams, and are not reimbursed for many of the services teams provide (e.g., spiritual counseling, social work) (Szabo 2007). Providing such services reduces future costs for the healthcare system, but the physicians themselves receive no financial benefits because they are not reimbursed for these activities. Providing coordinated care through a team of healthcare professionals would require changing the way Medicare, Medicaid, and private third-party insurance pay for care.

Changes in reimbursement to pay for the "softer side of healthcare" can significantly increase customer service, healthcare outcomes, and patient satisfaction. Whether such changes are incorporated in the final healthcare reform plan remains to be seen and may be difficult to implement in light of the current economic downturn. Thus far, health insurance reform has aimed to cover more people and to expand reimbursement for current procedures. Discussions about reimbursement for better communication, better clinical outcomes, and better customer service have not been as intense.

STRATEGY

Today, an amazing amount of information is available about patients and what the competition offers in providing services to those patients, and only the organizations that tap into that information to truly understand what their patients and other customers want will survive and prosper. They must use this information to design a corporate strategy, discover which of their competencies customers consider to be core, and then concentrate on making these core competencies better. For example, they use the customers' wants, needs, and expectations to sharpen their marketing strategies, budgeting decisions, organizational and production systems design, and human resources management strategy.

Southwest Airlines is an excellent example of a company that has used its understanding of the customer to discover and then provide what its passengers really want. Like most organizations, Southwest originally used customer surveys to ask what customers wanted and found customers wanted everything: cheap fares, on-time performance, great meals, comfortable seats, free movies, and more.

Southwest realized it could not give its customers everything, so it did additional research to dig deeper into customer preferences and learned that its customers really wanted low fares, reliable schedules, and friendly service. The Southwest product is now exactly what its target market wants and, more importantly, wants enough to pay for and return to again and again.

The point of this example for healthcare managers is that they must dig deeper than the simple market survey of patient preferences to understand what preferences actually drive patient behavior. The organization can use the results from deeper probing to match the organization's core competencies and mission with what the customers want.

Key Drivers

Outstanding organizations study their patients extensively to discover the key drivers of their healthcare experience. Some drivers are highly influential, and some seem relatively unimportant. Nonetheless, they all contribute to the impression the patient takes away from the healthcare experience and help determine whether or not that patient will be satisfied. A trip to a hospital, or a visit to a physician's office or clinic, is a holistic experience to most people; excellent customer service organizations do the research necessary to identify all the separate components of this whole experience. Then they carefully manage them all.

In a sense, key drivers can be divided into two categories. The first category consists of basic things patients expect the organization to offer its patients to operate in the particular market segment. For example, customers expect the following basics from a hospital: nice, clean rooms; acceptable food; appropriately trained and skilled medical and professional staff with a decent bedside manner; a caring attitude; efficient work systems; a clinical product of high quality; and no irritations in the environment.

The organization must meet these basic expectations, or customers will be dissatisfied. If the organization habitually fails to meet these basic expectations, it will fail altogether. Organizations must offer the basic characteristics if they seek to maintain a reputation and attract the repeat business that leads to long-term success.

The second category of key drivers encompasses the characteristics and qualities that make the experience memorable. These are the features that differentiate the experiences at an excellent organization. Benchmark organizations find a way to go beyond meeting the basic expectations with which patients arrive when they come in the door to have a medical need addressed. Outstanding organizations provide the key factors that make a difference, make the experience memorable, compel patients to return again and again, and even motivate patients to tell all their friends about these exceptional organizations.

The following organizations survey customers to determine how well they are providing the basics that patients need, want, and expect: Holy Cross Hospital in Chicago; Sharp HealthCare in San Diego, California; SSM Health Care in St. Louis, Missouri; Baptist Health Care in Pensacola, Florida; St. Mary's Hospital in Green Bay, Wisconsin; Parkland Health & Hospital System in Dallas, Texas; and Albert Einstein Healthcare Network in New York. These organizations also use a variety of techniques to identify the key drivers that determine how customers view the total healthcare experience.

The key drivers of patients and other customers will vary from one facility to another. For example, a managed care company may find that its customers want easy access online, responsive and knowledgeable customer service representatives, and an unchanging panel of providers. For a primary care physician practice, the key drivers might be the possibility of quick appointment scheduling, physician promptness in seeing the patient at the appointed time, and clear communication from the physician and nurse.

Generally speaking, the key drivers reflect expectations related to clinical outcomes, behaviors (i.e., being treated with respect and dignity), systems and processes (i.e., the way patients are scheduled for tests), and the environment (i.e., cleanliness and ease of navigation). Each organization needs to identify its customers' key drivers in general and then do the same for customers in each department and/or service/product line. Customers for certain services or products may have different expectations from customers for other services or products. An emergency department (ED) patient, for example, has expectations different from those of a maternity-ward patient.

An organization cannot know what factors in the service product, the environment, and the delivery system are key to patient satisfaction and intent to return until it carefully studies all of these drivers. Many times, what management learns in such studies is a surprise because what management thought were key drivers may not turn out to be so from the patient's point of view. This service gap is the difference between what the organization delivers and what the patient needs, wants, and expects. No matter how much patient data it collects and analyzes, the organization may still be surprised occasionally by what patients say are important to them.

Excellent organizations not only study their patients extensively but also accumulate the information they have learned about patients, individually and collectively. Computerized databases and sophisticated techniques of database analysis allow an organization to know a great deal about its patients—as a demographic, as a psychographic group, or as individuals. The best organizations mine these databases to dig up as much information as they can about what is important to their patients so they can ensure that they provide what is expected.

Extras

Outstanding organizations that attract repeat patients accumulate patient information that may be used to customize the service experience. In other words, these organizations know that the best get even better by wisely using customer databases to personalize each patient's healthcare experience according to her unique needs, wants, and expectations.

Some hospitals have developed systems for making each patient feel special by letting each manager view the service experience for a particular diagnosis from the patient's perspective. For example, a manager might follow a patient undergoing an MRI (magnetic resonance imaging) procedure so that he too can experience every step of the process. Within 24 hours, the manager calls staff to a debriefing session, during which participants discuss the experience and any problems encountered and then brainstorm solutions. Later, the manager documents the experience and the items discussed at the session, including key observations, improvement opportunities, and recommendations. In this way, not only does the organization get a chance to improve its service product and strengthen its managers' commitment to customer service, but the patient being observed and monitored also gets to feel special.

Knowing what makes each patient feel special enables organizations to add the differentiating factors and extras all excellent organizations want to provide to keep their patients so satisfied they will want to return if and when they need treatment again. The little bit more than the patient expected can make the difference; it can turn a satisfactory experience into a memorable one and can keep the organization at the top of the customer's mind when thinking about where to go the next time a particular patient service is desired or when making recommendations to others.

These extras can be built into the service product, the environment, the service delivery system, or across all parts of the service experience. Based on knowledge about patient key drivers and likes and dislikes, the designers of the experience can build in those things that will make a noticeable positive difference in the patient's mind. They should, however, always follow up to develop the metrics that will allow them to know if they were successful and, if not, they should initiate efforts to find out where and why they failed.

The extras do not have to be expensive, complicated, or elaborate, although they may be. Bedside manner does not cost anything, for example, but certain environmental features may be quite expensive. Florida Hospital in Orlando has created a staff position—concierge—for its orthopedics unit. This position involves being a contact person for each patient and making sure that each patient receives a seamless healthcare experience.

Planning

Providing the patient with both the expected parts of the healthcare experience and the extra or differentiating factors is the result of extensive planning. And this planning always starts with the patient. Capacity and location decisions, staffing plans, the design of personnel policies, and the selection of medical equipment must all be based on the organization's best information on what kind of experience the patient wants, needs, and expects from the organization.

If the organization's mission is to build a chain of freestanding "doc-in-the-boxes," then it must identify what staffing, locations, medical equipment, exterior appearances, and clinic sizes it should have. These decisions can be properly made if they are based on solid and extensive customer research. Organizations that understand the key drivers of a healthcare experience use the best data they can gather. Although many organizations still base these decisions on a variety of factors, benchmark institutions always start with the patient and make sure every decision is based on a thorough knowledge and understanding of the patient.

Feedback

Benchmark organizations also know that the discovery process is never ending, so they constantly seek feedback from their customers about what works and what does not. Patient needs, wants, and expectations change, and the best organizations change as well in response to evolving patient expectations. Those organizations that constantly seek to exceed patient expectations build in their own future challenges. Today's extras are tomorrow's standard patient expectations.

Outstanding organizations are constantly trying to outdo their present performance, and they survey customers constantly to determine how well they are satisfying their key drivers. For example, a medical group practice had a long history of complaints and frustrations associated with a paper scheduling system for patient appointments. As a result of survey data from three customer groups (i.e., physicians, staff, and patients), a new online appointment system was installed. Success indicators were then developed to evaluate the results of the new system, focusing on key drivers suggested by each of the three customer groups. Significant improvement in satisfaction of all three customer groups resulted from this process.

Culture

Managers of outstanding organizations should remember the importance of the organizational culture in filling in the gaps between what the organization can anticipate and train its people to deal with and what actually happens in the daily encounters with a wide variety of patients. Anticipating the many different things patients will do, ask for, and expect from the service provider is impossible.

Thus, the power of the culture to guide and direct employees to do the right thing for the patient becomes vital. Good managers know that the values, beliefs, and norms of behavior the culture teaches its employees are critical in ensuring that the patient-care staff do what the organization needs them to do in unplanned and unanticipated situations, even if the organization has no specific policies relevant to that situation.

The culture must be planned and carefully thought through to ensure that the message sent to all employees is the one the organization really wants to send. An important part of any strategy is to ensure that everything the organization and its leadership says and does is consistent with the culture it wishes to define and support. The more intangible the healthcare product, the stronger the cultural values, beliefs, and norms must be to ensure that the provider delivers the quality and value of healthcare experience the patient expects and the organization wants to deliver.

Service or Price

In the future, healthcare organizations will tend to compete on service or price even more than they do now. A successful group of organizations in every service sector will seek to add value to each customer service encounter (like the strategy of Pearle Vision) or seek to define value on price alone (like the strategy of discount opticals). By focusing on a particular niche of the market, advertising to that niche, and then serving that niche well, these companies (like Southwest Airlines and retail health clinics) will thrive. However, healthcare organizations typically market their services based on some combination of clinical effectiveness, service quality, and (possibly) price. In other words, they market based on value received rather than price alone.

Low-cost providers may appeal to price-conscious consumers by using technology to become more efficient. High-cost providers can increasingly customize the product to each patient's expectations at the price point plus offer a little bit more because they can provide their employees with the necessary information to personalize the service in a prompt, friendly, and efficient way.

The healthcare businesses between these two ends of the spectrum will have the most difficult challenge. They will be challenged to offer patient services that are as personalized as those offered by the high-cost organizations, while providing the low prices that the price-oriented firms offer. This middle group of organizations may do neither very well. They may find themselves in the position of overpromising and underdelivering, which is not the way to have satisfied, loyal, or repeat patients.

STAFFING

Staffing has become an increasingly important factor for all healthcare organizations as they realize that the most effective way to differentiate themselves from their competitors is through the quality of the service encounters the patient-contact staff provide. Competitors can readily imitate the service product, the physical elements of the environment, and the technical aspects of the delivery system, but not the people. For example, each hospital or clinic may have nearly the same physical equipment as every other hospital/clinic. It will not take long for one hospital or clinic to duplicate the factor that makes its competitor successful. Any new machine or system is an innovation only for as long as it takes the competition to replicate it.

Employee Engagement

People, not MRI technology, make the difference. If one clinic has friendly employees and another clinic does not, customers will go to the friendly one, unless their HMO requires the second. When all other factors are equal, or nearly so, the healthcare staff make the difference. The challenge for healthcare managers is to empower the service provider to engage each patient on a personal, individual basis while still maintaining production efficiency and consistent quality in the service delivery process.

For example, a pharmacist is responsible for filling prescriptions exactly as prescribed in an efficient fashion that respects a patient's time constraints. He can handle the transaction in an impersonal manner (barely speaking to the patient). Alternatively, the patient can be engaged in a conversation about other prescriptions, any allergic reactions to drugs, the weather, or inquiries about family members (if known to the pharmacist). If the pharmacist just processes people, he may become bored. If he engages them, the job becomes more interesting. The latter approach is much more likely to enhance the patients' relationship with the provider and to make way for a healthcare experience that exceeds expectations.

The division will widen between organizations that can engage all the capabilities of its employees and those who use employees only from the neck down. Value added to the healthcare experience through the skills of employees engaging in service encounters will become a more important differentiating strategy as the decreasing costs and increasingly available technology make the healthcare product and service delivery system components (except for people) increasingly easy to duplicate and emulate by all competitors. If all eye exams are essentially alike, the feel-good part of the eye exam becomes an increasingly important part of the total experience.

Advertising alone cannot provide this difference and, in fact, may be counterproductive if patients do not encounter what the glowing ads lead them to expect. Staff members can make the difference that patients remember. If your patients continue to think and speak well of you, you must be doing something right. If they do not speak well of you and do not hold your organization in high regard, then implementing the principles outlined in this book will move you toward healthcare excellence. If their continued high regard is vital to your organization's survival, you better find a way to keep it.

Selection and Training

Some employees figure it out, engage their customers, and actually do have fun. They are usually the ones who were selected properly in the first place. Finding the right people for patient-service jobs is an important responsibility of the selection process. Putting the right people in these jobs eliminates many of the problems in delivering high-quality healthcare experiences. Some people are just plain good at quickly establishing personal contact with patients, and they can be identified through effective selection techniques. Finding these people and training them in both the cultural values and the basic engagement skills necessary for effective service delivery are key responsibilities for healthcare human resources managers.

Recall that patient-contact employees have three responsibilities in the service encounter: They deliver the service (or in some cases create it on the spot), they manage the quality of the encounters or interactions between the patient and the organization, and they identify and fix the inevitable problems. Too many organizations train only for the first responsibility and neglect the other two. In many instances, receiving the service product is just one element in the patient's determination of the quality and value of the experience. Employees must also be trained to deal effectively with the variety of personalities and concerns that different patients will bring to the healthcare experience.

Selecting the right person for the job starts by clearly defining what the job requires. If you want a person to be a receptionist, who serves as a pleasant, reasonably informed first point of contact for new patients, then hire someone with a certain bundle of skills. If you want a person to be a triage decision maker, who not only serves as the first point of contact but also decides who needs immediate treatment and who does not, then hire someone with skills different from those of a good receptionist. Leaders should also allow peers to participate in selection interviews as these are the people who will be working with the new employee.

Studer (2008) has recommended re-recruiting new employees at 30- and 90-day intervals. The purpose of these 30- and 90-day interviews is to make sure that the employee is "on board," her expectations are being met, and the goals of both supervisor and employee are aligned. "On-board" means the employee has bought into the goals, requirements, and behavior of staff members necessary to implement a customer-service culture. A major purpose is also to enhance retention of new employees, as they often leave within the first three months.

The second part of the staffing issue is training. Studer (2008) recommends that leaders be trained first, because it makes no sense to train employees and align their behavior with the organization's mission, vision, values, and strategies if the top management team is not also aligned. The right person in the right job must be trained to do it the right way. Some jobs in the healthcare industry are repetitive, simple, and boring; others are also repetitive and boring but complex instead of simple. Both require incredible attention to detail and concentration on task performance so the employee provides the same healthcare experience in the same flawless way for each patient.

An employee can easily lose focus, daydream, or otherwise lose interest in taking blood from the 30th person of the day. By that time, his arms are tired, his attention span is short, and his interest in greeting one more patient with a friendly smile and positive eye contact is about zero. Part of that employee's training should include how to cope with the emotional labor that is part of these jobs (Larson and Yao 2005).

When the encounters are short—as in a visit to the lab or the billing office—the training challenge is particularly difficult because the staff member must know how to build a connection to the patient quickly. The use of scripts or scripted behaviors is one way organizations help employees respond appropriately to the different expectations of different patients, even when the employee may be bored, tired, or stressed out.

Rewards and Recognition

Service excellence requires that rewards and recognition be provided for leaders and staff who demonstrate high levels of service excellence. Studer (2008) recommends identifying low performers, middle performers, and high performers. For high performers, he suggests more training and development as well as more recognition and rewards. For low performers, he suggests conversations that identify deficiencies and possible ways the employee must enhance her performance. However, in some cases the person may have to be dismissed from the organization if performance does not improve. For the middle level of performers, he suggests continuing conversations, measuring performance, and rewarding performance as it improves.

The advantage service organizations like healthcare offer to employees over typical industrial settings is the positive feedback and stimulation that dealing with patients can bring, especially when employees know that what they do may make the difference between sickness and health or life and death. Once employees learn, through experience or training, how to derive some sense of satisfaction out of doing something that makes a patient happy, they enjoy their jobs and feel a sense of accomplishment.

In addition to their paid employees, benchmark organizations rely on volunteers to provide some of the patient contact. Volunteers may be better able to engage patients and their families because they have more time to do so. The only question is whether they are provided with appropriate rewards and recognition that motivate them to do so. Recent empirical research indicates that volunteers can and do make significant, positive contributions to patient satisfaction (Hotchkiss, Fottler, and Unruh 2009). Many healthcare organizations have discovered that some of their best volunteers are older, retired people who are often lonely, bored, and looking for something to do that will allow them to have positive contact with other people. Some organizations that originally recruited older people because of labor shortages have found to their pleasant surprise that many older people bring an enthusiasm for service that makes them great employees.

Obviously, all staff members are "volunteers" in the sense that they can choose to do more than the minimum required by their job description or not. They work under a wide variety of financial or nonfinancial rewards, including personal recognition. If organizations are able to identify and respond to these needs by providing valued rewards and recognition, they are more likely to achieve higher levels of customer satisfaction.

More and more healthcare employees are looking for job challenges and increased opportunities to be responsible for the patient encounter. The need to trust the employees and allow them to take on this responsibility will intensify as the competition for talented employees becomes greater. Good people want to take the responsibility, and successful organizations are those that find ways to preserve the quality and value of the healthcare experience while empowering their employees to be responsible for patient satisfaction.

Allowing playfulness is an important approach to reward and recognition that enables staff to release tension in stress-filled settings. Furthermore, most people like to celebrate, and employees are no different. Celebrations of success can take the form of parties, balloons, banners, pictures of the honored managers and staff, and recognition dinners. No success should be allowed to pass unnoticed.

Finally, a customer-focused reward and recognition system requires an excellent performance appraisal system. Because what is measured and rewarded is managed, leaders should be continually checking on the performance of their subordinates based on objective measures of the individual's customer service and other key performance attributes. In addition, the performance evaluation system needs to be tied to compensation and other rewards valued by the subordinates. Finally, the organization needs to continually monitor employee satisfaction and take steps to remedy any deficiencies to enhance employee retention and respond to employee concerns.

Standards of Behavior and Performance

One way to ensure understanding of and agreement with the organization's commitment to a customer service mission is to require that before being hired, all job applicants read and sign a performance standards agreement that specifies, among other things, the customer service standards expected by the organization. This performance standards agreement should be based on input from all employees, align individual behavior with strategic goals and mission, use specific language, hold people accountable, and be updated periodically.

A large part of a manager's job is to define employees' job responsibilities, goals, standards of performance, and management's expectations of what behaviors match the organization's culture. These must be clearly spelled out, defined with specific metrics, and reinforced and rewarded by managers every day.

Once a manager lets an employee provide service of less than outstanding quality or overlooks poor employee performance, the message goes out to everyone that managers do not always really mean what they say about providing high-quality customer service. Just as a patient has many "moments of truth" during the course of a single healthcare experience, employees have many moments of truth with every manager every day. What happens during these moments of truth tells the employees a great deal about what management really believes in. This is where the organizational mission statement, corporate culture, and corporate policies about customer focus become real.

Just as one employee at one moment of truth can destroy the patient's perception of the entire organization and what it stands for, so too can one supervisor overlooking one violation of patient-care quality standards or job performance change the way an employee looks at an organization. Although most organizations do a good job of developing selection techniques and providing the necessary job training, many fall short in the reinforcement area. When they let things slide, they miss the chance to reinforce the positive and coach away the negative aspects of employee performance.

Many outstanding organizations require their managers to be in their job areas "walking the walk and talking the talk"; it is a vital part of how the message is sent to employees that everyone is responsible for customer service, including the managers. This policy also builds a sense of community among the employees in that everyone is there to serve the customer.

Patient and Family

Just as organizations can benefit from thinking of their employees as customers, they can also benefit from thinking of their customers as employees. It gives the organization a different way of looking at and thinking about their customers if they define them as quasi-employees.

Customer-employees can serve several important functions. They can be knowledgeable unpaid consultants, as they give helpful feedback to the organization regarding their level of satisfaction with the healthcare experience. They can help create the service experience for other patients, as they are typically part of the service environment. If being surrounded by other patients is a necessary part of each patient's experience, then how these customer-employees are used to help create each other's experience becomes an important part of the management process.

Most important, with encouragement and training from the organization, customers can become coproducers of their own service experience. Coproduction benefits both the patient and the organization. It reduces the labor costs for the organization, and knowledgeable patients (perhaps with the help of their family and friends) are likely to receive a better healthcare experience because they helped produce it. In addition, patients do not have to wait for some services that they can do on their own.

SYSTEMS

The best, most thoroughly trained people in the world cannot satisfy a patient if they deliver the wrong medicine, operate on the wrong body part, or provide the wrong therapy perfectly. A huge, complex system (like a university teaching hospital) and a simple system (like a dental clinic) both have to be carefully managed so the right product is delivered to patients when they expect it to be.

Patients do not care that the room is not ready yet because the laundry broke down, or that the organization misplaced a medical shipment so they cannot get the drugs they need, or that the staff specialists are unavailable because someone forgot to schedule them. The patient just wants a clean room, the right medicine, and the right specialist, and the patient wants those now. If these things do not happen, then the production system, the support system, the information system, or the organizational system has failed, and someone needs to fix it—fast.

Models

The most highly developed applications related to providing an excellent healthcare experience can be found in the clinical systems area. Models of patient behavior in many situations can be built and used to understand and predict ways in which the organization can best treat the patient's medical condition. Such clinical models can be extended into modeling all aspects of the healthcare experience. Simulations are an important technique for doing this, and with the decreasing costs of computers and increasingly user-friendly software packages, simulations will become more available and relevant to all types of healthcare organizations.

Once the planning process has gotten the design right and the measurement systems are in place to get patient feedback, the stage is set to use simulations of the entire healthcare experience to see if it all works as a system. Organizations need to ensure that the right capacity has been built into their service delivery system. The design-day selection and the parameters used (such as maximum wait times) drive the rest of the capacity decisions.

Because customers are not impressed by excuses such as "the computer system is down today," backup systems need to be in place so that customers are not inconvenienced. Having managers go through the service delivery process like patients sensitizes them to potential problems. In many organizations, the most visible part of the healthcare experience is the wait for care. This wait system, therefore, requires extra organizational time and attention to ensure that the inevitable waits are tolerable and within the limits patients will accept without becoming dissatisfied.

Waiting Times

Waiting periods are easily modeled and studied with simulation techniques and easy-to-use computer software. Everything from the number of beds in a hospital to the number of physicians on duty in an ED to the number of phone lines needed at an HMO call center can be simulated based on patient demand data. If you know how many patients are coming to your place of business and can estimate a predictable distribution to represent their arrival patterns and times for service, modeling how the waiting experience can be managed and balanced against capacity is relatively simple.

Managing the waiting time is important from the capacity standpoint and the psychological standpoint. Because few can build enough capacity to serve peak demand periods, and few can stockpile their mostly perishable and intangible product, managing the patient's wait is critical for all organizations. The greater the perceived value of the healthcare experience, the longer the patient will wait. Again, this area is susceptible to empirical research; how long patients will wait for anything before they give up and leave can be studied, measured, and understood.

Measurement

The excellent organizations of the future will use every tool at their command to figure out what patients want and then provide it in a way that is consistent with the patient expectations of value and quality. If they promise a high-quality healthcare experience that includes friendly service, they better provide those features or patients with other options will not come back. Most organizations depend on the high regard of their patients, and disappointing them will cost dearly in a competitive marketplace.

Once you tell your customers what you will do for them, you have made a commitment and a promise. If the promise is broken or the commitment unrealized, patients will be unhappy and will tell everyone they know how unhappy they are. Few organizations can afford to break their promises, and the more an organization depends on a good reputation and positive word of mouth, the less chance it can take of violating that trust.

Information and opinions about service quality are freely and widely available now and will become even more so in the future. If a dissatisfied patient posts a negative comment on the Web about a service, that comment is readily accessible to anyone with Internet access. The more the Internet is involved in helping consumers select a healthcare provider, the more critical it becomes to avoid service failures.

Some major healthcare organizations now have an employee whose only job is to monitor discussion groups and blogs on the Internet to detect and hopefully correct patient complaints and false rumors that show up. A job classification that did not even exist ten years ago is becoming an increasingly important part of the organization's communication strategy as it seeks to monitor and address the negative word of mouth or misinformation that now travels instantly across cyberspace to the entire world.

Measurement is crucially important because what gets measured gets managed and improved. As noted earlier, feedback given in various forms from both employees and patients is critical. In this way, the total healthcare experience is transparent, individual behavior is aligned with strategic goals, people are held accountable for achieving these goals, and the organization is able to show progress over time.

Consistent Improvement

The future will be information management, people management, an increasing focus on understanding what each patient really wants (a "market niche of one" that allows the organization to build a relationship with each patient), and a focus on the organizational core competencies that satisfy these patient expectations. The future will also bring forth more knowledgeable customers with ever-rising expectations. The more competitors in a marketplace try to outdo each other in providing superb healthcare experiences, the more familiar these experiences will become.

Yesterday's exceptional experience becomes today's expected minimum level of service. Healthcare managers will need to engage the entire organization in constantly reviewing all aspects of the customer service product, strategy, environment, and staffing of the service delivery system to innovate new and not easily duplicated features that make the future patient experience as memorable as today's.

The easiest and most fruitful area in which to develop these features is in the interaction between staff and patients, where healthcare employees can elevate an expected experience into something that is truly memorable. The challenge here is to empower them to provide that unique extra touch without jeopardizing the quality and consistency of the clinical experience. Human error is inevitable, and the need to blend technology and people to provide a high-tech and high-touch experience of consistently high quality will be the biggest and most interesting challenge for the future healthcare manager seeking excellence in the healthcare experience provided.

Finally, service recovery is crucial. Because no organization is perfect, providing multiple methods for customers to communicate problems is necessary. The cost of losing a patient, as well as his family and friends, far exceeds the immediate costs of making things right.

THE ROLE OF LEADERS

We end this chapter by stressing an idea that has been implied throughout this book: Managers must lead staff toward excellence. The leader is the symbol and teacher of what the organization stands for and believes. If the leader does not lead, all the efforts to discover the key drivers that cause the customer to seek out a particular healthcare experience; the expense of designing a healthcare environment; the resources dedicated to building, maintaining, and constantly improving a service delivery system; and the effort to recruit and train the best people are wasted. Every day and in every way, the leaders must set the example and consistently communicate to all employees what their value is to the organization and to its mission of creating the healthcare experience.

Everyone wants to feel that what she does has value and meaning to a purpose larger than enriching a company's top executives and stakeholders. Leaders not only inspire their staff to realize their individual worth to the organization but also help staff see how they contribute to the greater good by doing their jobs with excellence. Telling people how important it is that they do their jobs well is not enough; all employees must understand and believe that their contributions make a difference and that doing well, whatever they do, is vital in making the world a better place.

Many organizations make efforts in this direction, but only a few succeed. These benchmark organizations inspire their employees to believe they are responsible for saving lives, relieving human suffering, and healing many who would not otherwise return to health. These organizations constantly remind all employees that what they are doing has a greater purpose than merely giving shots, cleaning rooms, or emptying bedpans.

Each job has value, and the person doing the job has value because of the contribution to the larger purpose. This is a vital part of inspiring people not only to do a job but to do it with pride and commitment. Not every employee will be deeply affected, but this idea is planted in so many healthcare employees' minds that it creates the strong cultural reinforcement that focuses everyone's attention on producing an excellent experience for each patient. This is a powerful leadership technique and a valuable way to ensure that everyone stays focused on the patient.

The commitment and enthusiasm of great organizational leaders is contagious and leads to involvement and passion among all organizational members. Leaders find ways to make employees feel that their jobs are fun, fair, interesting, and important. Leaders establish a culture of service excellence and reinforce it by word, deed, and celebration. Leaders give value to employees by showing them they are appreciated and respected for their contributions to the organization and to the larger purpose toward which the organization aspires. Leaders have the joy and the responsibility of making it all happen: happy, motivated staff members; outstanding healthcare experiences; and highly satisfied patients whose loyalty, goodwill, and positive word of mouth in the community form the foundation of organizational service and performance.

Common sense and research suggest that a relationship exists among the behavior of organizational leaders, how employees feel about their jobs, and how that feeling is translated into the level of service they provide. If staff members feel positive, they provide a high level of service. Creative, high-quality service for patients links directly to patient opinions, and these opinions are a key part of any organization's success. This chain reaction all starts with the leaders. In the organizational units where employees rate their leaders as outstanding in such behaviors as listening, coaching, recognition, and empowerment, the patient satisfaction ratings are invariably the highest.

Finally, the leader blends the strategy, staff, and systems so everyone knows he is supposed to concentrate on patients and other customers. The strategy, staffing, and systems must be carefully managed if the combined effort is going to succeed in providing an outstanding total healthcare experience. If the leader sees that any element is not contributing to the employee's ability to provide outstanding experiences, the leader will fix it or have it fixed.

Just as the organization wants to fix any patient problem that detracts from the healthcare experience, the outstanding leader wants to fix any staff member's problem that detracts from that person's ability to provide the outstanding healthcare experience. Vision, skills, incentives, delivery system, and measurement are leadership components that leaders must manage if they are to meet this challenge effectively. As noted in Exhibit 15.2, all must be present to produce and maintain highly satisfied customers. More specifically, leaders must do the following:

- Define an organizational vision of what patient segment is to be served and what service concept will best meet customer expectations (vision).
- Establish a customer-focused culture to enhance clinical excellence (vision).
- Communicate the organization's mission and vision to all customers on an ongoing basis through a wide variety of methods (vision).
- Select employees with service-oriented attitudes, and train them in the necessary clinical and customer service skills (skills).
- Train staff to exceed customer expectations on an ongoing basis using scripts, role playing, and other training methods (skills).
- Create standards of behavior and performance, and hold staff accountable for upholding these standards (incentives).
- Create and implement the incentives that will motivate empowered employees to provide unsurpassed customer service (incentives).
- Establish a service recovery system that empowers all staff to identify and rectify all customer service problems (incentives).
- Communicate and celebrate all individual and group successes (incentives).
- Ensure that employees have the proper resources to provide outstanding service (resources).
- Create a clean and attractive environment for all customers (delivery system).
- Design specific delivery systems that translate plans, employee skills, and resources into an experience that meets patient expectations and perhaps even wows the patient (delivery system).
- Focus on employee retention and patient retention (measurement).
- Provide the measurement tools that allow employees (and coproducing patients) to see how well they are doing in providing the targeted or desired healthcare experience (measurement).
- Use data generated from the measurement tools to continually identify and implement improvements in customer service, because success is never final (measurement).

Measurement is critical for ensuring that all factors of service are correctly focused on achieving the best for the patient. Simply, if you do not know how you are doing, you do not know if you need to do better, and you do not know how to do better. If you try to improve patient service, you do not know if you have succeeded unless you implement measurement techniques. Continual improvement is also necessary given that momentum can easily be lost.

Exhibit 15.2 Leadership Components

Skills + Incentives + Resources + Delivery System + Measurement − *Vision*
= Unfocused Employees = Unfocused Service = Confused Customers

Vision + Incentives + Resources + Delivery System + Measurement − *Skills*
= Untrained Employees = Probable Failed Service = Disappointed
Customers

Vision + Skills + Resources + Delivery System + Measurement − *Incentives*
= Unmotivated Employees = Lackluster Service = Disillusioned
Customers

Vision + Skills + Incentives + Delivery System + Measurement − *Resources*
= Unsupported Employees = Inadequate Service = Complaining
Customers

Vision + Skills + Incentives + Resources + Measurement − *Delivery System*
= Unreliable Employees = Unreliable Service = Unsatisfied Customers

Vision + Skills + Incentives + Resources + Delivery System − *Measurement*
= Uninformed Employees = Inconsistent Service = Unfulfilled
Customers

Vision + Skills + Incentives + Resources + Delivery System + Measurement
= Unsurpassed Employees = Superb Service = Highly Satisfied
Customers

Exhibit 15.2 shows how the customer and the customer's experience can be negatively affected when leaders fail to manage any one of these important leadership components. However, negative outcomes can be prevented. Just as service problems happen in the best-managed organizations, so can patient-contact staff of poorly managed organizations sometimes provide successful healthcare experiences in spite of the organization and its faults. When one or more leadership components are missing, however, the chances of consistent service success are reduced. The exact effect on the healthcare experience may not be predictable in precise terms, but it will not be a happy one.

Exhibit 15.2 also shows how a missing leadership element can affect employees. Although managers will do as good a job as they can of managing the nonhuman elements, their ability to change them may be limited. If the clinic is already constructed and the laboratory set up, the clinic manager may not be able to manage the service environment and the mechanical parts of the delivery system much.

In a way this is good news because it enables managers to focus on the people part of the healthcare experience: the patients as part of the environment for each other, the patients as they participate in creating their own experiences, the clinical and staff as they try to provide outstanding customer experiences, and all other support staff as they provide the assistance that their internal customers require. These many and ever-changing elements of the healthcare situation require and deserve each manager's attention.

If the organization's leaders lack an overall vision of the target market and its expectations, this lack will be communicated from the top throughout the culture and may lead to unfocused service. Staff members will not be sure exactly what they are trying to achieve, and patients will receive mixed messages and an inconsistent experience. If managers put untrained people in patient-contact positions, service failures and disappointed patients are the probable result. If incentives are lacking or inappropriate, unmotivated staff will simply go through the motions of providing lackluster healthcare experiences.

Failure to provide resource support for all staff—clinical and nonclinical—will prohibit even a motivated and patient-focused staff from providing adequate service. Similarly, flaws in the delivery system will keep even the best personnel from providing reliably satisfactory healthcare experiences, much less superb ones; as the saying goes, "A bad system will defeat a good person every time."

Finally, if levels of service quality and patient satisfaction are not measured, employees will be frustrated by not knowing whether the healthcare experiences they are providing are achieving the healthcare mission or not; so in a hit-or-miss fashion, they will continue to provide inconsistent service.

Only when these components are all in place can the leader be effective in enabling and empowering employees. Only then can empowered employees provide the outstanding healthcare experiences that fulfill the organizational vision of providing remarkable service that exceeds patient expectations. Every manager, from the chief executive officer to the frontline supervisor, must ultimately make sure that employees feel good about what they are doing, that they convey this feeling to patients, and that patients leave knowing the experience was worth every penny paid and maybe a little bit more. Leadership makes the difference between success and failure in today's healthcare organizations, and it will make the difference in the future.

CONCLUSION

The healthcare experience, despite all its components—service product, service setting, and service delivery system—is not complete without the patient. Without the patient, the carefully designed service product; the detailed and inviting setting; the highly trained, motivated staff; and the finest facilities and equipment are just part of an experience waiting to happen. Throughout this book, we have made the point that everything starts with the patient. We conclude by saying that everything ends with the patient as well.

Service Strategies

1. Start with the customer—both external patients and internal staff members.
2. Articulate a vision, transcending any single job, that gives all staff a sense of value and worth in what they do.
3. Manage all three parts of the organization's service system—strategy, staffing, and systems—and focus them on achieving strategic goals related to customer service.
4. Build a strong customer service culture and sustain it with stories, deeds, and actions.
5. Organize, staff, train, and reward around the patient's needs, wants, and expectations.
6. Train all staff to think of the people in front of them as their guests.
7. Ensure that jobs are fun, fair, and interesting to help employees provide superb experiences.
8. Keep in mind the strong relationship between highly satisfied employees and highly satisfied patients.
9. Incorporate customer satisfaction skills into employee training programs.
10. Never stop teaching; inspire everyone to keep learning.
11. Establish a standard of performance, measure it, and then manage it carefully.
12. Use information to improve strategy, staffing, and service elements identified by customers as deficient.
13. Link customer satisfaction scores to management and employee rewards and recognition.
14. Prevent every service problem you can, find every problem you cannot prevent, and fix every problem you find every time and, if possible, on the spot.

References

AARP. 2008. "Best Employers for Workers Over 50." [Online information; retrieved 5/29/09.] www.aarp.org/money/work/best_employers/Best_Employer_Winners/.

ACHe-news. 2001. "Dissatisfied Employees? Your Training Programs Could Be the Culprit." *ACHe-news* (April 16): 2.

AHRQ Health Care Innovations Exchange. 2009. "Rooftop Garden Provides Healing Environment, Enhancing Recovery for Rehabilitation Hospital Patients." [Online information; retrieved 5/29/09.] www.innovations.ahrq.gov/content.aspx?id=2143.

Airoldi, D. M. 2007. "JetBlue to Pay Bill of Rights." *Business Travel News* 24 (4).

Albrecht, K. 1988. *At America's Service: How Your Company Can Join the Customer Service Revolution.* New York: Warner Books.

———. 2004. "Take Time for Effective Learning." *Training* 41 (7): 38–42.

Albrecht, K., and R. Zemke. 2002. *Service America in the New Economy.* New York: McGraw-Hill.

Alliance. 1998. "Consumer Attitudes." *Alliance* (May–June): 11.

Alvarez, A. M., and M. A. Centeno. 2000. "Simulation-Based Decision Support for Emergency Room Systems." *International Journal of Healthcare Technology and Management* 2 (5–6): 523–38.

American Association of Colleges of Nursing (AACN). 2007. "Nursing Shortage." [Online news release; retrieved 1/29/08.] www.aacn.nche.edu/Media/FactSheets/NursingShortage.htm.

American Customer Satisfaction Index (ACSI).

2008. "Scores by Industry." [Online information; retrieved 7/09.] www.theacsi.org/index.php?option=com_content&task=view&id=148&Itemid=156.

American Hospital Association. 2007. "The 2007 State of America's Hospitals—Taking the Pulse: Findings from the 2007 AHA Survey of Hospital Leaders July 2007." [Online information; retrieved 1/31/08.] www.aha.org/aha/content/2007/ PowerPoint/StateofHospitalsChartPack2007.ppt.

Anderson, R.T., F. T. Camacho, and R. Balkrishnan. 2007. "Willing to Wait?: The Influence of Patient Wait Time on Satisfaction with Primary Care." *BMC Health Services Research* 7: 31–36.

Associated Press. 2009. "50 Million New Patients? Expect Doc Shortages." [Online article; retrieved 9/15/09.] www.msnbc.msn.com/id/32829974/ns/health-health_care/.

Arcspace. 2003. [Online information; retrieved 5/29/09.] www.arcspace.com/architects/gehry/maggies/.

Arnst, C. 2007. "The Doctor Will See You—In Three Months." *Business Week* (July 9/16): 100.

———. 2008. "If Healthcare Were Run Like Retail." *Business Week* (December 22): 66–67.

Atchison, T., and G. Carlson. 2009. *Leading Healthcare Cultures: How Human Capital Drives Financial Performance.* Chicago: Health Administration Press.

Athavaley, A. 2007. "Job References You Can Control." *Wall Street Journal* (September 27): D1–D2.

Atkins, P., B. S. Marshall, and R. G. Javalgi. 1996. "Happy Employees Lead to Loyal

Patients." *Journal of Healthcare Marketing* 16 (4): 14–23.

Auerbach, D. I., P. I. Buerhaus, and D. O. Staiger. 2007. "Better Late than Never: Workforce Supply Implications of Later Entry into Nursing." *Health Affairs* 26 (1): 178–85.

Baird, K. 2000. *Customer Service in Health Care*. San Francisco: Jossey-Bass.

Baker, G. R., A. MacIntosh-Murray, C. Porcellato, L. Dionne, K. Stelmacovich, and K. Born. 2008. *High Performing Healthcare Systems: Delivering Quality by Design*. Toronto: Longwoods Publishing Corporation.

Ball, M., C. Smith, and R. Bakalar. 2007. "Personal Health Records: Empowering Consumers." *Journal of Healthcare Information Management* 21(1): 76–86.

Baptist Health Care. 2009. "Awards." [Online information; retrieved 5/1/09.] www.ebaptisthealthcare.org/Awards.

Barr, C. K. 1999. "Mission Statement Content and Hospital Performance in the Canadian Not-for-Profit Health Care Sector." *Health Care Management Review* 24 (3): 18–29.

Barsky, A., and S. A. Kaplan. 2007. "If You Feel Bad, It's Unfair: A Quantitative Synthesis of Affect and Organizational Justice Perceptions." *Journal of Applied Psychology* 88 (3): 432–43.

Beach, M. C., E. G. Price, T. L. Gary, K. A. Robinson, A. Gozu, A. Palacio, C. Smarth, M. W. Jenckes, C. Feuerstein, E. B. Bass, N. R. Powe, and L. A. Cooper. 2005. "Cultural Competence: A Systematic Review of Health Care Provider Educational Interventions." *Medical Care* 43 (4): 356–73.

Beck, M. 2008. "Bedside Manner: Advocating for a Relative in the Hospital." *Wall Street Journal* (October 28): D1.

———. 2009. "Health Matters." *Wall Street Journal*. [Online information; retrieved 7/09.] http://online.wsj.com/article/SB123445381743877781.html.

Beckwith, D. 2008. "Influences of Color on Health Care." [Online information; retrieved 3/4/08.] www.contemporary.ab.ca/ke/content/pdf/colorinfludences1000.pdf.

Bellou, V. 2007. "Achieving Long Term Customer Satisfaction Through Organizational Culture: Evidence from the Health Care Sector." *Managing Service Quality* 17 (5): 510–22.

Belton, L. W., and S. R. Dyrenforth. 2007. "Civility in the Workplace." *Healthcare Executive* (Sept/Oct).

Bendapudi, N., L. Berry, K. Frey, J. Parish, and W. Rayburn. 2006. "Patient's Perspectives on Ideal Physician Behaviors." *Mayo Clinic Proceedings* 81 (3): 338–44.

Berkowitz, E. N. 2006. *Essentials of Health Care Marketing,* 2nd ed. Sudbury, MA: Jones and Bartlett.

Berry, L. L. 1995. *On Great Service: A Framework for Action*. New York: The Free Press.

———. 1999. *Discovering the Soul of Service*. New York: The Free Press.

———. 2009. "Competing with Quality Service in Good Times and Bad." *Business Horizons* 52 (4): 309–17.

Berry, L., and N. Bendapudi. 2003. "Cluing in Customers." *Harvard Business Review* 81 (2): 100–06.

———. 2007. "Health Care: A Fertile Field for Service Research." *Journal of Service Research* 10 (2): 111–22.

Berry, L., and K. D. Seltman. 2008. *Management Lessons from the Mayo Clinic: Inside One of the World's Most Admired Service Organizations*. New York: McGraw-Hill

Berwick, D. M., and M. Kotagal. 2004. "Restricted Visiting Hours in the ICU: Time to Change." *Journal of the American Medical Association* 292 (6): 736–37.

Beryl Institute. 2007. "Moments of Truth: Hospital Switchboards a Bottom-Line Issue." [Online information; retrieved 5/4/09.] www.theberylinstitute.net/publications.asp.

Bigelow, B., and M. Arndt. 1995. "Total Quality Management: Field of Dreams?"

Health Care Management Review 20 (4): 15–25.

Bitner, M. J., B. H. Booms, and M. Stanfield Tetreault. 1990. "The Service Encounter: Diagnosing Favorable and Unfavorable Incidents." *Journal of Marketing* 54 (1): 71–84.

Bitner, M. J., A. L. Ostrum, and F. N. Morgan. 2008. "Service Blueprinting: A Practical Technique for Service Innovation." *California Management Review* 50 (3): 66–94.

Bodnar, W. 2007. "Consumer-Centric Strategies." *Marketing Health Service* 27 (2): 38–39.

Boshoff, C., and B. Gray. 2004. "The Relationships Between Service Quality, Customer Satisfaction and Buying Intentions in the Private Hospital Industry." *South African Journal of Business Management* 35 (4): 27–37.

Bowen, D. E., and E. E. Lawler. 1992. "The Empowerment of Service Workers: What, Why, How, and When." *Sloan Management Review* 33 (1): 31–39.

Bowers, M. R., J. E. Swan, and W. F. Koehler. 1994. "What Attributes Determine Quality and Satisfaction with Health Care Delivery?" *Health Care Management Review* 19 (4): 49–55.

Brady Spellman, D., and D. Franke. 2007. "The Heart of Healing." [Online information; retrieved 5/21/09.] www. healthcaredesignmagazine.com/ME2/ dirmod.asp?sid=9B6FFC446FF7486981 EA3C0C3CCE4943&nm=Articles&type =Publishing&mod=Publications%3A%3 AArticle&mid=8F3A7027421841978F18 BE895F87F791&tier=4&i d=01557D1E BFAB42E3B65F183053BA0775.

Brinker, N., and D. T. Phillips. 1996. *On the Brink: The Life and Leadership of Norman Brinker.* Arlington, TX: The Summit Publishing Group.

Buckingham, M., and C. Coffman. 1999. *First Break All the Rules: What the World's Greatest Managers Do Differently.* New York: Simon and Schuster.

Buckley, L. 2007. "This Hospital Is a Top Patient Satisfaction Performer." *Quality Improvement Report.* [Online article; retrieved 4/08.] www.healthleadersmedia. com/content/87464/topic/WS_HLM2_ HOM/This-hospital-is-a-top-patient-satisfaction-performer.html.

Buckley, L., and M. O. Larkin. 2007. "Use Mystery Shoppers to Improve Your Scores." *Health Care Strategic Management* 25 (6): 1–3.

Bush, H. 2007. "Hospitals Embrace Hotel-Like Amenities." [Online article; retrieved 5/29/09.] www.hhnmag. com/hhnmag_app/jsp/articledisplay. jsp?dcrpath=HHNMAG/Article/ data/11NOV2007/0711HHN_InBox_ PatSatisfaction&domain=HHNMAG.

Business Performance. 2008. "Evaluating Training Effectiveness." [Online article; retrieved 4/08.] www.businessperform. com/html/evaluating_training_effectiven. html.

Business Research Lab. 2007. "Improving Customer Satisfaction Once a Customer Satisfaction Measurement Program Is in Place." [Online article; retrieved 5/29/09.] www.busreslab.com/tips/tip11. htm#Hiring.

Business Wire. 2008. "TheraDoc® Real Time Surveillance and Clinical Decision Support Technologies Adopted by Two Leading Health Systems." *Business Wire.* [Online article; retrieved 5/29/09.] www.biospace.com/news_story. aspx?NewsEntityId=104324.

Caldwell, D. F., J. Chatman, C. A. O'Reilly, M. Ormiston, and M. Lapiz. 2008. "Implementing Strategic Change in a Health Care System: The Importance of Leadership and Change Readiness." *Health Care Management Review* 33 (2): 124–33.

Cameron, S., M. Armstrong-Stassen, S. Bergeron, and J. Out. 2004. "Recruitment and Retention of Nurses: Challenges Facing Hospital and Community Employers." *Nursing Leadership* 17 (3): 79–92.

Cannon, M. F., and M. D. Tanner. 2005. *Healthy Competition: What's Holding Back Health Care and How to Free It.* Washington, DC: Cato Institute.

Carey, J. 2006. "Medical Guesswork." *Business Week* (May 29): 72–79.

Carlzon, J. 1987. *Moments of Truth.* New York: Ballinger.

Carpenter, M. 2009. "The New Children's Hospital: Design Elements Combine to Put Patients, Parents at Ease." [Online article; retrieved 5/29/09.] www.post-gazette.com/pg/09116/965608-114.stm.

Castle, N. G. 2007. "A Review of Satisfaction Instruments Used in Long-Term Care Settings." *Journal of Aging & Social Policy* 19: 9–41.

Chase, R. B., F. R. Jacobs, and N. J. Aquilano. 2006. *Operations Management for Competitive Advantage.* New York: McGraw-Hill/Irwin.

Clark, P. A., and M. P. Malone. 2005 *Making It Right.* South Bend, IN: Press Ganey Associates.

Cohen, E. 2008. "Is Boutique Medicine Worth the Price? [Online information; retrieved 5/4/09.] www.cnn.com/2008/HEALTH/09/18/ep.concierge.medicine/index.html.

Coile, R. 2000. "E-Health: Reinventing Healthcare in the Information Age." *Journal of Healthcare Management* 45 (3): 206–10.

Connell, J. 2006. "Medical Tourism: Sea, Sun, Sand, and Surgery." *Tourism Management* 27 (6): 1093–100.

Consumer Assessment of Healthcare Providers and Systems (CAHPS). 2009. "Overview." [Online information; retrieved 7/09.] www.cahps.ahrq.gov/content/cahpsOverview/OVER_Intro.asp?p=101&s=1.

Consumer Reports. 1996. "How Good Is Your Health Plan?" *Consumer Reports* 61 (8): 34–35.

Cooper, A. 2008. "The Nature of Design." *Miller-McClune* 1 (8): 22–24.

Correa, H. L., L. M. Ellram, A. J. Scavarda, and M. C. Cooper. 2007. "An Operations Management View of the Services and Goods Offering Mix." *International Journal of Operations and Production Management* 27 (5): 444–63.

Corvino, F. A. 2005. "Standards for Satisfaction." *Marketing Health Services* 25 (2): 45–47.

Cram, B. 2008. "GE Healthcare Life Systems Service Teams Wins NorthFace Award for 7th Consecutive Year." *DotMed News.* [Online information; retrieved 7/09.] www.dotmed.com/news.

Craven, E. D., J. Clark, M. Cramer, S. J. Corwin, and M.R. Cooper. 2006. "New York-Presbyterian Hospital Uses Six Sigma to Build a Culture of Quality and Innovation." *Journal of Organizational Excellence* 25 (4): 11.

Crosby, P. 1978. *Quality Is Free.* New York: McGraw Hill.

Crotts, J., D. Dickson, and R. C. Ford. 2005. "Aligning Organizational Processes with Mission: The Case of Service Excellence." *The Academy of Management Executive* 19 (3): 57.

Dagger, T. S., J. C. Sweeney, and L. W. Johnson. 2007. "A Hierarchical Model of Health Service Quality: Scale Development and Investigation of an Integrated Model." *Journal of Service Research* 10 (2): 123–42.

Dansky, K. H., and J. Miles. 1997. "Patient Satisfaction with Ambulatory Healthcare Services: Waiting Time and Filling Time." *Hospital & Health Services Administration* 42 (2): 165–78.

Danzinger, J., and D. Dunkle. 2005. *Methods of Training in the Workplace.* Irvine, CA: Center for Research on Information Technology and Organizations, School of Social Sciences, University of California. [Online information; retrieved 4/08.] www.crito.uci.edu/papers/2005/DanzigerDunkle.pdf.

Davidow, W. H., and B. Uttal. 1989. *Total Customer Service.* New York: Harper.

Davidson, J. 2007. "Caring and Daring to Complain: An Examination of UK

National Phobic Society Members' Perceptions of Primary Care." *Social Science and Medicine* 65 (3): 560–571.

DDI. 2008. "Targeted Selection." [Online information; retrieved 3/08.] www. ddiworld.com/ products_services/ targetedselection.asp.

Decker, P. J. 1999. "The Hidden Competencies of Healthcare: Why Self-Esteem, Accountability, and Professionalism May Affect Hospital Customer Satisfaction Scores." *Hospital Topics* 77 (1): 14–26.

DeMan, S., P. Vlerick, P. Gemmel, P. De Bondt, D. Matthys, and R. A. Dierckx. 2005. "Impact of Waiting on the Perception of Service Quality in Nuclear Medicine." *Nuclear Medicine Communications* 26 (6): 541–47.

Denove, C., and J. D. Power. 2006. *Satisfaction.* New York: Penguin Group.

Dickson, D., R. C. Ford, and B. Laval. 2005. "Managing Real and Virtual Waits in Hospitality and Service Organizations." *Cornell Hotel and Restaurant Administration Quarterly* 46 (1): 52–68.

Dilchert, S., C. Viswesveran, and T. A. Judge. 2007. "In Support of Personality Assessment in Organizational Settings." *Personnel Psychology* 60 (4): 995.

Donahue, K., E. Ashkin, and D. Pathman. 2005. "Length of Patient–Physician Relationship and Patient's Satisfaction and Preventive Service Use in the Rural South." *BMC Family Practice* 6 (1): 40–48.

Donnelly, L. F., and J. L. Strife. 2006. "Establishing a Program to Promote Professionalism and Effective Communication in Radiology." *Radiology* 238 (8): 773–79.

Dreachslin, J. L., P. L. Hunt, and E. Sprainer. 1999. "Key Indicators of Nursing Care Team Performance: Insights from the Front Line." *The Health Care Supervisor* 17 (4): 70–76.

Dube, L. 2003. "What's Missing from Patient-Centered Care?" *Marketing Health Services* 23 (1): 30–38.

Duffy, J. A., M. Duffy, and W. E. Kilbourne.

2001. "A Comparative Study of Resident, Family, and Administrator Expectations for Service Quality in Nursing Homes." *Health Care Management Review* 26 (3): 75–85.

East, R., K. Hammond, and P. Gendall. 2006. "Fact and Fallacy in Retention Marketing." *Journal of Marketing Management* 22: 5–23.

El Camino Hospital. 2009. "Healing Arts Program." [Online information; retrieved 5/29/09.] www.elcaminohospital.org/ Patient_Services/Patient_Resources/ Healing_Arts/.

Elwyn, G., A. Edwards, P. Kinnersley, and R. Grol. 2000. "Shared Decision Making and the Concept of Equipoise: The Competencies of Involving Patients in Healthcare Choices." *British Journal of General Practice* 50 (460): 892–99.

Encinosa, W. E., and F. J. Hellinger. 2008. "The Impact of Medical Errors on Ninety-Day Costs and Outcomes: An Examination of Surgical Patients Health Services Research Early View." *Health Services Research* 43 (6): 2067–80.

Encyclopedia of Small Business. 2007. "Training and Development." [Online information; retrieved 3/08.] www. referenceforbusiness.com/small/Sm-Z/ Training-and-Development.html.

Eubanks, P. 1991. "Retreats Advance Corporate Culture." *Hospitals* 65 (18): 58.

Evanschitzky, H., and M. Wunderlich. 2006. "An Examination of Moderator Effects in the Four-Stage Loyalty Model." *Journal of Service Research* 8 (4): 330–45.

Fabien, L. 2005. "Design and Implementation of a Service Guarantee." *Journal of Services Marketing* 19 (1): 33–38.

Fantin, L. 2006. "Wealth Care Is Shaking Up Medicine." [Online information; retrieved 5/4/09.] www.scrippsnews.com/ node/13268.

Faust, D. 2007. "Diagnosis: Identity Theft."

Business Week (January 8): 30–32.

Fiorito, J., D. P. Bozeman, A. Young, and J. A. Meurs. 2007. "Organizational Commitment, Human Resource Practices, and Organizational Characteristics." *Journal of Managerial Issues* 19 (2): 186–207.

Ford, R. C., S. A. Bach, and M. D. Fottler. 1997. "Methods of Measuring Patient Satisfaction in Health Care Organizations." *Health Care Management Review* 22 (2): 74–89.

Ford, R. C., and D. P Bowen. 2008. "A Service-Dominant Logic for Management Education: It's Time." *Academy of Management Learning and Education* 7 (2): 224–43.

Ford, R. C., and D. D. Dickson. 2008. "Executive Voice Interview: Bruce Laval." *Journal of Applied Management and Entrepreneurship* 13 (2): 80–99.

Ford, R. C., and C. P. Heaton. 2000. *Managing the Guest Experience in Hospitality,* 99–100. Albany, NY: Delmar Thomson Learning.

———. 2001. "Managing Your Guests as a Quasi-Employee." *Cornell Hotel and Restaurant Administration Quarterly* 42 (1): 46–54.

Ford, R. C., C. P. Heaton, and S. W. Brown. 2001. "Delivering Excellent Service: Lessons from the Best Firms." *California Management Review* 44 (1): 39–56.

Ford, R. C., F. S. McLaughlin, and J. W. Newstrom. 2004. "Questions and Answers About Fun at Work." *Human Resource Planning* 26 (4): 18–33.

Ford, R. C., S. A. Sivo, M. D. Fottler, D. Dickson, K. Bradley, and L. Johnson. 2006. "Aligning Internal Organizational Factors with a Service Excellence Mission: An Exploratory Study in Healthcare."*Health Care Management Review* 31 (4): 259–69.

Foster, D. 2001. "California Man Finds Comfort, Solace in ER." *The Gainesville Sun,* 10A.

Fottler, M. D., J. D. Blair, C. L. Whitehead, and M. J. Laus. 1989. "Who Matters to Hospitals and Why? Assessing Key Stakeholders." *Hospital & Health Services Administration* 34 (4): 525–46.

Fottler, M. D., D. Dickson, R. C. Ford, K. Bradley, and L. Johnson. 2006. "Comparing Hospital Staff and Patient Perceptions of Customer Service: A Pilot Survey Utilizing Survey and Focus Group Data." *Health Services Management Research* 19 (1): 52–66.

Fottler, M. D., R. C. Ford, V. Roberts, and E. Ford. 2000. "Creating a Healing Environment: The Importance of the Service Setting on the New Customer Oriented Healthcare System." *Journal of Healthcare Management* 45 (2): 91–106.

Fottler, M. D., and D. M. Malvey. 2010. *The Retail Revolution in Healthcare.* Westport, CT: Greenwood Press.

Frampton, S. B., and P. A. Charmel (eds.). 2008. *Putting Patients First: Designing and Practicing Patient-Centered Care,* 2nd ed. San Francisco: Jossey-Bass.

Francis, T. 2006. "Spread of Records Stirs Patient Fears of Privacy Erosion." *Wall Street Journal,* pp. A1, A8.

———. 2008. "Wait Times Lengthen at Emergency Rooms." *Wall Street Journal,* p. D2.

Free Library. 2004. "Program Continues to Improve Patient Care and Lower Costs." [Online information; retrieved 5/1/09.] www.thefreelibrary.com/Baptist+Hospital, +Pensacola,+Florida,+Reports+$2.56+Million+Savings...-a0114058016.

Freudenheim, M. 2009. "And You Thought a Prescription Was Private." *New York Times.* [Online information; retrieved 4/26/09.] www.nytimes.com/2009/08/09/business/09privacy.html.

Fried, B. 2007. "Congress Moves on Health IT: One Step Forward, A Few Steps Back." [Online information; retrieved 4/26/09.] www.ihealthbeat.org/Perspectives/2007/Congress-Moves-on-Health-IT-One-Step-Forward-A-Few-Steps-Back.aspx?topic=Policy.

Fried, B. J., and M. Gates. 2008.

"Recruitment, Selection and Retention."
In *Human Resources in Healthcare:
Managing for Success,* 3rd ed., edited by
B. J. Fried and M. D. Fottler, 197–235.
Chicago: Health Administration Press.

Friedewald, V. E. 2000. "The Internet's
Influence on the Doctor-Patient
Relationship." *Health Management
Technology* 21 (11): 79–80.

Fulford, M. D. 2005. "That's Not Fair!: The
Test of a Model of Organizational Justice,
Job Satisfaction, and Organizational
Commitment Among Hotel Employees."
*Journal of Human Resources in Hospitality
& Tourism* 4 (1): 73–84.

Gallup Management Journal. 2006. "Gallup
Study: Feeling Good Matters in the
Workplace." [Online article; retrieved
3/8/08.] http://gmj.gallup.com/content/
20770Gallup-Study-Feeling-Good-
Matters-in-the.aspx?verysi.

Garman, A. N., J. Garcia, and M. Hargreaves.
2004. "Patient Satisfaction as a Predictor
of Return-to-Provider Behavior:
Analysis and Assessment of Financial
Implications." *Quality Management in
Healthcare* 13 (1): 75–80.

Geboy, L. 2007. "The Evidence-Based Design
Wheel: A New Approach to Understanding the Evidence in Evidence-Based Design." [Online article; retrieved 5/29/09.]
www.healthcaredesignmagazine.com/
ME2/dirmod.sp?sid=&nm=&type=Publis
hing&mod=Publications%3A%3AArticle
&mid=8F3A7027421841978F18BE895F
87F791&tier=4&id=2153E8F25630409
18EFAEEF4ED22BE3.

Geggis, A. 2008. "Report Shows How Patients
Rate Hospitals." *Daytona Beach News
Journal* (May 24): 1c, 4c.

Gelade, G. A., and S. Young. 2005. "Test
of the Service Profit Chain Model in
the Retail Banking Sector." *Journal
of Occupational and Organizational
Psychology* 78 (1): 1–22.

Girard-DiCarlo, C. B. 1999. "The Importance
of Leadership." *Healthcare Executive* 14
(6): 48.

Gittell, J. H. 2003. *The Southwest Airlines Way:
Using the Power of Relationships to Achieve
High Performance.* New York: McGraw-
Hill.

Glebbeck, A. C., and E. H. Box. 2004.
"Is High Employee Turnover Really
Harmful?" *Academy of Management
Journal* 47 (3): 266–86.

Goldman, E. F., and K. V. Corrigan. 1998.
"Thinking Retail in Health Care: New
Approaches for Business Growth."
Alliance (May/June): 9–11.

Goldstein, S. M., and S. B. Schweikhart. 2002.
"Empirical Support for the Baldridge
Award Framework in U.S. Hospitals."
Health Care Management Review 27 (1):
62–75.

Goodman, E. 2008. "Self-Serve and Slave."
Orlando Sentinel (July 23): A9.

Goodman, J. C. 2007. "Perverse Incentives in
Healthcare." *Wall Street Journal* (April 5):
A13.

Greene, J. 2007. "Microsoft Wants Your
Health Records." *Business Week* (October
15): 44–46.

Green, H., and C. Himmelstein. 1998. "A
Cyber Revolt in Health Care." *Business
Week* (October 19): 154–56.

Greengard, S. 2003. "Gimme Attitude."
Workforce Management 81 (7): 56–60.

Gross, S. 2004. *Positively Outrageous Service:
How to Delight and Astound Your
Customers and Win Them for Life.*
Chicago: Dearborn Trade Publishing.

Grugal, R. 2002. "66 Steps to Cleanliness."
Investor's Business Daily (March 11): A4.

Guenther, R. 2008. "Why Should Health
Care Bother?" *Frontiers of Health Services
Management* 25 (1): 25–32.

Guenther, R., and G. Vittori. 2008. *Sustainable
Healthcare Architecture.* Hoboken, NJ:
John Wiley and Sons.

Gupta, H. D. 2008. "Identifying Health Care
Quality Constituents: Service Provider
Perspective." *Journal of Management
Research* 8 (1): 311–24.

Guth, L., and D. Deems. 2008a. "Exceptional
Care: World Class Service." *AGD Impact*
36 (1): 24–25.

———. 2008b. "Exceptional Care: Which Brand Are You?" *AGD Impact* 36 (2): 24–25.

Halbesleben, J. R. B. 2009. *Managing Stress and Preventing Burnout in the Healthcare Workplace,* 88–91. Chicago: Health Administration Press.

Hamel, G., and C. K. Prahalad. 1994. *Competing for the Future.* Boston: Harvard Business School Press.

Hanaman, J. C. 2006. "Going Retail." *Healthcare Executive* 21 (3): 49–50.

Hansemark, O., and M. Albinsson. 2004. "Customer Satisfaction and Retention: The Experiences of Individual Employees." *Managing Service Quality* 14 (1): 40–57.

Harkey, J., and R. Vraciu. 1992. "Quality of Health Care and Financial Performance: Is There a Link?" *Health Care Management Review* 17 (4): 55–63.

Hart, C. W. L. 1988. "The Power of Unconditional Service Guarantees." *Harvard Business Review* 66 (4): 54–62.

Hart, C. W. L., J. L. Heskett, and W. E. Sasser, Jr. 1990. "The Profitable Art of Service Recovery." *Harvard Business Review* 68 (4): 153.

Hays, J. M., and A. V. Hill. 2006. "An Extended Longitudinal Study of the Effects of a Service Guarantee." *Production and Operations Management* 15 (1): 117–31.

The Healthcare Advisory Board (HCAB). 2002. *Hardwiring for Right Retention: Best Practices for Retaining a High Performance Workforce.* Washington, DC: The Advisory Board Company.

Healthcare Financial Management. 2008. "Emergency Department Waits Increase Nationwide, Says Study." *Healthcare Financial Management* 62 (2): 8.

Health Resources and Services Administration (HRSA). 2006a. "The Registered Nurse Population: Findings from the 2004 National Sample Survey of Registered Nurses." [Online information; retrieved 1/29/08.] http://bhpr.hrsa.gov/healthworkforce/rnsurvey04.

———. 2006b. "What Is Behind HRSA's Projected Supply, Demand, and Shortage of Registered Nurses?" [Online information; retrieved 1/29/08.] http://bhpr.hrsa.gov/healthworkforce/reports/behindrnprojections/index.htm.

Heathfield, S. 2008. "How to Conduct a Simple Training Needs Assessment." About.com. [Online information; retrieved 1/29/08.] http://humanresources.about.com/od/trainingneedsassessment/ht/training_needs.htm.

Heckscher, C., and P. S. Adler (eds.). 2006. *The Firm as a Collaborative Community: The Reconstruction of Trust in the Knowledge Economy.* Oxford, UK: Oxford University Press.

Henricksen, K., S. Isaacson, B. L. Sadler, and E. M. Zimring. 2007. "The Role of the Physical Environment in Crossing the Quality Chasm." *Journal of Quality and Patient Safety* 33 (11): 68–80.

Henry Ford West Bloomfield Hospital. 2009. "How We Are Different." [Online information; retrieved 5/29/09.] www.henryfordwestbloomfield.com/body_wbloomfield.cfm?id=50423.

Herzlinger, R. 1997. *Market-Driven Healthcare: Who Wins in the Transformation of America's Largest Service Industry?* Reading, MA: Addison-Wesley.

———. 2007a. "Where Are the Innovators in Healthcare?" *Wall Street Journal* (July 19): A15.

———. 2007b. *Who Killed Healthcare?* New York: McGraw-Hill.

Heskett, J. L., W. E. Sasser, Jr., and C. W. L. Hart. 1990. *Service Breakthroughs: Changing the Rules of the Game.* New York: The Free Press.

Heskett, J. L., T. O. Jones, G. W. Loveman, W. E. Sasser, and L. A. Schlesinger. 1994. "Putting the Service Profit Chain to Work." *Harvard Business Review* 72 (2): 105–11.

HGA. 2006. "New Facility for Iowa's Orange City Area Health System Incorporates Site Sensitivity, Natural Materials,

Daylighting Strategies, Patient Privacy and a Spiritually Uplifting Central Chapel for Rural Healthcare Organization." [Online information; retrieved 5/21/09.] www.hga.com/the_latest/press_releases/orange_city_122006.html#home.

Hill, C. J., and K. Joonas. 2005. "The Impact of Unacceptable Wait Time on Health Care Patients' Attitudes and Actions." *Health Marketing Quarterly* 23 (2): 69–87.

Hindo, B. 2006. "Satisfaction Not Guaranteed." *Business Week* (June 19): 32–36.

Hoffman, B. J., and D. J. Woehr. 2006. "A Quantitative Review of the Relationship Between Person–Organization Fit and Behavioral Outcomes." *Journal of Vocational Behavior* 68 (3): 389–99.

Horburgh, R. C. 1995. "Healing by Design." *New England Journal of Medicine* 333 (11): 735–41.

Hotchkiss, R. B., M. D. Fottler, and L. Unruh. 2009. "Valuing Volunteers: The Impact of Volunteerism on Hospital Performance." *Health Care Management Review* 34 (2): 119–28.

Huelat, B. 2009. "The Healing Experience." [Online information; retrieved 5/29/09.] www.healthcaredesignmagazine.com/ME2/dirmod.asp?sid=9B6FFC446FF7486981EA3C0C3CCE4943&nm=Articles&type=Publishing&mod=Publications%3A%3AArticle&mid=8F3A7027421841978F18BE895F87F791&tier=4&id=CDF5EC75765B434C98A1A6CAB1969A1C.

Huerta, S. 2003. "Recruitment and Retention: The Magnet Perspective." Chart. *Journal of Illinois Nursing* 100 (4): 4–6.

INTEGRIS. 2009. [Online information; retrieved 5/29/09.] www.integris-health.com/INTEGRIS/en-US/AboutUs/Newsroom/2009/05May09/campFunnybone2009.htm.

Institute of Medicine. 2000. *To Err Is Human: Building a Safer Hospital System.* Washington, DC: National Academies Press.

———. 2001. *Crossing the Quality Chasm: A New Health System for the 21st Century.* Washington, DC: National Academies Press.

The Joint Commission. 1991. *Quality Improvement Standards.* Oakbrook Terrace, IL: The Joint Commission.

———. 2007. *Assessing Hospital Staff Competence*, 2nd ed. Oakbrook Terrace, IL: The Joint Commission.

———. 2008. "Facts About ORYX® for Hospitals: National Hospital Quality Measures." [Online information; retrieved 12/08.] www.jointcommission.org/AccreditationPrograms/Hospitals/ORYX/oryx_facts.htm.

Jones, T. O., and W. E. Sasser. 1995. "Why Satisfied Customers Defect." *Harvard Business Review* 73 (2): 88–101.

Joseph, A. 2006. "The Impact of Light on Outcomes in Healthcare Settings." [Online information; retrieved 10/8/08.] www.healthdesign.org/research/reports/light.

Joy, M., and S. Jones. 2005. "Transient Probabilities for Queues with Applications to Hospital Waiting List Management." *Health Care Management Science* 8: 231–36.

Kacmar, K. M., M. C. Andrews, D. L. Van Rooy, R. C. Steilberg, and S. Cerron. 2006. "Sure Everyone Can Be Replaced … But at What Cost? Turnover as a Predictor of Unit-Level Performance." *Academy of Management Journal* 49 (1): 133–44.

Kalogredis, V. 2004. "Should You Consider Concierge Medicine?" [Online information; retrieved 5/4/09.] www.physiciansnews.com/business/204.kalogredis.html.

Kapp, M. B. 2007. "Consumer-Driven Healthcare: Implications for the Physician–Patient Relationship." *The Pharos: Alpha Omega Alpha's Quarterly Journal* 70 (2): 12–15.

Keeler, G. 2008. "Soothing Sounds Help Patients Heal." *Orlando Sentinel* (May 20): E3.

Kerry, J., and N. Gingrich. 2007. "E-Prescriptions." *Wall Street Journal* (November 16): A20.

Killian, S. 2009. "What Percentage of Salary Should Go to Training?" The Effective Leadership Development Community. [Online information; retrieved 8/4/09.] http://effective.leadershipdevelopment.edu.au/what-percentage-of-salary-should-go-to-training/general.

Kim, D. 2005. "An Integrated Supply Chain Management System: A Case Study in the Healthcare Sector." In *Lecture Notes in Computer Science*. Berlin: Springer.

Kornblum, J. 2008. "Medical Records a Click Away." *USA Today* (June 12): 1D–2D.

Kouzes, J. M., and B. Z. Posner. 1995. *The Leadership Challenge: How to Keep Getting Extraordinary Things Done in Organizations*. San Francisco: Jossey-Bass.

Kreindler, S. A. 2008. "Watching Your Wait: Evidence-Informed Strategies for Reducing Health Care Wait Times." *Quality Management in Health Care* 17 (2): 128–35.

Kristof-Brown, A. L., R. D. Zimmerman, and E. C. Johnson. 2005. "Consequences of Individuals' Fit at Work: A Meta-Analysis of Person–Job, Person–Organization, Person–Group, and Person–Supervisor Fit." *Personnel Psychology* 58 (2): 281–342.

Kroll, K. 2005. "Evidence Based Design in Healthcare Facilities." [Online information; retrieved 5/29/09.] www.facilitiesnet.com/healthcarefacilities/article/Better-Health-From-Better-Design--2425.

Kronstadt, J., A. Moiduddin, and W. Sellheim. 2009. *Consumer Use of Computerized Applications to Address Health and Health Care Needs*. [Online report; retrieved 8/14/09.] http://aspe.hhs.gov/sp/reports/2009/consumerhit/report.shtml.

Kumar, V., P. A. Smart, H. Maddern, and R. S. Maull. 2008. "Alternative Perspectives on Service Quality and Customer Satisfaction: The Role of BPM." *International Journal of Service Industry Management* 19 (2): 176–87.

Laborwitz, G. 2005. "Well-Aligned: Using Alignment to Achieve Extraordinary Results." *Builders and Leaders* 12 (1): 24–25.

LaGanga, L. R., and S. R. Lawrence. 2007. "Clinic Overbooking to Improve Patient Access and Increase Provider Productivity." *Decision Sciences* 38 (2): 251–76.

Laing, A., G. Hogg, and D. Winkleman. 2004. "Healthcare and the Information Revolution: Reconfiguring the Healthcare Service Encounter." *Health Services Management* 17 (3): 188–200.

Lake, L. 2009. "Why Word of Mouth Marketing?" [Online article; retrieved 9/9/09.] http://marketing.about.com/b/2009/08/24/why-word-of-mouth-marketing.htm.

Landro, L. 2006a. "Hospitals Open Up Space in ER." *Wall Street Journal* (October 18): D16.

———. 2006b. "Cutting Waits at the Doctor's Office." *Wall Street Journal*, pp. D1–D3.

———. 2007a. "Hospital Food That Won't Make You Sick." *Wall Street Journal* (September 19): D1, D9.

———. 2007b. "Keeping Patients From Landing Back in Hospital." *Wall Street Journal* (December 12): D1, D7.

———. 2007c. "ICU's New Message: Welcome Families." *Wall Street Journal* (July 12): A1, A12.

———. 2007d. "The Growing Clout of Online Patient Groups." *Wall Street Journal* (June): DI.

———. 2008. "A Treatment Room with a View." *Wall Street Journal* (August 20): D1–D2.

Lane, L. 2007. "Jet Blue Customers Stand by their Carrier." *Business Week* (March 26): 20–22.

Larson, E. B., and X. Yao. 2005. "Clinical Empathy as Emotional Labor in the Patient–Physician Relationship." *Journal of the American Medical Association* 293 (9): 1100.

Latham, G. P., and S. Mann. 2006.

"Advances in the Science of Performance Appraisal: Implications for Practice." In *International Review of Industrial and Organizational Psychology,* Vol. 21, edited by G. P. Hodgkinson and J.K. Ford, 295–337. Hoboken, NJ: Wiley.

Lau, G. 2000. "A Training Program Must Zero in on What Your Staffers Must Know." *Investor's Business Daily* (June 18): A1.

Lawson, B., and M. Phiri. 2000. "Hospital Design: Room for Improvement." *Health Services Journal* 110 (5688): 24–26.

Lee, F. 2004. *If Disney Ran Your Hospital: 9 1/2 Things You Would Do Differently.* Bozeman, MT: Second River Healthcare Press.

Leggitt, M. S., V. N. Potrepka, and T. J. Kukolja. 2003. "Le Bistro Serves Up Cultural Change." *Nursing Administration Quarterly* 27 (4): 318–23.

Lemieux-Charles, L. and W. L. McGuire. 2006. "What Do We Know About Health Care Team Effectiveness? A Review of the Literature." *Medical Care Research and Review* 63 (3): 1–38.

Lenaghan, J. A., and A. B. Eisner. 2006. "Employers of Choice and Competitive Advantage: The Proof of the Pudding Is in the Eating." *Journal of Organizational Culture, Communications and Conflict* 10 (1).

Lethlean, J. 2009. "Fast Care: FHN Partners with Shopko to Meet Health Care Needs." *The Journal-Standard.* [Online information; retrieved 9/2/09.] www.journalstandard.com/homepage/x594731498/Fast-care-FHN-partners-with-Shopko-to-meet-health-care-needs.

Levine, L. 2008. "Strengthing Your Business by Developing Your Employees." [Online information; retrieved 4/2/09.] www.allbusiness.com/human-resources/employee-development/1240-1.html.

Levitt, T. 1972. "Production-Line Approach to Service." *Harvard Business Review* 50 (5): 50.

Liebowitz, R. 2008. "Putting Patients First." *Healthcare Executive* 23 (4): 42–44.

Lin, B. Y., N. J. Leu, G. M. Breen, and W. H. Lin. 2008. "Service Scape: Physical Environment of Hospital Pharmacist's Work Outcomes." *Health Care Management Review* 33 (2): 156–68.

Lohr, S. 2009. "G.E. and Intel Working on Remote Monitors to Provide Home Health Care." *New York Times.* [Online information; retrieved 4/2/09.] www.nytimes.com/2009/04/03/health/03health.html?ref=business.

Lutz, S. 2008. "What Do Consumers Want?" *Journal of Healthcare Management* 53 (2): 83–87.

MacStravic, S. 2005. "High Expectations." *Marketing Health Services* 25(1): 200–24.

Magid, D. J., A. F. Sullivan, P. D. Cleary, S. R. Rao, J. A. Gordon, R. Kaushal, E. Guadagnoli, C. A. Camargo, and D. Blumenthal. 2009. "The Safety of Emergency Care Systems: Results of a Survey of Clinicians in 65 US Emergency Departments." *Annals of Emergency Medicine* 53 (6): 715–23.

Malkin, J. 1992. *Hospital Interior Architecture: Creating Healing Environments for Special Patient Populations.* New York: Van Nostrand Reinhold Company.

Malloch, K. 1999. "A Total Healing Environment: The Yauapal Regional Medical Center Story." *Journal of Healthcare Management* 44 (6): 495–512.

Malvey, D., and M. D. Fottler. 2006. "The Retail Revolution in Health Care." *Health Care Management Review* 31 (3): 168–78.

Manion, J. 2004. "Nurture a Culture of Retention." *Nursing Management* 35 (4): 28–39.

Marberry, S. O. (ed.). 2006. *Improving Healthcare with Better Building Design.* Chicago: Health Administration Press.

Marketing Health Services. 2004. "Keeping Happy." *Marketing Health Services* 24 (1): 6.

Marley, K., D. A. Collier, and S. M. Goldstein. 2004. "The Role of Clinical and Process Quality in Achieving Patient Satisfaction in Hospitals." *Decision Sciences* 35 (3): 349–69.

Marrow, P., and J. McElroy. 2007. "Efficiency as a Mediator in Turnover–Organizational Performance Relations." *Human Relations* 60 (6): 827–49.

Masselink, L. E. 2008. "Globalization and the Healthcare Workforce." In *Human Resources in Healthcare: Managing for Success,* 3rd ed., edited by B. J. Fried and M. D. Fottler, 47–70. Chicago: Health Administration Press.

MassLongTermCare.org. 2009. "Oversight of Nursing Homes." [Online information; retrieved 7/09.] www.masslongtermcare.org/index.php?option=com_content&task=view&id=19&Itemid=81.

Mathews, A. W. 2008. "Consumers Union to Rate Hospitals." *Wall Street Journal* (May 29): D6.

Mayer, T., R. Cates, M. J. Mastorovich, and D. Royalty. 1998. "Emergency Department Patient Satisfaction in Customer Service Training Improves Patient Satisfaction and Ratings of Physician and Nurse Skill." *Journal of Healthcare Management* 43 (5): 427–38.

McCann, M. 2009. "Fun at Work Helps Retain Employees." [Online information; retrieved 8/17/09.] http://EzineArticles.com/?expert=Michael_McCann.

McCaughey, B. 2007. "Our Unsanitary Hospitals." *Wall Street Journal* (November 29): A18.

McGregor, J. 2007. "Customer Service Champs." *Business Week* (March 5): 50–64.
———. 2008. "Consumer Vigilantes." *Business Week* (March 3): 38–42.

McKim, R., S. Warren, C. Montgomery, J. Zaborowski, C. McKee, D. Towers, and B. H. Rowe. 2007. "Emergency Department Patient Satisfaction Survey in Alberta's Capital Health Region." *Healthcare Quarterly* 10 (1): 34–42.

McMillan, C. 2007. "In the Wait-Times Guarantee, We Trust; Canada's Health Care Problems Can Be Conquered Using Incremental Steps." Canadian Medical Association. [Online newsletter; retrieved 5/29/09.] http://www.cma.ca/index.cfm/ci_id/52188/la_id/1.htm.

McPherson, H. 2007. "Hospitals Add Restaurant Flair to Patient's Fare." *Orlando Sentinel* (July 19): A1, A2.

Medical News Today. 2006. "Methodist Healthcare Opens Wellness Room. Demonstration Room Showcases Home-Like Healing Environment." [Online article; retrieved 5/29/09.] www.medicalnewstoday.com/articles/41441.php.

Mercy Health System. 2007. [Online information; retrieved 9/8/09.] www.mercyhealthsystem.org/default.cfm.

Michel, S., D. Bowen, and R. Johnston. 2008. "Making the Most of Customer Complaints." *Wall Street Journal* (September 22): R4, R11.

Mittal, B., and W. Lassar. 1998. "Why Do Customers Switch? The Dynamics of Satisfaction Versus Loyalty." *Journal of Services Marketing* 12 (1): 177–91.

Montague, J. 1995. "Family Designs." *Hospitals & Health Networks* 69 (11): 94.

Moore, J. 2009. "Experiences at Cleveland Clinic with HealthVault." *Healthcare IT News.* [Online article; retrieved 5/29/09.] www.healthcareitnews.com/blog/experiences-cleveland-clinic-healthvault.

Mullaney, T. 2006. "The Doctor Is Plugged In." *Business Week* (June 26): 56–58.

Nadler, D. A., and M. L. Tushman. 1997. *Competing by Design.* New York: Oxford University Press.

Nathan, S. 2000. "Hospital Mends Customer Service." *USA Today* (May 5): 7B.

National Coalition on Health Care. 2008. "Consumers Lose Confidence in Health Care Systems." [Online article; retrieved 8/20/08.] www.nchc.org.

National Committee for Quality Assurance (NCQA). 2009. "What Is HEDIS?" [Online article; retrieved 3/10/09.] www.ncqa.org/tabid/187/Default.aspx.

National Institute of Business Management. 2001. "Good HR Boosts Customer Retention." *Success in Recruiting and Retaining* 1 (1): 8.

National Partnership for Women and Families. 1998. "A Study of Women's Attitudes Toward Health and Healthcare." [Online article; retrieved 8/20/08.] www.nationalpartnership.org.

National Quality Forum. 2005. *Standardizing*

a *Measure of Patient Perspectives of Hospital Care.* Washington, DC: National Quality Forum.

Naveh, E., and Z. Stern. 2005. "How Quality Improvement Programs Can Affect General Hospital Performance." *International Journal of Health Care Quality Assurance* 18 (4): 249–70.

Nelson, E. C., R. T. Rust, A. Zahorok, R. L. Rose, P. Batalden, and B. A. Siemanski. 1992. "Do Patient Perceptions of Quality Relate to Hospital Financial Performance?" *Journal of Health Care Marketing* 12 (4): 6–13.

Noor, A. 2007. "Re-Engineering Healthcare Mechanical Engineering." *Mechanical Engineering Magazine*, 22–27.

Northwest Business Press. 2005. "New Women's Health Center Has Spa Atmosphere." [Online article; retrieved 8/20/08.] www.redorbit.com/news/health/151412/new_womens_health_center_has_spa_atmosphere/index.html.

O'Connor, M. 2007. "Omaha Hospitals Ease Waiting Room Anxieties." Alegent Health in the News. [Online article; retrieved 4/21/08.] www.alegent.com/blank.cfm?print=yes&id=7&action=detail&ref=197.

Okrent, D. 2000. "Twilight of the Boomers." *Time* (June 12): 72.

O'Malley, J. 2004a. "The Caring Before the Care." *Marketing Health Services* 24 (2): 12–13.

———. 2004b. "The Total Service Experience." *Marketing Health Services* 24 (3): 12–13.

Online Search Authority. 2009. "Bank Systems and ATM Technology." [Online information; retrieved 4/2/09.] www.onlinesecurityauthority.com/banking-security/bank-systems-and-atm-technology.

Orlando Sentinel. 2001. "Consumers Use Web to Fight Back." *Orlando Sentinel* (May 23): E1.

Otani, K., R. S. Kurz, and L. F. Harris. 2005. "Managing Primary Care Using Patient Satisfaction Measures." *Journal of Healthcare Management* 50 (5): 311–24.

Ottenheimer, D. 2008. "On the Tracks of Medical Data: Electronic Records Pressure." *SC Magazine.* [Online information; retrieved 5/10/09.] www.scmagazineus.com/On-the-tracks-of-medical-data-Electronic-records-pressure/article/111447.

Pakdil, F., and T. Harwood. 2005. "Patient Satisfaction in a Preoperative Assessment Clinic: An Analysis Using SERVQUAL Dimensions." *Total Quality Management & Business Excellence* 16 (1): 15–30.

Palfini, J. 2008. "Even Brainstorms Should Have a Forecast." [Online information; retrieved 5/10/09.] http://blogs.bnet.com/teamwork/?p=161.

Parasuraman, A., V. A. Zeithaml, and L. L. Berry. 1988. "SERVQUAL: A Multiple-Item Scale for Measuring Consumer Perception of Service Quality." *Journal of Retailing* 64 (1): 38–40.

Parchman, M., and S. Burge. 2004. "The Patient–Physician Relationship, Primary Care Attributes and Preventive Services." *Family Medicine* 36 (1): 22–27.

Parrish Medical Center. 2008. "About the Healthy Environment." [Online information; retrieved 5/10/09.] www.parrishmed.com/about_us/about.cfm#color.

Parthasarathy, S. 2004. "Sleep in the Intensive Care Unit." *Intensive Care Medicine* 30 (2): 197–206.

Patientprivacyrights.org. 2009. "HIPAA—The Intent vs. The Reality." [Online information; retrieved 4/8/09.] www.patientprivacyrights.org/site/PageServer?pagename=HIPAA_Intent_Vs_Reality.

Pearce, J. A., and R. B. Robinson. 2005. *Formulation, Implementation, and Control of Competitive Strategy.* Chicago: Irwin.

Peltier, J. W., J. A. Schibowsky, and C. R. Cochran. 2002. "Patient Loyalty that Lasts a Lifetime." *Marketing Health Services* 22 (2): 29–33.

Petersen, A. 1997. "Restaurants Bring In Da Noise to Keep Out Da Nerds." *Wall Street*

Journal (December 30): B-1.

———. 2007. "Uprooted: When Patients Seek Treatment Far From Home." *Wall Street Journal* (October 9): D1.

Pfeffer, J. 1998. *The Human Equation: Building Profits by Putting People First.* Boston: Harvard Business School Press.

Pho, K. 2008. "Shortage of Primary Care Threatens Healthcare System." *USA Today* (March 13): 11A.

Pine, B. J., and J. H. Gilmore. 1998. "Welcome to the Experience Economy." *Harvard Business Review* 78 (4): 97–105.

———. 1999. *The Experience Economy.* Cambridge, MA: Harvard Business School Press.

———. 2009. "Orthopedists Should Strive to Offer an Experience in Health Care." [Online information; retrieved 4/8/09.] www.orthosupersite.com/view. asp?rID=36750.

Pink, G. H., and M. A. Murray. 2003. "Hospital Efficiency and Patient Satisfaction." *Health Services Management Research* 16 (1): 24–39.

Planetree. 2009. "About Planetree." [Online information; retrieved 7/18/09.] www. planetree.org/about.html.

Platonova, E. A., K. N. Kennedy, and R. M. Shewchuk. 2008. "Understanding Patient Satisfaction, Trust and Loyalty to Primary Care Physicians." *Medical Care Research and Review* 65 (6): 696–712.

Porter, M. E. 1996. "What Is Strategy?" *Harvard Business Review* 74 (6): 61–78.

Porter, M. E., and E. O. Teisberg. 2006. *Redefining Health Care: Creating Value-Based Competition on Results.* Boston: Harvard Business School Press.

Powers, T. L., and E. P. Jack. 2008. "Using Volume Flexible Strategies to Improve Customer Satisfaction and Performance in Health Care Services." *Journal of Services Marketing* 22 (2–3): 188–97.

Prahalad, C. K., and V. Ramaswamy. 2004a. "Co-Creating Unique Value with Customers." *Strategy and Management* 32 (3): 4–10.

———. 2004b. *The Future of Competition.* Boston: Harvard Business School Press.

Prajogo, D. C. 2006. "The Implementation of Operations Management Techniques in Service Organizations." *International Journal of Operations & Production Management* 26 (12): 1374–90.

Press, I. 2003. "Patient Satisfaction with the Outpatient Experience." *Healthcare Executive* 18 (3): 94–95.

Press Ganey. 1997. National Priority List-Medical Practices. South Bend, IN: Press Ganey Associates.

———. 2007a. "Physician's Office and Outpatient Pulse Report." [Online article; retrieved 8/20/08.] www.pressganey.com/ outpatient-report.pdf.

———. 2007b. "Press Ganey Releases Comprehensive National Report on Patient Perspectives of Their Experience in Emergency Rooms." [Online article; retrieved 8/20/08.] www.pressganey.com/ erreport.pdf.

PricewaterhouseCoopers Health Research Institute. 2007. "Top Eight Health Industry Issues in 2008." [Online article; retrieved 8/20/08.] www.pwc.com/ extweb/pwcpublications.nsf/docid/7d3a3 531588fa044852573b0006b9020.

Pruitt, S. D., and J. E. Epping-Jordan. 2005. "Preparing the 21st Century Global Healthcare Workforce." *British Medical Journal* 330: 637–39.

Pullman, M. E., and G. Thompson. 2003. "Strategies for Integrating Capacity With Demand in Service Networks." *Journal of Service Research* (5) 3: 15.

QMS Partners. 2009. "Understanding Customer Retention and Switching Behavior in the Healthcare Sector." [Online article; retrieved 9/9/08.] www. marketresearchbulletin.com/2009/01/ understanding-customer-retention-and-switching-behavior-in-the-healthcare-sector.

Ramsaran-Fowdar, R. R. 2005. "Identifying Health Care Quality Attributes." *Journal of Health & Human Services Administration* 27 (4): 465–43.

Reichheld, F. F., and W. E. Sasser, Jr. 1990. "Zero Defections: Quality Comes to Services." *Harvard Business Review* 68 (5): 105–11.

Rohini, R., and B. Mahadevappa. 2006. "Service Quality in Bangalore Hospitals— An Empirical Study." *Journal of Services Research* 6 (1): 59–84.

Romana, H. W. 2006. "Is Evidence-Based Medicine Patient Centered and Is Patient Centered Care Evidence-Based?" *Health Services Research* 41 (1): 1–8.

Rosse, J. G., and R. A. Levin. 2003. *The Jossey-Bass Academic Administrator's Guide to Hiring.* San Francisco: Jossey-Bass.

Rubin, R. 2008. "Primary Care Doctors in Short Supply." *USA Today* (November 18): 7D.

Ruohonen, T., P. Neittaanmaki, and J. Teittinen. 2006. "Simulation Model for Improving the Operation of the Emergency Department of Special Health Care." Simulation Conference, WSC 06. Proceedings of the Winter, December 3–6, pp. 453–58.

Rust, R. 1998. "What Is the Domain of Service Research?" *Journal of* Service Research 1 (2): 107.

Rust, R.T., B. Subramanian, and M. Wells. 1992. "Making Complaints: A Management Tool." *Marketing Management* 3 (1): 40–45.

Rutledge, E. 2001. "The Struggle for Equality in Healthcare Continues." *Journal of Healthcare Management* 46 (5): 313–24.

Rynes, S. L., and D. M. Cable. 2003. "Recruitment Research in the Twenty-First Century." In *Handbook of Psychology: Industrial and Organizational Psychology,* Vol. 12, edited by W. C. Borman, D. R. Ilgen, and R. J. Klimoski, 55–76. Hoboken, NJ: John Wiley & Sons Inc.

Sack, K. 2009. "Despite Recession, Personalized Health Care Remains in Demand." *New York Times.* [Online information; retrieved 5/4/09.] www.nytimes.com/2009/05/11/health/policy/11concierge.html.

Sadler, B. L. 2006. "The Business Case for Building Better Buildings." *Trustee* 59 (10): 35–36.

Sadler, B. L., R. F. DuBose, and E. H. Zimring. 2008. "The Business Case for Building Better Hospitals Through Evidence-Based Design." *Health Environments Research and Design Journal* 1 (3): 22–39.

Saranow, J. 2006. "Selling the Special Touch." *Wall Street Journal* (July 11): B1, B8.

Sashin, D. 2007. "Hospitals Act More Like Hotels." *Orlando Sentinel* (May 18): C1, C3.

Saultz, J., and W. Albedaiwi. 2004. "Interpersonal Continuity Care and Patient Satisfaction: A Critical Review." *Annals of Family Medicine* 2 (4): 445–51.

Schein, E. 1985. *Organizational Culture and Leadership: A Dynamic View.* San Francisco: Jossey-Bass.

Schneider, B., and D. E. Bowen. 1995. *Winning the Service Game.* Boston: Harvard Business School Press.

Schneider, B., W. H. Macey, and S. A. Young. 2006. "The Climate for Service: A Review of the Construct with Implications for Achieving CLV Goals." *Journal of Relationship Marketing* 5 (2–3): 111–32.

Schneider, B., and S. S. White. 2004. *Service Quality: Research Perspectives.* Thousand Oaks, CA: Sage Publications.

Schneider, B., S. White, and M. Paul. 1998. "Linking Service Climate and Customer Perceptions of Service Quality." *Journal of Applied Psychology* 83 (2): 150–63.

Scott, G. 2001. "Accountability for Service Excellence." *Journal of Healthcare Management* 46 (3): 152–54.

Scott, J. 2006. "Eastern North Carolina Community Takes Radical Approach to Fight Nation's Top Two Health Problems." *Business Wire*, October 2. [Online information; retrieved 5/4/09.] www.redorbit.com/news/health/677537/eastern_north_carolina_community_takes_radical_approach_to_fight_nations/index.html.

Scott, J. G., J. Sochalski, and L. Aiken.

1999. "Review of Magnet Hospital Research: Findings and Implications for Professional Nursing." *Journal of Nursing Administration* 29 (1): 9–19.

Scotti, D. J., A. E. Driscoll, J. Harmon, and S. J. Behson. 2007. "Links Among High-Performance Work Environment, Service Quality, and Customer Satisfaction: An Extension to the Health Care Sector." *Journal of Healthcare Management* 52 (2): 109–24.

Sewell, C., and P. B. Brown. 1990. *Customers for Life*. New York: Pocket Books.

Sharp HealthCare. 2007. "Malcolm Baldridge National Quality Award Application: Health Care Category." [Online information; retrieved 8/25/08.] www.sharp.com/uploadedFiles/About_Us/Baldrige/2007_Baldrige_application.pdf.

———. 2009. "Pillars of Excellence." [Online information; retrieved 5/18/09.] www.sharp.com/choose-sharp/sharp-experience/pillars-excellence.cfm.

Shaw, J. D., N. Gupta, and J. E. Delery. 2005. "Alternative Conceptualizations of the Relationship Between Voluntary Turnover and Organizational Performance." *Academy of Management Journal* 48 (1): 50–68.

Sherman, S. G. 1999. *Total Customer Satisfaction: A Comprehensive Approach for Health Care Providers*, pp. 26–27. San Francisco: Jossey-Bass.

Sherman, S. G., and V. C. Sherman. 1998. *Total Customer Satisfaction: A Comprehensive Approach for Health Care Providers*. San Francisco: Jossey-Bass.

Singh, J. 1990. "A Multifacet Typology of Patient Satisfaction with a Hospital Stay." *Journal of Health Care Marketing* 10: 8–21.

Slowiak, J. M., B. E. Huitema, and A. M. Dickinson. 2008. "Reducing Wait Time in a Hospital Pharmacy to Promote Customer Service." *Quality Management in Health Care* 17 (2): 112–27.

Smith, S. 2009. "Winning True Customer Loyalty and Trust in a Recession." [Online article; retrieved 5/4/09.] www.mycustomer.com/cgi-bin/item.

cgi?id=134190.

Smith, C. H., C. Francovich, and J. Geiselman. 2000. "Pilot Test of an Organizational Culture Model in a Medical Setting." *Health Care Supervisor* 19 (2): 68–77.

Smith, H. L., J. D. Waldman, J. N. Hood, and M. D. Fottler. 2007. "Strategic Management of Internal Customers: Building Value Through Human Capital and Culture." *Advances in Health Care Management* 6: 99–126.

Stavins, C. 2004. "Developing Employee Participation in the Patient Satisfaction Process." *Journal of Healthcare Management* 49 (2): 135–39.

Stefl, M. 2008. "Common Competencies for Healthcare Managers: The Healthcare Leadership Alliance Model." *Journal of Healthcare Management* 53 (6): 360–74.

Stencel, C. 2006. "Medication Errors Injure 1.5 Million People and Cost Billions of Dollars Annually." *The National Academies*. [Online article; retrieved 5/4/09.] www.nationalacademies.org/onpinews/newsitem.aspx?RecordID=11623.

Stengle, J. 2008. "ER Patients Check in at Computer Kiosks." ABC News. [Online article; retrieved 5/4/09.] http://abcnews.go.com/print?id=3598505.

Stenz, J. 2008. "Creating a Truly Healing Environment with LEED Hospitals." [Online article; retrieved 5/4/09.] www.greenbiz.com/news/reviews_third.cfm?newsid=35708.

Stockholm Challenge Event. 2008. "Digital Hospital—SingHealth's Journey Towards Digitization of Healthcare." [Online article; retrieved 5/4/09.] http://event.stockholmchallenge.se.

Stone, V. 2009. "Discovery: Healing Environments." [Online article; retrieved 5/4/09.] www.stonecircledesign.com/dsc_environ_healing.html.

Strack, G., and M. D. Fottler. 2002. "Spirituality and Effective Leadership in Healthcare: Is There a Connection?" *Frontiers of Health Services Management*

18 (4): 3–19.

Strack, G., M. D. Fottler, and A. O. Kilpatrick. 2008. "The Relationship of Health Care Managers' Spirituality to their Self-Perceived Leadership Practices." *Health Services Management Research* 21 (4): 236–47.

Stroisch, T., and S. Creaturo. 2002. "Essential Elements of Effective Classroom Training." [Online article; retrieved 4/9/08.] www.techsoup.org/learningcenter/training/page5113.cfm.

Studer, Q. 2004. "The Value of Employee Retention." *Health Care Financial Management* (1): 52–57.

———. 2008. *Results That Last.* Hoboken, NJ: John Wiley and Sons.

Studdert, D. M., M. Melo, and T. A. Brennen. 2004. "Medical Malpractice." *New England Journal of Medicine* 350 (3): 283–92.

Sung-Eui, C. S. 2005. "Developing New Frameworks for Operations Strategy and Service System Design in Electronic Commerce." *International Journal of Service Industry Management* 16 (3): 294–314.

Swan, J. E., L. Richardson, and J. D. Hutton. 2003. "Do Appealing Rooms Increase Patient Evaluations of Physicians, Nurses and Hospital Services?" *Health Care Management Review* 28 (3): 254–64.

Szwarc, P. 2005. *Researching Customer Satisfaction and Loyalty.* Sterling, VA: Kogan-Page Limited.

Szabo, L. 2007. "Teaming Up to Ease the Pain." *USA Today* (April 26): D1–D2.

Tang, P., and D. Lansky. 2005. "The Missing Link: Bridging the Patient–Provider Health Information Gap." *Health Affairs* 24 (5): 1290–95.

Tax, S. S., and S. W. Brown. 1998. "Recovering and Learning from Service Failure." *Sloan Management Review* 39 (3): 80.

Taylor, S. A. 1994. "Distinguishing Service Quality from Patient Satisfaction in Developing Health Marketing Strategies." *Hospital & Health Services Administration* 39 (2): 221–36.

Taylor, D. M., R. Wolfe, and P. A. Cameron.

2002. "Complaints from Emergency Department Patients Largely Result from Treatment and Communication Problems." *Emergency Medicine* 14 (1): 43–49.

Technical Assistance Research Program (TARP). 1986. *Consumer Complaint Handling in America: An Update Study.* Washington, DC: Department of Consumer Affairs.

Tesoriemo, H. W. 2008. "Aetna, Cigna, Rank Highest in Efficiency." *Wall Street Journal* (May 29): D6.

Thomas, R. K. 2005. *Marketing Health Services.* Chicago: Health Administration Press.

Thompson, A., G., and R. Sunol. 1995. "Expectations as Determinants of Patient Satisfaction: Concepts, Theory, and Evidence." *International Journal for Quality in Health Care* 7 (2): 127–41.

Thompson, J. 2009. "Patients Appreciate the Transparency of Critical Incident Disclosure." [Online article; retrieved 5/4/09.] www.hiroc.com/AxiomNews/2009/April/April02.html.

Tracey, J. B., M. C. Sturman, and M. J. Tews. 2007. "Ability Versus Personality: Factors that Predict Employee Job Performance." *Cornell Hotel and Restaurant Administration Quarterly* 48 (3): 313.

Tu, H. T., and G. Cohen. 2008. "Striking Jump in Consumers Seeking Health Care Information." Center for Studying Health System Change, Tracking Report No. 20. [Online article; retrieved 8/26/09.] www.hschange.org/CONTENT/1006/.

Ulrich, R. S. 2006. "The Environment's Impact on Stress." In *Improving Healthcare with Better Building Design,* edited by S. O. Marberry, 37–61. Chicago: Health Administration Press.

Ulrich, R. S, J. A. Zimring, X. Quan, and R. Choudhary. 2004. "The Role of the Physical Environment in the Hospital of the 21st Century: A Once-in-a-Lifetime Opportunity." Center for Health Design. [Online article; retrieved 3/5/08.] www.

rwjf.org/files/publications/other/roleof
thephysical environment.pdf.

United Healthcare. 2009. "UnitedHealthcare,
IBM, and Arizona Physicians to Launch
Groundbreaking Patient-Centered
Healthcare Initiative." [Online article;
retrieved 7/18/09.] www.uhc.com/
news_room/2009_news_release_archive/
launch_of_groundbreaking_patient_
centered_healthcare_initiative.htm.

Unruh, L., and M. D. Fottler. 2005.
"Projections and Trends in RN Supply:
What Do They Tell Us About the
Nursing Shortage?" *Policy, Politics and
Nursing Practice* 63 (3): 171–82.

Upenieks, V. 2002. "Assessing Differences in
Job Satisfaction of Nurses in Magnet
and Non-Magnet Hospitals." *Journal of
Nursing Administration* 32 (11): 564–76.

VanBerkel, P., and J. Blake. 2007. "A
Comprehensive Simulation for Wait
Time Reduction and Capacity Planning
Applied in General Surgery." *Health Care
Management Science* 10 (4): 373–85.

Van der Wiele, T., M. Hesselink, and J. van
Iwaarden. 2005. "Mystery Shopping: A
Tool to Develop Insight into Customer
Service Provision." *Total Quality
Management & Business Excellence* 16 (4):
529–41.

Vega, V., and S. J. McGuire. 2007. "Speeding
Up the Emergency Department: The
RADIT Emergency Program at St. Joseph
Hospital of Orange." *Hospital Topics* 85
(4): 17–24.

Vernon, W. 2009. "Keeping Green: Reducing
Energy Consumption Without Harming
the Budget." *Journal of Healthcare
Management* 54 (3): 159–62.

Volzer, R. 2006. "West Indies Panache."
Nursing Homes. [Online article; retrieved
5/4/09.] http://findarticles.com/p/articles/
mi_m3830/is_3_55/ai_n16118932/.

Wall Street Journal. March 26, 2001, p. B13.

Wallauer, J., D. Macedo, R. Andrade, and
A. von Wangenheim. 2008. "Building a
National Telemedicine Network." *IT Pro*
(March/April): 12–17.

Wang, S. S. 2006. "To Improve Service,
Hospitals and Doctors Hire Spies to Pose
as Patients and Report Back." *Wall Street
Journal* (August 8): D1.

Washington State Hospital Association
(WSHA). 2009. [Online information;
retrieved 5/18/09.] www.wsha.org/page.
cfm?ID=core_competencies.

Weiss, G. G. 2003. "How to Cut Patient Wait
Time." *Medical Economics,* pp. 75–82.

Wessel, H. 2008. "Doctor's In—Online."
Orlando Sentinel (April 28): 17–18.

Whittmore, C. B. 2007. "Flooring the Customer."
Disneyworld. [Online information; retrieved
5/18/09.] http://flooringtheconsumer.
blogspot.com/2007/05/story-brings-brands-
to-life.html.

Wiley, J. P. 1999. "Help Is on the Way."
Smithsonian 30 (4): 22.

Wilicox, S., M. Seddon, S. Dunn, R. T.
Edwards, J. Pearse, and J. V. Tu. 2007.
"Measuring and Reducing Waiting
Times: A Cross-National Comparison
of Strategies." *Health Affairs* 26 (4):
1078–87.

Williams, M. E., J. Latta, and P. Conversano.
2008. "Eliminating the Wait for Mental
Health Services." *Journal of Behavioral
Health Services & Research* 35 (1): 107–
14.

Willis, R. W. 2000. "Positive Paradigm Shifts
in Health Care." *Journal of Religion and
Health* 39 (4): 355–65.

Wilper, A. P., S. Woolhandler, K. E. Lasser, D.
McCormick, S. L. Cutrona, D. H. Bor,
and D. U. Himmelstein. 2008. "Waits to
See an Emergency Department Physician:
U.S. Trends and Predictors." *Health
Affairs* 27 (1/2): pw84–pw95.

Wrzesniewski, A., and J. E. Dutton. 2001.
"Crafting a Job: Revisioning Employees as
Active Crafters of Their Work." *Academy
of Management Review* 26: 179–201.

Wrzesniewski, A., J. E. Dutton, and G. Debebe.
2003. "Interpersonal Sensemaking and
the Meaning of Work." *Research in
Organizational Behavior* 25: 93–135.

Wyckoff, D. D. 1984. "New Tools for Achieving Service Quality." *Cornell Hotel and Restaurant Administration Quarterly* 25 (3): 89–99.

Zborowsky, T., and M. J. Kreitzer. 2008. "Creating Optimal Healing Environments in a Health Care Setting." [Online information; retrieved 5/4/09.] www.minnesotamedicine. com/PastIssues/March2008/ ClinicalZborowskyMarch2008/ tabid/2489/Default.aspx.

Zeithaml, V. A., L. L. Berry, and A. Parasuraman. 1996. "The Behavioral Consequences of Service Quality." *Journal of Marketing* 60 (2): 31–46.

Zeithaml, V. A., M. J. Bitner, and D. Gremler. 2008. *Services Marketing.* New York: McGraw-Hill.

Zhao, H., and S. E. Seibert. 2006. "The Big Five Personality Dimensions and Entrepreneurial Status: A Meta-Analytical Review." *Journal of Applied Psychology* 91 (2).

Zibriskie, K. 2009. "Customer Service Tips for Healthcare Professionals, Rx for Pleasing Patients: Ten Things They Don't Need to Hear." [Online article; retrieved 5/4/09.] www.businesstrainingworks.com/ Onsite%20Training%20Web/Free%20 Articles/08%20Tips%20for%20 Better%20Healthcare%20Service%20 -%20Free%20Article.html.

Zimmer, D., P. Zimmerman, and C. Lund. 1997. "Customer Service: The New Battlefield for Market Share." *Health Care Financial Management* 51 (10): 51–53.

Zizzo, D. 2008. "Researchers Track Role of Laughs." [Online information; retrieved 5/4/09.] http://newsok.com/ article/3213471/1205148347.

Zomerdijk, L. G., and J. D. Vries. 2007. "Structuring Front Office and Back Office Work in Service Delivery Systems." *Production Management* 27 (1): 108–31.

Zuger, A. 2005. "For a Retainer, Lavish Care by 'Boutique Doctors'." *New York Times* (October 30).

Additional Resources

The Cochrane Collaboration. 2009. See www. cochrane.org/reviews/clibintro.html.

Dickson, D., R. C. Ford, and B. Laval. 2005. "The Top 10 Excuses for Bad Service and How to Avoid Needing Them." *Organizational Dynamics* 34 (2): 168–84.

Gehant, D. P. 2008. "Hospitals and the Environment." *Frontiers of Health Services Management* 25 (1): 3–10.

Green, L. 2000. "He Who Laughs, Lasts." *Spirit* 16 (2): 74–78.

Hall, A. G. 2008. "Greening Health Care: 21st Century and Beyond." *Frontiers of Health Services Management* 25 (1): 37–43.

Health Care Without Harm. 2008. *Menu of Change: Healthy Food in Healthcare: A 2008 Survey of Healthy Food in Health Care Pledge Hospitals.* Arlington, VA: Health Care Without Harm.

Katz, G. 2003. *The Costs and Benefits of Green Buildings: A Report to California's Sustainable Buildings Task Force.* Sacramento, CA.

LiJen, J. H., A. Eves, and T. Delsombre. 2003. "Gap Analysis of Patient Service Perceptions." *International Journal of Health Care Quality Assurance* 16 (2): 143–51.

Mittal, S. 2009. "Developing a Vision in Health Care," Part 1 and Part 2. [Online information; retrieved 5/1/09.] http:// ezinearticles.com/?Developing-Vision-in-Health-Care-(Part-1)&id=2291316.

Ridley, K. 2006. "Healing by Design." *Ode Magazine.* [Online article; retrieved 8/20/08.] www.odemagazine.com/ doc/35/healing_by_design.

Seward, Z. M. 2007. "Doctor Shortage Hurts a 'Coverage for All' Plan." *Wall Street Journal* (July 25): B1–B2.

Will, T. J. 2003. "Online CRM: On to the Next Level." *Medicare on the Net.* [Online article; retrieved 5/4/09.] www.hcpro. com/services/corhealth/index.cfm.

Winslow, R., and C. Gentry. 2000. "Medical Vouchers: Health Care Trend—Give Workers Money, Let Them Buy a Plan." *Wall Street Journal* (February 8): A1, A12.

Index

Consumer: confidence of, 5; informing, 240–41; role changes, 217–18

Consumer-driven healthcare: market trends, 16–17; reform and, 384, 386–87

Content mastery testing, 174

Continuous quality improvement. See CQI

Control, 7

Control factors, 231–32

Convenience, 7–8

Coproduction: advantages/disadvantages, 224–28, 230; cost–benefit analysis, 232–33; determinants, 230–35; patient roles, 222; perspective on, 228–29; reasons for, 231–32; service excellence model, 400–401

Core competencies: culture and, 114; definition, 60; internal assessment, 60–61

Cost–benefit analysis, coproduction, 232–33

Cost: evidence-based design, 83; savings, 247; total healthcare experience, 48

CQI: accreditation criteria, 12

Critical incident: explanation, 46; skills, 151; survey technique, 352–53

Critical path, 288, 289

Critical skills, 168

CRM, 31–32

Cross-functional organization, 293–95, 296

Cross-functional training, 181

Cues, 71, 73

Cultural competence, 8

Cultural norms, 107–8

Culture: basic elements, 106–10; changing, 124–26; communication of, 117–20; conversions, 125–26; definition, 105; importance of, 113–17; leaders' role, 110–13; patient-centered, 112–13; practicing, 112–13; reinforcement, 121–23; teaching, 120–24; translating, 112

Customer: defection, 363–64; definition of, 4; expectations, 12; focus, 21–22; information, 241; loyalty, 9–11; types, 13

Customer contact: group, 253; improvement strategies, 45; scheduled time for, 124

Customer relationship management. See CRM

Customer service: chain, 28–30; expectations, 13; fundamentals, 19; mission statement and, 64; retreats, 180; Web-based technology, 242

Customization, 8

Decision making: culture and, 116; facilitating, 257–58; Internet and, 245–46; process stages, 209–11

Decision modeling, 256

Decision systems, 255–56

Delphi technique, 58

Demand management, 306–7, 369

Design day, 56, 310–11

Distributive fairness, 378

Diversity training, 181–82

Econometric models, 55

ED: triage, 306–7; wait time, 302

Electronic medical record: breach of, 262–63; Web-based technology, 241–42

Emergency department. See ED

Emotional commitment, 146–47

Emotional response, 102–3

Employee: acknowledgment of, 190; behavior, 70, 399–400; coaching, 196; contributions of, 132–35; desires, 194; development programs, 184–87; empowering, 132, 207–14; engagement, 395–98; feedback, 337–38; general abilities, 146–47; healing environment, 88–89; job analysis process, 135–38; job crafting, 147–48; mission-focused, 192–94; motivation of, 189–94; output–input ratio, 192–93; performance rewards, 198–99; performance standards, 399–400; person–organization fit, 148–49; recruitment process, 138–44; retention, 153–56; rewards/recognition, 398–99; satisfaction, 117, 153–54, 194–98; screening methods, 149–53; selection, 144–49, 396–98; service delivery, 43; service lovers, 134–35; shortages, 133–34; survey, 196–98; training, 396–98; work teams, 201–7

Empowerment: benefit, 207; degrees of, 208; electronic recordkeeping, 247; explanation, 208; job content/context grid, 208–11; organizational limitations, 213; Point B strategy, 210–12; potential,

213–14; program implementation, 212–13

Environment: assessment, 52, 59; dimensions of, 94–100; factors, 81–82; sounds, 95–96

Evangelist, 364

Evidence-based databases, 252–53

Evidence-based design, 82–83, 83–84

Expectations: awareness of, 12; external customers; 30–35; internal customers', 35; management of, 32–33; variability, 33

"Experience economy," 24, 40–42

Expert systems, 256–59

External assessment, 54–59

External customer, 30–35

External environment, 114–15

External training, 173–74

15-foot rule, 107

Family: role of, 219

Feedback: employee, 337–38; service excellence model, 393–94; training, 172–73

Fellowship program, 186–87

Financial compensation policies, 200

Finder's fee, 141

Fishbone analysis, 283–85

Flowchart, 280

Focus group: coproduction strategy, 221; qualitative assessment, 58, 338; recruitment, 141

Folkways, 109

Food service: trends, 91

Forecasting, 54–59, 369

Formalized learning, 169

Functional congruence, 97

General abilities, 146–47

General education, 185–86

Globalization, 17–18

Green movement, 92–93

Guestology, 26–27

Guest service representatives, 90

Healing environment: creation approaches, 86; effects of, 83; elements conducive to,

84–85; employees and, 88–89; family-friendly designs, 85; humor and, 87–88; nature and, 85, 87

Health advice: Web-based technology, 241–42

Healthcare database, 243

Healthcare Effectiveness Data and Information Set. See HEDIS

"Healthcare hours," 151

Healthcare organization, as information system, 264–68

Healthcare support group, 253

Health information systems. See Information systems

Health insurance: rating service, 15; Web-based technology, 241

Healthplexes, 93–94

Healthscape, 43

HEDIS, 14

Heroes, 118–19

High-involvement work environment, 117

Homelike design, 85

Hospital: rating service, 14–15

Hotel-style amenities, 90–91

Human resources system: organizational culture and, 123

Humor, 87–88

Individual needs assessment, 171

Inducements, 200–201

Information: bad, 261; confidentiality, 261–63; electronic expertise, 252–53; level-to-level flow, 253–55; overload, 260–61; primacy of, 265; security, 261–63; service delivery system, 351; service environment, 250–51; service product, 249–50; on service quality, 251–52; sharing, 247

Information flow: increasing, 265–66; intranet utilization, 266–67; reducing need, 266

Information system: advantages/disadvantages, 260; customer-contact group, 253; decision systems, 255–56; expert systems, 256–59; healthcare organization as, 264–68; healthcare support group, 253; information flow, 253–55; interconnectivity, 267–68; learning cost, 264; problems with, 259–64; service delivery, 43; value of, 240–41; value

Total healthcare experience: cost, 48; quality of, 47–48; service delivery system, 43–46; service product, 42–43; service setting, 43; value of, 48–49

Total quality management. See TQM

TQM: goal, 274; lessons learned, 272

Training: attitudinal, 181–82; barriers, 166; benefits, 163, 166, 184; classroom presentation, 175–76; components, 162; computer-based learning, 178–79; cost analysis, 184; cross-functional, 181; customer service retreats, 180; diversity, 181–82; external versus internal, 173–74; feedback, 172–73; frontline staff, 163; job instruction technique, 178; leaders, 160–62; measurements, 174–75, 183–84; methods, 175–83; objective, 172, 183; on-the-job supervision, 177–78; orientation, 181; patients, 165; problems/pitfalls, 183–84; retention impact, 164–66; roleplaying method, 180–81; service excellence model, 396–98; service recovery strategy, 369–70; special competencies, 181; staff, 162–66; turnover impact, 164–66; video instruction, 176–77

Training program: big picture reinforcement, 168–69; components, 170–75; continuous improvement, 170; development guidelines, 167–68; formalized learning, 169; multiple learning approaches, 170

Transactional administrators, 191

Transactional leaders, 111

Transactional skill, 199

Transformational leaders, 111–12, 191

Transformational leadership skill, 200

Trend analysis, 55

Triage, 306–7

Tuition reimbursement policy, 185

University collaboration, 141

Value: congruence, 148; differential, 11; equation, 48; of total healthcare experience, 48–49; perceived, 9; service

strategy factor, 66–67;

Values: customer-focused, 106–7; examples of, 52; cultural reinforcement, 115–16

Video training, 176–77

Virtual wait strategy, 308

Vision, 52

Vision statement, 62–64, 123

Wait management: perceived service value, 327–28; perceptions, 323–28; practices, 322

Wait time: for appointment, 303; capacity decision, 304–12; definition, 300; diversions, 307–8; ED, 302; importance of, 300–303; management, 312–23; organizational options, 305–12; patient dissatisfaction with, 301–2; physician, 302–3; queuing theory, 313–19; service time versus, 324; solo versus group, 326; standards, 309–10; tracking, 310; for treatment, 303; uncertain lengths, 325; uncomfortable waits, 326; unexplained waits, 325; unfair, 325–26; uninteresting, 326; virtual strategy, 308; capacity–demand balance, 319, 321–23; service excellence model, 402

Waiting area: hotel-style amenities, 90–91; improvements, 308–9

War gaming, 58–59

Web-based survey, 353

Word of mouth, 365–66

Work team: benefits of, 201–4; characteristics, 202; nursing care, 204; problems, 204–5; self-directed, 204; utilization, 206–7

Yield management, 57

About the Authors

Myron D. Fottler, PhD, is a professor and executive director of the Health Services Administration Programs in the College of Health and Public Affairs at the University of Central Florida, where he teaches courses in healthcare human resources management, service management and marketing, and dissertation research. His research interests include all aspects of human resources management, service management, stakeholder management, strategic management, integrated delivery systems, and healthcare report cards. He has won awards from the American College of Healthcare Executives, American Association of Medical Administrators, and the Healthcare Management Division of the Academy of Management for his research. His publications include 18 books and more than 100 journal articles.

Previously, Dr. Fottler was professor and director of the PhD program in Administration—Health Services, with a joint appointment in both the School of Health Related Professions and the School of Business at the University of Alabama at Birmingham. He completed his MBA at Boston University and his PhD in business at Columbia University. He has been active in both the Academy of Management and the Association of University Programs in Health Administration. He has also served on several editorial review boards and is a founding coeditor of *Advances in Health Care Management,* an annual research volume published by JAI/Elsevier.

Dr. Fottler has served as a member of the editorial boards for *Medical Care Research and Review, International Journal of Applied Quality Management, Journal of Health Administration Education* and *Health Care Management Review.* He has served as a reviewer for *Industrial and Labor Relations Review, Industrial Relations, Academy of Management Review, Medical Care, Journal of Management, Journal of Occupational Behavior, Health Services Research, Hospital & Health Services Administration, Health Care Financing Review, Journal of Management Studies, Journal of Healthcare Management, Journal of Labor Studies,* and *Academy of Management Journal.* He has been listed in numerous biographical publications, including *Dictionary of International Biography, Who's Who in The World, Outstanding Young Men in America, Who's Who in the East, Contemporary Authors, International Directory of Business and Management Scholars and Research, American Men and Women of Science, International Writers and Author's Who's Who,* and *Directory of American Scholars.*

Robert C. Ford, PhD, is a professor of management in the College of Business Administration at the University of Central Florida (UCF). He joined UCF in 1993 as chair of the Department of Hospitality Management, and, until 2003, he was associate dean for Graduate and External Programs. He also served on the management faculty of the University of North Florida and was management department chair and a member of the faculty at the University of Alabama at Birmingham.

Dr. Ford has authored or coauthored more than 100 articles, books, and presentations on organizational issues, human resources management, and services management, especially as it relates to healthcare and hospitality applications. He won the 2001 Sodexho Marriott Health Care Division Faculty Publication of the Year for a coauthored article with Myron Fottler. He has published in a wide variety of academic and practitioner journals, including the *Journal of Applied Psychology, Academy of Management Journal, Organizational Dynamics, Health Care Management Review,* and *The Academy of Management Executive.* His books include *Principles of Management, Organization Theory, Managing the Guest Experience in Hospitality, Achieving Service Excellence, Leading with a Laugh,* and *Managing Destination Marketing Organizations.*

Dr. Ford was editor of the *Academy of Management Executive* and chair of both Management History and Management Education and Management Development Divisions of the Academy of Management. In addition, he has been the chair of the Accreditation Commission for Programs in Hospitality Administration. He is a Fellow and former dean of the Southern Management Association.

Cherrill P. Heaton, PhD, was a professor of organizational communications at the University of North Florida. In addition to teaching organizational and business communications in the MBA and M.Acc. programs, he taught more than 100 short courses for business and industry in these areas. He was editor of *Management by Objectives in Higher Education* and was coauthor of *Essentials of Modern Investments* and several articles and three books (with Robert Ford): *Principles of Management, Organization Theory,* and *Managing the Guest Experience in Hospitality.* In addition, Dr. Heaton was managing editor of the *Academy of Management Executive.* He is now retired.